Flesh and Blood

Flesh and Blood

Organ Transplantation and Blood Transfusion in Twentieth-Century America

Susan E. Lederer

OXFORD
UNIVERSITY PRESS
2008

OXFORD
UNIVERSITY PRESS

Oxford University Press, Inc., publishes works that further
Oxford University's objective of excellence
in research, scholarship, and education.

Oxford   New York
Auckland   Cape Town   Dar es Salaam   Hong Kong   Karachi
Kuala Lumpur   Madrid   Melbourne   Mexico City   Nairobi
New Delhi   Shanghai   Taipei   Toronto

With offices in
Argentina   Austria   Brazil   Chile   Czech Republic   France   Greece
Guatemala   Hungary   Italy   Japan   Poland   Portugal   Singapore
South Korea   Switzerland   Thailand   Turkey   Ukraine   Vietnam

Published by Oxford University Press, Inc.
198 Madison Avenue, New York, New York 10016
www.oup.com

Oxford is a registered trademark of Oxford University Press

Lederer, Susan E.
Flesh and blood: organ transplantation and blood
transfusion in twentieth-century America/
Susan E. Lederer.
p.; cm.
ISBN: 978-0-19-516150-2
1. Transplantation of organs, tissues, etc.—United States—History—20th century.
2. Blood—Transfusion—United States—History—20th century.
[DNLM: 1. Organ Transplantation—history—United States.
2. Blood Transfusion—history—United States.
3. Blood Transfusion—psychology—United States.
4. History, 20th Century—United States.
5. Organ Transplantation—psychology—United States.
6. Social Change—history—United States.
WO 11 AA1 L473f 2008]
I. Title.
RD120.7.L42 2008
362.17'84—dc22

2007038548

9 8 7 6 5 4 3 2 1

Printed in the United States of America
on acid-free paper

For Emma, Eric, and Gregory,
my own flesh and blood

Contents

Introduction

Organ transplantation is one of the most dramatic interventions in modern medicine. Since the 1950s, thousands of people have lived with "new" hearts, kidneys, lungs, corneas, and other organs and tissues transplanted into their bodies. But, even before the 1950s, American surgeons had attempted to treat catastrophic disease or injuries using tissues and organs retrieved from the bodies of other people and other species. Long before the success of kidney transplantation in the 1950s and heart transplantation in the 1960s, many Americans looked to the potential of these new surgeries to restore lost function and repair the ravages of illness and injury.

The contrast of surgical reality with the "surgical imaginary"—namely, the prospect of replacing old organs with new ones retrieved or purchased from another person—is a major focus of this book, which explores how the body and its parts—organs, tissues, cells, and fluids—possess not just medical and surgical significance, but complex political and cultural meanings as well. By focusing on the earlier "pre-history" of organ transplantation, as well as the successes of the 1950s and 1960s, *Flesh and Blood: Organ Transplantation and Blood Transfusion in Twentieth-Century America* argues that the so-called failures of organ transplantation have much to tell us about the ways in which Americans experienced the conceptual development of organ transplantation in twentieth-century America and the social and cultural implications of remaking American bodies through the harvest of other bodies—animal and human, living and dead.

The dramatic expansion of surgery in the late nineteenth century encouraged American surgeons to extend and explore the boundaries of the body, using a variety of new materials and new techniques. One of the most potent illustrations of innovation in American surgery was the development of blood transfusion. First introduced in the seventeenth century and periodically revived over the next two centuries, blood transfusion became, in the hands of twentieth-century American surgeons, a life-extending therapeutic intervention useful in the treatment of a broad array of injuries and diseases. Although several historians have written about the checkered development of blood transfusion, they have focused, for the most part, on the various techniques and indications for the procedure, rather than on the cultural implications of the practice.[1] In the early twentieth century, moving blood between bodies required much more than a willing surgeon, scalpel, and syringe; transfusion could only be effectively accomplished by physically uniting the exposed blood vessels of donors and recipients. The invasive intimacy of such transfusions made it difficult to ignore the social and material realities of the individual bodies and bloods involved.

Both the movement of blood between bodies and organ transplantation entail a supply problem. Then, as now, surgeons often encountered shortages of people willing and able to supply blood. Obtaining solid organs like ovaries, testes, skin, thyroid glands, bone, nerves, and other materials from human sources posed immediate challenges for surgeons during the first part of the twentieth century. In the face of these shortages, surgeons helped to broker financial arrangements between families and friends to acquire the tissues and blood for the necessary surgeries. Almost from the start, the commodification of the body, its fluids, and parts coexisted alongside a "gift exchange" in which no money changed hands. Although surgeons occasionally expressed concern about the "traffic in organs" and "blood money," there was little or no public criticism about compensating individuals for their "parts and labor." The status of blood and organs as commodities became increasingly contested in the second half of the twentieth century, and this sacralization of human flesh and blood is one focus of this book.

A second major focus of *Flesh and Blood* is how Americans responded to therapeutic interventions—blood transfusion and organ transplantation—that literally redrew the lines between self and nonself, between someone and a stranger, between spouses and family members, between the living and the dead, and between humans and animals. Most commentators who have studied the cultural status of organ transplantation have focused on resistance to organ donation. Some have drawn parallels between biologic resistance (an organism's immune-mediated response to foreign tissue) and cultural resistance to organ donation. This idea has a becoming and attractive symmetry, but there is a danger that this attraction can obscure a more important truth: namely, the rapid embrace of organ transplantation by a large segment of the American public. Drawing on newspapers, magazines, legal cases, films, and the papers and correspondence of physicians and surgeons, *Flesh and Blood* challenges the assumptions, offered by bioethicists, anthropologists, and policy makers, that popular fears about organ transplantation necessarily reflect timeless human concerns and preoccupations with the body.[2] It provides a compelling illustration of how notions about the body—intact, in parts, living, and dead—are shaped by the particular culture and society in which they are embedded and articulated. It also suggests the process whereby medical knowledge offered new conceptions of individual bodies and their relationships to others through sharing the "gift of life" via donations of flesh and blood.

The first two chapters of the book explore the early development of the surgical transfer of skin, bone, nerves, organs, and blood between bodies. Not least among the challenges facing surgeons performing skin grafting was locating suitable sources for tissue. Living human donors presented a number of difficulties; the pain associated with the procedure of shaving off pieces of skin to be donated to another person troubled donors, as did the psychological dimension of being "flayed alive." In light of these problems, surgeons looked to alternative sources. Surgeons harvested skin from pigeons, dogs, cats, chickens, rabbits, and frogs for application to their patients. Doctors also retrieved human skin from the bodies of the dead, amputated limbs, and stillborn infants. Chapter 1 considers what it meant for physicians and patients in the first part of the twentieth century to administer and receive physically intimate materials from others—animal and human. It explores the role of the news media in shaping expectations about the procedure and its results, and in influencing ideas about altruism, self-sacrifice, and heroism involving the donation of one's skin or other body part. Drawing on early twentieth-century letters from individuals seeking transplantation for themselves or for a family member, the chapter contends that, just as such basic human instincts as hunger and appetite are influenced by social and cultural factors, so too conceptions of the intact and dismembered human body—dead and alive—are transformed in particular cultural settings.

The second chapter examines the reintroduction of blood transfusion during the early twentieth century. Performed only sporadically in the nineteenth century, the transfusion of blood became a significant surgical intervention in the first part of the twentieth century. In the era before blood could be safely stored, surgical transfusion offered a dramatic, technically demanding method to treat hemorrhages and other blood conditions. Surgical practices, as historian Christopher Lawrence has argued, "are never mere empirical procedures. Even the most simple of them employ a theory of the body, either explicit or implicit."[3] *Direct transfusion*, as surgically achieved blood transfusion became known, was neither a simple procedure nor a merely empirical one. Instead, the physically intimate contact between the veins of two different individuals entailed a radical reconceptualization of the body, its fluids, and its parts.

Focusing on Crile's clinical tests of surgical transfusion involving 55 patients, Chapter 2 examines the American development of direct transfusion as a means to restore life to the nearly dead. Essential to the success of the procedure was the availability of suitable donors willing and able to endure the physical and psychological rigors of donation, including the incision made on the arm or leg to expose a blood vessel and the surgical union with a dying recipient. Part of the compensation for this participation was the lionization of donors in the popular press. Almost from its introduction in 1906, blood transfusions engaged newspaper reporters attracted by the drama and mystery of these miracles of resurrection. Chapter 2 explores the medical and cultural implications of moving blood between bodies, from Crile's pioneering efforts to the advent of blood banking in the 1930s.

The third chapter, Banking on the Body, considers the contested commodification of the human body, its fluids, and parts. Almost from the inception of surgical transfusion, a market for human blood developed in the United States. By the 1930s, when the American Federation of Labor recognized a "blood seller's union," obstetricians were turning to such professionals to serve as "ghost fathers" for artificial insemination. The rigors of early blood transfusion made financial incentives necessary to obtain sufficient donors in time of need. Doctors and surgeons often brokered the transactions between blood suppliers and the patient's friends or family members to ensure that blood would be available. This chapter considers how the buying and selling of blood influenced the American experience of transfusion from the earliest payments to blood suppliers, through the development of networks of professional blood sellers, to the large-scale reliance on blood from prison inmates and the residents of Skid Row. The chapter explores how money shaped interactions between donors, recipients, and surgeons, and how systems for paying blood suppliers coexisted, at times uneasily, with a new "philanthropy of the body" and its fluids.

Chapter 3 also probes the power and significance of the "banking" metaphor for both blood transfusion and organ transplantation. In the 1930s, physicians in Spain and Russia developed systems for preserving and storing blood in a central facility, but it was the American physician Bernard Fantus who coined the word "blood bank" when he opened the first such facility at Chicago's Cook County Hospital in 1937. In an era notable for bank failure and economic collapse, American surgeons became blood "bankers," who discussed loans, deposits, and balance sheets. Physicians borrowed this usage in developing storage facilities for other body fluids (sperm) and tissues (bone banks, eye banks). This chapter considers alternative concepts of blood and tissue storage and the implications of selecting a financial institution as the model for the storage and distribution of blood and other tissues.

During the first half of the twentieth century, occasional reports surfaced about the selling of solid tissue—skin, ears, and especially male generative glands. This prompted, in the 1920s, the first expressions of concern about "traffic in organs." Long before the late 1960s, when the scarcity of donor organs for heart transplantation fostered speculation about a black market in hearts, authors and film makers incorporated the sale of body parts into fiction and film. In 1984, the United States Congress passed the National Organ Transplantation Act, which outlawed the buying and selling of human organs. Organ sales remain illegal in 2007, but despite critics of international organ selling by historian David J. Rothman and anthropologist Nancy Scheper-Hughes, among others, proposals for the legalization of organ selling have increased in light of the intensifying shortage of donor organs.[4] Chapter 3 examines the social and cultural implications of the incomplete and contested transformation of body parts into marketable goods and services.

The fourth chapter, Lost Boundaries, focuses on some of the dynamics of "blood mixing" in the twentieth century. Recent works by historians Keith Wailoo and Spencie Love have documented how, in 1941, the American National Red Cross assumed supervision of a massive blood-collection effort for American military personnel.[5] Amid concerns that blood donation would be adversely affected by rumors of racially mixed blood, officials of the Red Cross announced that blood from African American donors would not be accepted for collection. In the face of protests by organizations such as the National Medical Association, the American

Medical Association, and the American Public Health Association, and the personal intervention of First Lady Eleanor Roosevelt, the Red Cross reversed its policy; "Negro blood" would be accepted. However, this blood would be collected and labeled separately from that of white donors. This chapter emphasizes how experience with "transfusion accidents" involving donors infected with syphilis shaped popular and professional fears about "Negro blood," fears that had been largely absent through several previous decades of blood transfusion.

Chapter 4 extends into the postwar decades the history of moving blood between people of different races. Since the early twentieth century, the popular association of blood with an individual's ethnic, racial, religious, and even political identity made transfusion between dissimilar donors noteworthy. Newspapers reported, for example, that seven Republican legislators in Utah donated blood to their lone Democratic colleague (he died), how six white college students in Georgia donated blood to save the life of "a Negro servant" (he lived), and how an Orthodox Jewish woman refused any blood from gentile donors. By the 1940s, however, as the changing technology of transfusion cloaked the identity of donors, fears about the safety and purity of the nation's blood prompted segregation of the blood supply and the stigmatization of African American donors. Although the Red Cross and the American armed forces desegregated the blood supply on the eve of the Korean War, the racially charged politics of the 1950s and 1960s prompted legislators in southern states to enact laws for racial labels on blood and required notification when patients received racially dissimilar blood. This legislation represented only a minor skirmish in the larger battles over civil rights, but illustrates the enormously powerful symbolic role of blood in American culture and politics.

Chapter 5 examines how biomedical science differentiated blood not on racial grounds but on the knowledge of immunologic specificity. In the early twentieth century, Austrian pathologist Karl Landsteiner observed what he later labeled "the unexpected existence of clearly demonstrable differences between the bloods within one animal species." In 1900, he discovered that human blood could be differentiated into three distinct groups; his colleagues, repeating the work, added a fourth group in 1901. At first, these groupings represented more of an immunologic curiosity than a finding with clinical significance. Although Reuben Ottenberg introduced cross-matching for blood transfusion in 1912, routine pretransfusion blood typing did not take place in the United States until after World War I. In the 1920s, as more physicians practiced blood transfusion, efforts to educate Americans about blood groups introduced confusion about "blood relationships" in families. Why a father or mother would not be a suitable candidate for a blood transfusion to a child, for example, violated longstanding conceptions of "familial closeness" and relationships. Ideas about immunologically unsuitable blood, sometimes labeled "bad blood," resonated with older ideas about blood purity and pollution and were intensified during an era of acute anxiety about syphilis.

Chapter 5 examines the cultural history of the blood groups in twentieth-century America, especially Landsteiner's ABO system and his subsequent discovery with Alexander Weiner of the Rh blood factor. (In present-day Japan, many people believe that blood type determine an individual character; media profiles of Japanese politicians, for example, often disclose the individual's blood type.) Blood groups offered one avenue for a biomedical transformation of cultural knowledge of the self and self-identity over the course of the twentieth century. In the 1960s, the advent of tissue typing based on human leukocyte antigens offered another way to understand the extent to which humans were both different from and similar to one another. One of the major problems in organ and tissue transplantation continues to be the biologic rejection of foreign tissue. In the 1960s, the discovery of tissue groups promised to resolve this longstanding issue of incompatible donors and recipients, and to inaugurate a new era in transplantation. However, the nonrandom distribution of these tissue types—the fact that whites and African Americans had different antigen profiles—raised new questions about fairness and equity in the allocation of scarce cadaveric kidneys and other organs. More than that, the tissue types represented another means to understand differences and similarities among human beings and their families.

Some of these factors are considered in Chapter 6, Medicalizing Miscegenation, which focuses on the ways in which assumptions about race and value influenced the transfer of solid body parts. When South African surgeon Christiaan Barnard transplanted the heart of a "Cape coloured man" into the body of a white, Jewish, retired dentist in 1968, African American magazines such as *Ebony* noted the irony that the "colored man's heart" could now enter literally hundreds of places restricted to whites only. In the United States, African Americans expressed concern that white doctors—already feared for using black patients as experimental subjects—would hasten the deaths of black patients so that their bodies could be harvested for organs intended for white recipients. This chapter analyzes the role of race in the growth and diffusion of organ transplantation since the 1960s, and the efforts of African American transplant surgeons to raise the level of organ donation in the African American community, where donor rates remain low.[6]

"Blood is the life" reads the passage from the Biblical book Leviticus. The Judeo-Christian tradition brims with blood. In the eucharistic doctrine of the Catholic Church, bread and wine become transubstantiated into the body and blood of Jesus Christ. The complex cultural and spiritual associations of blood as a vital fluid, a source of life-sustaining, mystical power and essence, retained their potency in the twentieth century. New scientific findings about blood and its components did not strip blood of these mystical and spiritual meanings. Chapter 7 considers the controversial stance of the Jehovah's Witnesses about the acceptability of blood transfusion. Grounded in verses from Genesis, Leviticus, and the New Testament book of Acts, the sect ruled in 1945 that transfusion violated God's law and that Jehovah's Witnesses could not accept blood transfusion even if death was the alternative. The prohibition on blood transfusion troubled physicians and surgeons. In the 1950s, the Jehovah's Witnesses problem sparked renewed attention to medical ethics; in the 1960s, the issue moved into state and federal courts as hospitals pursued court orders to permit transfusions against the explicit wishes of patients and in spite of their firmly held religious beliefs.

Transplantation, even more than the transfusion of blood, raised fundamental religious questions about bodily integrity and identity. The potential violations of long-sacred boundaries between bodies and souls troubled many of the major religious groups in the twentieth century. Catholic theologians, already animated by the moral dimensions of birth control, abortion, and eugenic sterilization, helped to structure public discourse about the morality of "organic transplantation" long before transplantation achieved its first significant successes in the 1950s. Chapter 7 revives the religious dimensions of public response to transplanting body parts taken from human and animal donors, both living and dead, and argues that religion played a crucial role in the reception of medical advances in twentieth-century America.

The last chapter, Organ Recital, examines the cultural and social implications of transplantation and transfusion and how it established a trajectory for thinking about the developments of the 1950s, when a new generation of surgeons, building on extensive experience with animal models and galvanized by discoveries in immunology, prepared to reanimate transplantation. In 1954, surgeons at Harvard Medical School and the Peter Bent Brigham Hospital in Boston performed the first "successful" human organ transplant when they took one kidney from a healthy man and placed it into the body of his sick twin brother. The success of this surgery, and efforts to resolve the ongoing problems of immune response to foreign tissue, sparked intense activity on the part of surgeons, who quickly moved from kidneys, to lungs, to what *Life* magazine dubbed "the ultimate operation," the transplantation of the human heart. This chapter explores the changing fortunes of transplantation from the 1950s through the 1980s.

As it had in an earlier era, the large-scale advent of transplantation renewed old problems of how to locate suitable sources of tissue and raised new issues of morality and medical ethics. The introduction of heart transplantation prompted intense debate about the traditional conceptions of life and death and the need for a new, legal definition of brain death. Concerns about organ transplantation and fears that doctors would allow some patients to die in order to enhance the lives of others played a significant role in the development of a new public discourse about medical morality—bioethics.

Since the 1980s, American investment in organ transplantation has grown dramatically. Although the supply of organs available for transplantation has remained roughly the same, the medical indications for transplant have expanded. In 2007, more than 97,000 people in the United States are currently listed as waiting for one or more donor organs, but only 20,000 or so are expected to become available. The disparity between supply and demand has fostered intense interest in increasing the supply of organs, through xenotransplantation, through such political solutions such as laws for "presumed" consent to donate organs, and through economic plans of private insurers and state laws to pay organ suppliers or their families for tissue. The final chapter of *Flesh and Blood* explores how the problems of allocation and scarcity have influenced public responses to organ transplantation and donation by placing the issue in the context of larger societal concerns about the integrity of the body.

In the 1980s and 1990s, one profound challenge to bodily integrity was the advent of a new blood-borne and sexually transmitted agent, the human immunodeficiency virus (HIV). The outbreak of the acquired immune deficiency syndrome (AIDS) pandemic and the profound compromise of the American blood supply stirred new concerns about the violation of natural boundaries and the issue of self-protection. These boundary transgressions have intensified following publicity surrounding such emerging diseases as Ebola and "mad cow disease" (bovine spongiform encephalopathy), and the fears about crossing the species barrier in transplantation.

The issue of bodily integrity, as *Flesh and Blood* argues, is neither simple nor straightforward. Instead, the meanings of self, identity, and integrity reflect particular historical situations and contingencies. Throughout the twentieth century, the technologies of transfusion and transplantation offered new opportunities and novel interfaces for probing the limits of biomedical innovation, reconsidering the nature of heroism and altruism, reconceptualizing human individuality and community, and for understanding the nature of what it means to be flesh and blood.

Notes

1. The classic history is Max Wintrobe, ed. *Blood, Pure and Eloquent: A Story of Discovery, of People, and of Ideas* (New York: McGraw-Hill, 1980). For an excellent survey of blood transfusion over four centuries, see Douglas Starr, *Blood: An Epic Story of Medicine and Commerce* (New York: Knopf, 1998), and the significant contributions of historians William C. Schneider and Kim Pelis discussed elsewhere in this book.

2. See Donald Joralemon, "Organ Wars: The Battle for Body Parts," *Medical Anthropology Quarterly 9 (1995)*: 335–356.

3. Christopher Lawrence, ed. *Medical Theory, Surgical Practice: Studies in the History of Surgery* (New York: Routledge, 1992), 15.

4. See, for example, David J. Rothman, "Ethical and Social Consequences of Selling a Kidney," *JAMA* 288 (2002): 1640–1641, and David J. Rothman and Sheila M. Rothman, "The Organ Market." *The New York Review of Books* 50 (2003): 49–50. See Nancy Scheper-Hughes, *The Ends of the Body: The Global Traffic in Organs* (Farrar, Straus & Giroux, forthcoming).

5. Keith Wailoo, *Dying in the City of the Blues: Sickle Cell Anemia and the Politics of Race and Health* (Chapel Hill: University of North Carolina Press, 2001); and Spencie Love, *One Blood: The Death and Resurrection of Charles Drew* (Chapel Hill: University of North Carolina Press, 1997).

6. For the classic work on social aspects of transplantation, see Renée C. Fox and Judith P. Swazey, *Spare Parts: Organ Replacement in American Society* (New York: Oxford University Press, 1992). For recent work on heart transplants, see Nicholas L. Tilney, *Transplant: From Myth to Reality* (New Haven: Yale University Press, 2003); Donald McCrae, *Every Second Counts: The Race to Transplant the First Human Heart* (New York: Simon & Schuster, 2006); and the superb book by anthropologist Margaret Lock, *Twice Dead: Organ Transplants and the Reinvention of Death* (Berkeley: University of California Press, 2002).

Flesh and Blood

1

Living on the Island of Dr. Moreau
Grafting Tissues in the Early Twentieth Century

In his 1896 novel, *The Island of Doctor Moreau*, English novelist H. G. Wells created a memorable and influential portrait of a surgeon, forced to leave London after the press reported the escape of dogs mutilated in his experiments. Far away in the South Seas, Doctor Moreau performs surgery in what the island inhabitants call the "House of Pain." These surgeries produce "humanized animals"—wolf-hyena-man, ox-hog-man, and puma-woman—which Moreau regards as "triumphs of vivisection." The surgical manipulation of the flesh and blood, as he informs a hapless, shipwrecked visitor to the island where he conducts his dark science, could accomplish many things:

> You have heard, perhaps, of a common surgical operation resorted to in
> cases where the nose has been destroyed: a flap of skin is cut from the
> forehead, turned down on the nose, and heals in the new position. This is
> a kind of grafting in a new position of a part of an animal upon itself.

Moreau explains that tissue could also be transferred from one animal to another: "Grafting of freshly obtained material from another animal is also possible—the case of teeth, for example. The grafting of skin and bone is done to facilitate healing: the surgeon places in the middle of the wound pieces of skin snipped from another animal, or fragments of bone from a victim freshly killed."[1]

Wells knew that such surgical techniques were no scientific romance. Moreau's reference to teeth invoked the classic experiments in transplantation undertaken by surgeon John Hunter. In his 1771 *Treatise on the Natural History of Human Teeth*, Hunter had described how he successfully implanted a human tooth in a rooster's comb, and transferred the spur from a young cock onto a hen, and the spur of a hen onto a cock, in an effort to determine the influence of sex on the movement of these body parts. Hunter's experiments stimulated a vogue in England for "live tooth transplantation," in which healthy teeth removed from the mouths of poor children were implanted into the mouths of wealthy men and women who paid both the dentist and the donors.[2] *The Island of Doctor Moreau* also invoked the classic experiments of the French physiologist Paul Bert, who manufactured "monsters" by transporting animal parts to other animals or to different areas of the body. Moreau's description of "rhinoceros rats" echoed studies in which Bert implanted the tip of the tail of a rat under the skin of its back. The transplanted tail grew, forming new bone and establishing circulation. Bert also created such "double monsters" as the rat-cat by surgically uniting two different animals.[3]

Grafts involving both animal and human tissues became more common in the late nineteenth and early twentieth centuries. The expansion of surgery in the late nineteenth century encompassed considerable efforts to transfer skin, bones, nerves, muscles, tissue, and organs taken from both animal and human bodies—living and dead—in efforts to restore the appearance, structure, and function of human bodies.[4] Some of the human tissue was donated by friends, family members, and strangers, but, in other cases, surgeons salvaged tissue from the birthing-room, the anatomy laboratory, and the surgery. In some exceptional cases, doctors and patients purchased body parts from individuals seeking financial compensation for their tissue, discomfort, and potential risk. When human tissue was not available, patients and physicians used tissue taken from animals. Stories of these surgical exploits appeared frequently in the popular press and in the medical literature, and provided plot devices for some popular films of the early twentieth century.

This chapter examines the extensive use of grafting as a surgical therapy in the late nineteenth century, exploring the meaning of such surgeries for physicians and patients when they administered and received the physically intimate materials from others—animal and human. Surgeons adopted the term *grafting* from botanists and horticulturalists, who used the word to describe the process of joining two plants or plant parts together in such a way that the plant parts united and continued to grow. The propagation of fruit trees, for example, dated from the time of the Romans, who were credited with being the first to develop the technical skills of fruit cultivation, including grafting techniques. In the nineteenth century, surgeons generally used the term to refer to the transfer of tissues to the exterior of the body. Although some surgeons used the word *transplantation* as a synonym for grafting, other physicians and surgeons preferred to reserve that word to refer to the transfer of interior tissues, including pieces and parts of internal organs such as the thyroid, kidney, and ovary. Some surgeons also used the word *implantation* to mean "practically the same as transplantation," although again, some practitioners sought to reserve the term *implant* for the introduction of inorganic materials (ivory, rubber) into the body.

In the early twentieth century, the press sensationalized the transplantation of tissue and played a role in shaping popular expectations about grafting and its results. Reporters celebrated those donors willing to undergo the knife and those recipients whose misfortunes required extensive surgical repair. At the same time, novels, plays, and popular films of the early twentieth century explored the darker side of what came to be called "spare parts surgery." Just as Wells pursued the dire consequences of Doctor Moreau's "Beast Folk," some American writers and film-makers exploited the possibility of unusual surgical unions between humans and animals, between living and dead bodies. Many of these productions pressed the issue of the transmission of more than body parts or fluids; in these novels and films, when the surgeon transfers the hand of a murderer, the hand retains its desire to kill. In these stories, the horror of such transgressive surgical procedures was intensified by the corrupting role that the ample funds of the recipient and the financial need of the donor played in the endeavor. American critics of medical research, especially antivivisectionists and antivaccinationists, used such depictions to further their indictment of such practices.

These critics and these cultural productions should not obscure the apparent willingness of many Americans to pursue methods that transgressed the conventional boundaries of the human body in the name of restoring its appearance and function. Drawing on letters and other materials from individuals seeking graft surgery for themselves or for a family member, it becomes apparent that we need a more nuanced understanding of the cultural reception of transplantation in the first half of the twentieth century. Early twentieth-century Americans, like their twenty-first-century descendants, were willing to try radical methods if they promised relief from suffering and the prospect of bodily improvement. They were willing to obtain the necessary tissues given or taken from other people and to supply, if needed, the animals whose bodies could provide material. The threat to the donor's intact body posed by grafting and transplantation coexisted alongside the promise that the damaged bodies of recipients could be made whole. Just as the experience of such basic human instincts as hunger and appetite are influenced by social and cultural factors, so too conceptions of the intact and dismembered human body—dead and alive—are transformed in particular cultural settings. For many Americans in the twentieth century, the prospect of living on the Island of Doctor Moreau was no horror story. Instead, it promised a vista of healing disfigured bodies and reshaping broken lives.

Skin and Bones

In his 1897 address on surgery to the American Medical Association, Philadelphia surgeon William Williams Keen celebrated American contributions to the enormous strides being made in surgery during the second half of the nineteenth century. Ether, Keen noted, was discovered by an American dentist; it was first used by an American surgeon, and it was broadcast to the world in an American medical journal. So rapidly had surgical progress come in the late nineteenth century that the surgical giants of the preceding generation would neither be able to teach modern surgical principles nor to perform a modern surgical procedure. "Even our everyday surgical vocabulary," observed Keen, "staphylococcus, streptococcus, infection, immunity, antisepsis, toxin and antitoxin—would be unintelligible jargon to him; and our modern operations on the brain, the chest, the abdomen, and the pelvis would make him wonder whether we had not lost our senses."[5] The "magical, nay such almost divine power" of the modern surgeon encouraged them to undertake a variety of new procedures, techniques, and materials to repair bodies and restore lost function.

The interest in grafting skin accompanied the general expansion of surgery in the second half of the nineteenth century. The transfer of skin from one part of the body to another was not new; nineteenth-century medical writers religiously recorded the ancient pedigree of grafting by physicians in India as early as 2500 B.C., where "the barbarous custom" of cutting off noses encouraged the practice of rhinoplasty (grafting skin from the forehead onto the nasal area). These writers similarly acknowledged the Renaissance physician Gasparo Tagliacozzi's efforts at nasal reconstruction. Working in Bologna in the late sixteenth century, the Italian physician had introduced a method of using skin from more distant body parts (such as the forearm) to repair the damaged or missing nose.[6] Even a pioneering American surgeon merited respectful remembrance. American physicians cited the work of New York surgeon Frank Hamilton, who in the 1850s developed what he called "elkoplasty," a method of taking skin from one part of a patient's body to treat other badly ulcerated areas.[7] But the revolution in "epidermic grafting" followed the 1869 demonstration by Jacques Louis Reverdin, an intern at the Hôpital Necker in Paris, of a simple and reliable method for repairing ulcerated skin.[8]

Reverdin's method involved picking up small pieces of skin with a sharp hook and snipping them off with a pair of sharp scissors. These pieces, taken either from the patient or from another body, were then transferred to the injured area. If successful, the grafts served as islands of new growth on the skin surface. Other techniques for grafting skin quickly developed, including the Thiersch method, named for the Leipzig physician Carl Thiersch. His method involved splitting the skin with a razor and removing strips of epidermis (outer skin) and dermis 1–2 inches wide and 3–4 inches long. These strips were applied directly to the surface of the wound and strapped into position with gutta-percha (a resin produced by evaporating the milky fluid from the gutta-percha tree, native to the Malay peninsula).[9] Other significant grafting techniques included the Wolfe-Krause method (named for Glasgow ophthalmologist, J.R. Wolfe, and greatly improved by Berlin neurosurgeon Fedor Krause), which entailed the use of grafts from the full thickness of the skin (with fat) to fill in a defect or wound.[10] Spurred by the work of Reverdin, American surgeons adopted these methods and reported their results in the medical press. In 1871, Rafael Morales, the resident surgeon at the Charity Hospital on Blackwell's Island in New York, treated Bridget O'Connor's recurring leg ulcer using skin transplantation. He transferred 18 small pieces of skin from the 43-year-old Irish immigrant's left thigh to her ankle, successfully healing the ulcerated area after 48 days.[11] At St. Vincent's Hospital in New York, "indolent ulcers" prompted surgeons there to perform skin grafts on Ellen Wilson, a 29-year-old Irish laundress, and Mary Wilson, a 30-year-old immigrant employed as a domestic servant. Both women had undergone treatment with poultice and tonics, but the ulcers on their legs failed to heal. After years of unsuccessful treatment, both women agreed to undergo the attempt at skin grafting.

Chronic ulcers prompted much of the early efforts at skin grafting. "To the general practitioner," Georgia physician B.M. Cromwell noted in 1876, "an old ulcerated leg is the very *bete noir* of his profession; his spirit dies within him when one presents itself, and if, with a generous donation of 'salve' he can be rid of his patient and quiet his conscience, he rejoices at the thought of how much time, annoyance, and ultimate disappointment have been spared him."[12] The beleaguered surgeon found that the Reverdin method offered a gratifying solution to this problem. Cromwell described his success in treating a "colored" man who developed a large leg ulcer after he was kicked by a horse on the shin. The doctor applied skin grafts the size of "canary seed" and "barley corn" to the surface of the deep ulcer (the rotted shin bone was visible in the ulcer) and, after 2 months, reported the healing of the man's leg.

Industrial accidents and injuries provided many candidates for skin grafting. To read the surgical case reports of the late nineteenth century is to be reminded of the risks that workers incurred in a host of different occupations and settings. The cases at St. Vincent's Hospital, where grafting was attempted in 1871, included two such injured workers—a 22-year-old Norwegian laborer and a 29-year-old Irish laborer, who had both experienced trauma in the workplace. Olof Thostenson had his left thigh crushed by a falling bank of clay; John Cullen received extensive burns on his left thigh when he fell into a burning lime kiln. Both men were considered successfully treated by the skin grafts.[13] In 1878, Samuel Root, an iron moulder, underwent skin grafting after a stream of melted iron ran over his foot, incinerating his sock, boot, and badly burning his foot and leg.[14] In 1895, a 33-year-old "German laborer" employed in a bicycle factory had his clothes torn off in a revolving shaft. The machine also ripped away the entire skin covering his external genitals; two months after his injury, he left the hospital "highly pleased" with the grafting efforts to restore his appearance and function.[15]

Among the injured that physicians increasingly encountered were women factory workers, whose long hair became entangled in machinery. American surgeons had occasionally treated scalp avulsion (the extensive laceration and separation of the scalp) that resulted from "Indian scalpings." The mechanization of farming and factory work increased the numbers of women patients with this injury. In 1872, Miss M.N., a 16-year-old girl working at a bench in a shoe shop, caught her long hair in one of the revolving belts. Her scalp, forehead skin, and part of her right cheek were entirely torn off. Her physician immediately attempted to reattach her scalp. When the reattachment proved unsuccessful, her physician performed a series of skin grafts once a week over a period of 3 years. For the donors, the procedure involved lifting the skin with a pair of forceps and cutting out a piece of skin about one-eighth by one-sixteenth of an inch. During the 3 years in which Miss M.N. underwent skin grafting, her physician removed over 1300 grafts from 128 different people, many of them "mere children."[16] In 1874, Miss Hattie Thomas, working in a factory in Naugatuck, Connecticut, similarly caught her hair in a revolving shaft, which removed her entire scalp from her head, including her left ear. Although her physician attempted to reattach her scalp, the wounds were too extensive, and it failed to adhere. Doctor S. C. Bartlett removed skin for grafting from the young woman "until the excessive discharge from these additional wounds made it necessary to desist." He then removed 64 pieces of skin from many of her friends, and considered the treatment satisfactory for the slow process of recovering her scalp.[17] In 1902, when a 19-year-old woman caught her long hair in her mechanical loom at the American Felt Company, more than 200 of her fellow employees supplied skin to repair the area where she had lost her scalp and part of an ear.[18]

As these cases make clear, one of the issues immediately confronting surgeons was obtaining tissue for grafting. When the injury was extensive, much tissue was required to repair the damage. Who would serve as the source of the necessary tissue? Physicians identified three principal options: *autoplasty* (using the patient's own skin), *heteroplasty* (using another person's skin), or *zooplasty* (using skin taken from animals).[19] Most physicians looked first to the injured person to serve as a source of grafts. There were several reasons for doing so. Since Reverdin's "revolution," some physicians had noted that grafts using skin taken from the patient were often more successful than those taken from another person. Although they lacked a persuasive explanation of the phenomenon, the success was seen as the result of "the difficulty that sometimes accrues from a want of power in the new graft to assimilate itself to the tissues on which it is placed."[20] These early observations about the likely failure of grafts from another person remained little understood in the nineteenth century and were by no means universally shared. After World War I, the blood types discovered by Karl Landsteiner would be introduced into the process of skin grafting.[21] The immunologic specificity of the human body (the idea that distinct types of proteins exist in skin and other tissue) would be established in the 1940s, most notably through the work of English researcher Sir Peter Medawar.

Another reason for the preference for using skin from the patient's own body was fear of transmitting disease. This "risk of introducing into the blood of the living subject some new or poisonous element" inspired caution in some physicians.[22] Medical practitioners discussed the possibility that syphilis, smallpox, tuberculosis, and cancer could be transmissible through grafting.[23] Syphilis created the most concern. But reports of surgeons who developed cancers on their hands after performing surgeries to remove cancer also prompted speculation. In one notorious case, a German surgeon, Eugen Hahn conducted "an experiment for which he was severely censured"; he removed skin from a cancerous growth on a patient, then intentionally implanted the cancerous tissue into a wound in another part of the patient's body. At this point of implantation, a new cancer grew.[24] The fear of such diseases—incurable and fatal—made some, but not all, surgeons reluctant to use random volunteers as skin sources. But, despite this concern about disease transmission (and as the cases of Hattie Thomas and Miss M.N., who received grafts from 64 and 128 people, respectively, show), many physicians did not confine their grafting efforts to using only the patient as the source of tissue.

For many American physicians, asking the patient to undergo extensive removal of skin was not always feasible or acceptable. "To take large pieces of skin from the patient's own body is an objectionable practice on account of the large wound it creates," noted surgeon Thomas Bryant in 1872. In the case of young children, already traumatized by severe burns, shaving portions of skin from uninjured parts of the child's body was unacceptable to both physicians and parents. "The surface was so extensive, and the boy in such a weak and nervous condition," explained Boston physician George Seeley Smith in 1891, "that any attempt to have taken the necessary epidermis from him would have been imprudent."[25] When he treated 3-year-old Jacob Weisenfeld, badly burned after playing with matches, Buffalo surgeon Herman Mynter described how the hospital house staff "kindly consented to give the little patient some of their superfluous cuticle" when the boy himself could not supply the necessary skin. Mynter also called on 10 medical students to supply 20 large flaps of skin to treat 6-year-old Regina Meier, whose clothes had caught fire, leaving her badly burned.

Using the patient as the source of skin also entailed seeking permission from the individual or his family. In the late nineteenth century, the status of patient permission for surgery remained muddled in both law and practice. Surgeons were sometimes sued for "battery" when they performed surgery without the patient's consent; in the early twentieth century, lawsuits like that brought by Mrs. Mary Schloendorff in 1911 for an unauthorized hysterectomy (*Schloendorff v. Society of New York Hospital*) encouraged surgeons and hospital administrators to urge that doctors obtain written consent for surgical procedures. (This should not be understood as "informed consent," but only as recognition that the patient authorized some sort of surgical procedure.)[26] In the late nineteenth century, as skin grafting developed, surgeons discussed the need to obtain consent from the patient or guardian. "The consent of the patient is the first thing to be secured," M. Donelly, house surgeon at New York's St. Vincent's Hospital, explained in 1872, "but it is generally given when the advantages of this mode of treatment are properly represented."[27] Donelly's case reports illustrated that some patients resisted. It took 7 months before he was able to persuade his patient Olof Thostenson to allow the surgeon to draw blood to obtain skin for the grafts after his leg failed to heal. A railway surgeon echoed Donelly's experience. "I find much difficulty," he noted in 1894, "in getting patients to consent to the operation because of the pain it causes. Many persons will suffer from open sores for a long time rather than to have skin grafting performed."[28]

Failure to obtain consent could result in legal problems. Surgeon Leonard Freeman offered two cases in which legal complications resulted from skin grafting. In Atlanta a 13-year-old boy brought his cousin to a physician's office, where he agreed to have skin shaved from his arm to aid his cousin. According to Freeman, the father of the boy donor immediately brought suit against the physician on the grounds that the surgery was both "unjustifiable and brutal" and not authorized by the parent. In the second case, a Cincinnati man sued a physician after donating some of his skin. Although he received payment for his donation, the donor claimed that the surgeon took more skin than he had authorized. In these two cases, the physicians, rather than the patients, prevailed.[29]

One of the reasons physicians sought consent from their grafting patients was the need for the patient's cooperation with a demanding regimen. When Chicago surgeon Nicholas Senn proposed a daring new method to treat the hand of a man catastrophically burned in a wreck of the Chicago, Rock Island and Pacific Railway in 1894, he suggested a therapeutic experiment in which the man's hand ("like a piece of mangled beef") was inserted into a sling fashioned of skin sliced from his stomach. E. E. Lyday (the patient) reportedly "shuddered at the suggestion but pluckily agreed to the test." His hand was placed in the stomach flap until the skin adhered to the burned flesh; after detachment, he was once again able to use the injured part.[30]

When physicians sought to locate friends and family members for skin for grafting, they faced questions about the pain and risk. How painful was skin donation? To some extent, it depended on the technique used for removing the skin. For the Reverdin method, the surgeon used scissors to remove small "barley corn" sized pieces; in others, the surgeon employed a razor to remove larger pieces. Many surgeons dismissed as minor the pain associated with shaving a portion of the skin with a common or section razor. Eminent New York surgeon George R. Fowler, for example, observed that any pain was "really slight"; his donors described the donation procedure as "accompanied only by a peculiar burning sensation."[31] Another surgeon noted the transience of the pain associated with taking the skin; cutting the donor's skin "causes in nearly all of the patients only a sharp indrawing of the breath, 'sss,' for the few seconds to remove the graft."[32] Other surgeons scoffed at the "peculiar ideas" of some surgeons about foregoing anesthesia and the "needless torture" of patients when the grafts were taken.[33]

Watching the procedure may have alarmed some potential donors; for this reason, Brooklyn surgeon Julius Rose advised covering the eyes of "hysterical adults" and "very nervous children" with a bandage, so they could not "see the pain."[34] If surgeons dismissed the pain as minor, some patients certainly did not. When Rose treated a 7-year-old boy whose thumb and metacarpal bone were blown off by the explosion of a cannon firecracker, he explained that "grafts were taken from his thigh without anesthesia. He made quite a fuss, but then, he always did whenever the wound was dressed."[35]

The problem of pain introduced a new wrinkle into the skin grafting procedure: how to balance the risk and benefit from using anesthetics to make the procedure easier and more acceptable to donors. As historian Martin Pernick has argued, from its very introduction, the use of anesthesia raised ethical issues for physicians and surgeons. By the 1870s and 1880s, spurred by the adoption of antiseptic surgery and the introduction of cocaine, the practice of selective anesthesia—choosing patients suitable for anesthesia—was gradually being superseded by a process of tailoring anesthetic choice to individual patients.[36] In the case of skin grafting, the risks and discomforts of anesthetics for the "secondary wound" in a donor now had to be balanced against the need to obtain sufficient skin for a third party. Because many potential donors apparently feared the "choking and subsequent vomiting" associated with inhaling ether anesthesia, some physicians tried to dispense with anesthetics altogether, to develop alternative methods of applications (colonic anesthesia, for example), or to administer regional agents like cocaine.[37] But practical concerns also existed. In cases where large numbers of individuals donated small amounts of skin, it was problematic to administer anesthesia. "Where a number of individuals volunteer to furnish the skin for transplantation, and but a single strip is taken from each," Fowler noted in 1889, "it will be obviously impracticable to administer an anesthetic to each donor. On the other hand, but few will be found to volunteer to give a large amount of skin, and endure the inconveniences and risks of an anesthetic; nor yet to allow themselves to be flayed alive, with all that the term implies."[38] In addition to apprehension about being "flayed alive," physicians and patients worried about scarring when donating skin. Concern about the visible results of donating skin prompted some physicians, when possible, to remove skin only from areas where the scars could be covered by clothing–from the leg and thigh instead of the arm.[39]

These difficulties were even greater when surgeons proposed a more radical solution to the need for skin. When Johns Hopkins surgeon John M. T. Finney treated a badly burned 5-year-old, he removed skin from the thigh of her older sister. After donating a graft from her thigh, the young woman agreed to undergo a direct transplantation of skin, in which she and her sister were physically linked. Under ether, a 5-by-7-inch flap of skin was raised from her thigh and her sister's injured foot inserted between the flap and the leg. The two girls were placed in the same bed and were "surprisingly comfortable." But the surgical bond between the two sisters did not end well. The restless movements of the small child led Finney to end the procedure earlier than he had planned. "She was a spoiled child and willfully added to the pain and discomfort of her older sister by moving her foot as much as possible when she felt so disposed." After 10 days in which the two sisters were linked

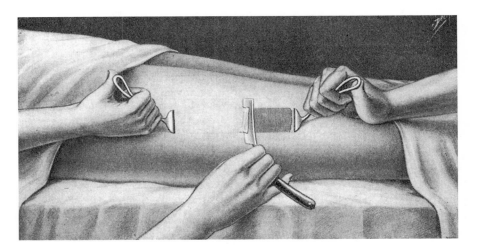

Figure 1.1 Physicians seeking skin for grafting sometimes encountered reluctance from those individuals who feared pain, scarring, or worse from skin donation (R. Fowler, *The Operating Room and the Patient*. Philadelphia: WB Saunders, 1913).

and placed in the same bed, Finney could not justify maintaining their bond any longer, "owing to the needless pain inflicted by the patient upon her sister, who bore it most heroically."[40] Finney was fortunate that the girls were able to stay linked for 10 days. When a Boston surgeon surgically linked the foot of one brother to a raised abdominal flap on his brother, he encountered worse problems. As soon as the boys recovered from the ether, "they began to be very uncomfortable and used language of the most violent kind toward each other, and almost came to blows." After only 6 days, he was forced to sever the flaps. The difficulties were not unpredictable. That same year, Finney's surgical colleague, William Halsted, described the problems he had encountered in uniting the muscles in one dog to another dog. "The experiments had finally to be given up because of the impossibility of keeping the dogs quiet."[41]

The difficulties associated with finding live human donors—the issue of consent, the concern about anesthesia—encouraged some surgeons to look for alternative sources. "Most individuals object to furnishing skin for grafting either onto their own body or any other person's body," observed Oshkosh physician F. Gregory Connell, "and this trait of human nature has led the surgeon to utilize any possible source of material that calls for little or no pain or sacrifice."[42] Among these human materials were the "waste products" of surgery, the "refuse of nature" from the birthing room, and skin from amputated limbs, the stillborn, and the newly dead. Skin from amputated limbs and the bodies of the newly dead were quickly appropriated for skin grafting. In 1874, Philadelphia surgeon David Hayes Agnew used skin from amputated limbs, although he noted that using such skin was "usually repugnant to a patient's feelings."[43] This early use of amputated skin and skin taken from the bodies of the newly dead excited editorial comment. In 1881, an editorial in the *New York Times* described a "plastic surgical operation that will strike most persons as revolting in its details, however successful its results."[44] The editorial described a recent claim by the surgeon John H. Girdner that he was the first to remove skin from a cadaver for grafting onto a living subject. The New York physician removed skin from the dead body of "a healthy young German, who had attempted suicide by cutting his throat," and placed it on a 10-year-old boy, badly burned when lightning struck his body.[45] Girdner did not indicate that the boy or his family were informed that the skin for the grafting came from a suicide victim. If they had not been informed by the physician, it is possible that they learned of it once the newspaper published the editorial about the doctor's practice. It is not possible to know whether they would have been repulsed by the practice.

Certainly, physicians did not express revulsion when they explored the possibility of using such tissue. In 1882, a Norwich, Connecticut physician reported his experiments on the limits of viability for skin taken from amputated limbs or the bodies of the dead. He conducted eight studies in which he used grafts taken from a newly amputated leg, a newly amputated foot, and the skin from a "still-born babe at full term," 36 hours after its death.[46] In some cases, patients or families were certainly aware of the source of skin. In 1895, physician C. F. Timmerman picked up a leg amputated at the Amsterdam City Hospital and drove to the home of his private patient, where, assisted only by the patient's sister, he made 22 "irregular clippings" from the leg and applied them to the severe burn on the chest of his patient.[47] By 1909, however, the potential supply of skin from amputated limbs had apparently diminished. "Fortunately for humanity," noted F. Gregory Connell, "even if unfortunate for the individuals in need of skin, amputations are becoming comparatively uncommon, so much so that they offer but a very uncertain source of material." In light of this growing scarcity, Connell recommended additional sources. These tissues included such "waste products from surgery" as the skin removed in the process of circumcision, and placental and fetal tissues. Connell recommended that patients undergoing laparotomy (a surgery that involved opening the abdomen) be asked for permission to use the skin removed during their surgery. Consent should always be secured, Connell argued, "otherwise misunderstandings with more or less annoying consequences might arise."[48]

One potential source of skin available in the hospital was the excised foreskin removed in the circumcision procedure. The "suppleness, thinness and vascularity" of this tissue made it especially attractive for grafting purposes.[49] Two developments in early twentieth-century America made such tissue increasingly available to grafters: hospital-based birth and the transformation of circumcision from a religious ritual to a commonly performed surgical procedure.[50] Grafts made from the foreskin, surgeon Leonard Freeman explained, "could be obtained in abundance in children's hospitals, just where it was most needed."[51] In addition to skin taken from newborns or from infants treated for phimosis (a tightness at the end of the foreskin which hinders the retraction of the penis), surgeons sometimes asked adults to undergo circumcision to aid a friend or family member. In 1909, when Stephen Calabro, a 19-year-old Italian man, was severely burned in an explosion in a fireworks factory, he developed massive scarring on his face, hands, and arms. To correct the defect, surgeons at the Massachusetts General Hospital performed numerous grafting operations, using skin from his uninjured legs, thigh, and chest. When more skin was needed, two of his brothers and a friend agreed to be circumcised and their donated prepuces were used for grafts to his face.[52] In another case, a New York surgeon unable to locate suitable tissue for grafting "advised circumcision" to a 16-year-old boy who had ripped off the end of his finger on a fence post. The tissue from the prepuce was used to graft the injured finger.[53] Richmond surgeon Stuart McGuire used tissue taken from the scrotum of a man undergoing an operation for varicocele as a graft on a woman who had surgery for cancer.[54]

The transfer of birth from the home to the hospital also provided physicians with a dependable supply of other tissue; namely, the placenta expelled after childbirth and fetal tissues obtained from miscarriages and stillbirths. In 1913, New York physician Nicholas Sabella began praising the use of fetal membranes as a source for skin grafting. When one of his burn patients, fearing the pain of the procedure and the resulting scarring, refused to allow the taking of skin, he began using tissue from the placenta available after childbirth.[55] Retrieving grafts from the fetal membranes eliminated "the use of the razor and anesthetic as well as the entailed secondary wound with its numerous inconveniences."[56] Did the source of tissue matter to the patients? Patients like the boy with the injured finger certainly knew the source of the tissue and its use on the body. But what of the woman whose face was repaired with scrotal tissue? We have no record that she knew the source of tissue, nor whether she had any objections to it. And the physicians left few, if any, records about how their patients responded to the use of these tissues.

In the continuing search to locate useable materials in sufficient quantity, surgeons turned to animals as a source of tissue for skin grafting. Using the tissue of pigs, dogs, rabbits, frogs, and other animals presented both opportunities and challenges. Pigeon-skin grafting, as one Massachusetts physician explained in 1893, offered several advantages. Removing skin from the bird did "not necessitate an anesthetic; its failure does not discourage because squabs come as cheap as a can of ether, and you can graft without even the consent of the patient, or in fact, the patient hardly realizing what you are doing."[57] Pigeon skin did raise the issue of feathers. N.B. Aldrich advised fellow surgeons that this prospect could be avoided by selecting young squabs whose feathers had not developed under the wings and half-grown birds, which he plucked after killing.

American surgeons attempted a bewildering array of procedures using parts taken from animals, both living and dead. As in the case of the linked children, some surgeons attempted skin grafting using a living animal, despite the difficulties this posed for the patient and the staff. The belief that skin that remained partially attached to its blood supply promised better results when grafted onto the recipient was grounded in a number of animal experiments in which surgeons surgically joined dissimilar animals.[58] Putting this into practice presented a number of obstacles for both patients and doctors. In 1880, when E. W. Lee, a physician at the County Hospital in Chicago, grafted skin flaps from a live lamb onto the back of a badly burned 10-year-old girl, he found it necessary to place the lamb in a wooden cage and fix its limbs into position by bandages and plaster of Paris to achieve the animal's complete immobilization. Maintaining the child's immobility presented less difficulty as her condition was already failing when the procedure was undertaken, and she died before the lamb skin was detached. When Lee repeated the procedure on a man with a large ulcer on his leg, he found it more difficult to achieve the desired immobilization. The animal's constant movement prevented adhesion of the flap, and he was compelled to dissolve their union.[59] In 1889, surgeons at the Grace Hospital in Detroit similarly attempted to treat the massive scalp injury of a 9-year-old girl with grafts from a live animal. They sutured a partially detached flap from the side of a live dog to the girl's head. (The dog was tied to the child's bed.) This graft failed.

In the first decade of the twentieth century, a "rising young surgeon at a well known New York medical school" attempted a similar experiment in the treatment of a socially prominent woman, whose severely burned thigh had failed to heal. According to New York physician Samuel Lambert, the surgeon dissected a 6-inch square of skin from the back of a young male white pig, leaving one 6-inch side still intact on the animal. He then attached the living pigskin to the woman's thigh. Although both the patient and the pig recovered from the anesthesia, complications soon developed. Nursing care provided "to care for the calls of nature for the Lady" did not meet the needs of the pig. Special arrangements, including tissue paper products from the Star Pulp Mills, the predecessors of Scott Tissue, were implemented with little success. In addition to the pig's eliminatory problems, the animal's constant movement of the skin flap caused the patient considerable pain. The surgeon was able to recruit several undergraduate students to maintain the pig in a constant state of etherization. After several days, however, the enthusiasm of the students waned; the surgeon decided to sever the pig' spinal cord to paralyze the animal. The incision, instead of immobilizing the animal, killed it. The pig was detached from the woman, who subsequently received Thiersch grafts with both her own skin and that of other human donors.[60] These grafts were understandably less common than simply removing the desired tissue from the animal body and transplanting it onto a patient.

Most physicians preferred to use skin wholly separated from the animal body. They attempted grafts with a number of animal species, including dogs, frogs, pigeons, chickens, cats, and rabbits. Availability and the absence of hair and fur (achieved by using young animals) generally influenced animal selection. In using dogs as skin donors, for example, physicians generally selected young animals or only certain breeds. In 1890, when M.E. Van Meter, a physician in Red Bluff, Colorado, wanted to apply skin grafts to treat the severe burns of a 14-year-old boy, he first took grafts from the boy's father and brother. Needing even more skin, however, the physician removed grafts from two young puppies of the "Mexican hairless breed," and applied them to the boy's arm, achieving a "superior result."[61] As one surgeon noted, dogs could be readily obtained by either the doctor or the patient's family.[62] When Richmond surgeon Stuart McGuire treated a badly burned African American child in 1903, he explained that the child was too feeble to provide skin. Not only did the child's relations refuse to donate material, but "no jail bird would volunteer as a victim" even with the prospect of parole. McGuire purchased a chocolate-colored pig for grafting. "The pig was brought in on one table, the pickaninny on another. Grafts were taken from the belly of the pig and planted on the back of the child." The pig skin graft was only partly successful because the child removed the dressing and disturbed the new skin.[63]

Perhaps the most commonly selected animal for grafting was the frog. Like dogs, frogs were easily acquired (although less available in winter months). Surgeon George Fowler recommended using large, healthy frogs that could be maintained for several days in a container containing clean water. When the animal was needed, Fowler explained how the amphibian was "held by an assistant by grasping its extremities and head while the operator, pinching up a fold of skin, snips it through transversely to the long axis of the frog's body, and just behind its eyes, for from a quarter to half an inch, according to the size of the frog."[64] Fowler predicted that the size of the strips would reflect the steadiness on the part of the assistant holding the animal.

What did patients or their families make of the reconstitution of the human body with tissue from nonhuman animals? Although some British and French patients apparently refused to accept skin from frogs, American physicians did not discuss the prospect of frogskin as a potential problem.[65] American surgeons who used frog grafts noted that the pigment in frog skin disappeared after 7–10 days; this may have served to reassure anxious patients about the resulting appearance of their grafts. Some physicians apparently shared concerns about the subsequent life of the transplanted skin. When he introduced chicken-skin grafting, for example, one physician assured readers that the new skin did not "show any signs that would excite the fear of a growth of feathers."[66] When he described the case of the woman surgically joined to the pig, surgeon Samuel Lambert informed the fellow members of the Charaka Club (an association for literary and historically minded physicians) that the appearance of the graft "really looked not unlike a bristleless pig skin." This may explain why the lady continued to believe that her skin had in fact united with that of the pig—that and the fact that her surgeon failed to disclose that "the pig experiment was an entire failure." Perhaps it was the wonder of the surgical union of woman and pig that prompted her to insist on exhibiting the resulting scar tissue to interested women physicians. (Lambert did not see the actual scar; he received that intelligence from a female colleague.)[67] We have no direct information about how patients regarded the union of their skin with animal skin. Some individuals, like this lady and the boy who received skin from a Mexican hairless dog, were aware of the source of grafts. Some learned about their surgery after their recovery, like John Doughtery, who "was greatly surprised" to hear that he had a chicken bone engrafted in his shinbone in 1891, after being injured working on the Wabash Railroad.[68] Some patients, because of their age or serious injury, no doubt never realized the nature of their surgery. When Adele Robertson attempted suicide in 1923, she underwent a surgical procedure in which a kidney taken from a lamb was placed in her thigh in an effort to rid her body of the toxin. But Robertson never regained consciousness and died shortly after, unaware of the nature of her surgery.

Given the catastrophic nature of their injuries, the source of the material used to treat wounds, burns, and ulcerations may have seemed the least of one's concerns. Horace Packard, a Massachusetts homeopathic physician, published his patient's own account of her extensive injuries following a fire in 1892. "I came down four stories from a burning apartment by means of a rope suspended from a window one story higher than my own. My hands simply clasped the rope, and as it was very rough, . . . the palms of my hands and my fingers were completely denuded of skin." The young woman's hands were so badly damaged that doctors initially believed that they would have to be amputated. "The agony that I suffered," wrote Miss R.H., "was intense. The nerves were exposed, and although the boracic acid ointment that was applied after the first week proved most healing, I felt much of the time as if the pangs of hell had verily 'got hold upon me,' and part of the time I was delirious with the horrible suffering." Once the swelling went down, her fingers contracted, making her hands unusable. Her physician cut away the scar tissue and applied skin grafts taken from the young woman's thigh. After several operations and weeks of recovery, her fingers "which were hopelessly crippled for all necessary uses, such as attention to personal necessities," remained crooked but regained their usefulness.[69] Given the nature of the injuries these patients experienced, it seems reasonable to infer that their primary concern was to regain the semblance of human appearance and function. The fact that the skin used to treat their injuries came from their own body or that of another—living or dead, animal or human—may not have registered as a cause for anxiety or concern.

Going Under the Knife

Skin grafting was more than a surgical procedure in the late nineteenth and early twentieth century; it was a dramatic event. Like surgical blood donation (which is discussed in Chapter 2), stories about giving and receiving skin often appeared in the popular press, despite physician concerns about the "theatrical and sensational aspect" that reporters accorded the operation.[70] In the case of skin grafting, the usually brief reports identified the patient, doctor, and donor. In addition, reports often described the nature of the injury to the patient, and the heroism associated with the gift of skin. The *New York Times* published scores of brief reports in which men, women, and children volunteered to donate skin to family members and even strangers in need. "This is genuine devotion," read the headline in January 1891, when Minnie Emma Wilck's husband offered to provide skin to his wife. Mrs. Wilck lost her scalp when her hair became caught in an industrial laundry machine, and she was taken to Bellevue Hospital. Her husband, according to the report, "was a big sturdy fellow and the operation will not be particularly painful to him as the scalpel will only remove the outer skin. He will carry the scars always, however, to remind him of his devotion to his young wife."[71] In 1891, when a Manhattan trainman was struck by a moving freight train and badly injured his thigh, the *Times* reported the "surgeon's sacrifice." Although some grafts were removed from the patient's healthy leg, he "strenuously objected" to additional removal of his skin; a senior surgeon, Dr. Bates, volunteered "to undergo the pain and inconvenience for the wounded man and in the interests of science and humanity."[72]

What made skin grafting attractive to the press? In some cases, the nature of the injury made the grafting of interest. In 1897, surgeons at the Charity Hospital in Cleveland described their need for 6 square feet of skin to treat Mrs. Angeline Davidson, who had been burned so extensively that she needed grafts over her entire body. The first graft came from the amputated hand of a man injured in an accident, but the surgeons sought additional skin to treat her burns. In 1902, Rufus Janman, a train engineer, who had lost his nose, chin, eyes, ears, eyelids, and scalp in a train wreck, endured 200 consecutive days of surgery in which skin from his legs was used to provide him with "a new face."[73] But some grafts were notable in light of the large numbers of skin donors. In 1903, over 200 friends of William S. Frederick donated 2400 grafts when he was badly scalded in the wreck of a New Jersey Central Westfield train. Still other grafts appeared in the press as "surgical triumphs," including the creation of new eyelids for patients who lost theirs to burns and other injuries.[74] Some skin grafts appeared in the newspaper as "human interest stories," illustrating quaint aspects of the surgery. In this perhaps apocryphal story from a San Francisco newspaper, a San Rafael girl appeared in the newspaper after she underwent grafting for extensive burns. The so-called "human crazy quilt" could identify the various donations she had received from her chums: "This is Jennie's hide; that's a piece of Willie's skin; here's a freckle off Charlie's shoulders; and this is a piece of Bessie's arm—you can tell because it is so white."[75]

In some cases, species difference made the tissue graft newsworthy. In November 1890, a surgical procedure involving a dog and a 14-year-old boy named John Gethins attracted enormous press coverage. In an effort to avoid amputation of his malformed leg, the boy and his parents agreed to allow surgeon A.M. Phelps to graft 2 inches of the dog's foreleg onto the boy's exposed shin bone. This procedure required that the boy and the dog remain surgically linked for 12–14 days to promote the growth of the graft. Firmly encased in a plaster jacket to prevent movement of the graft, the dog, a black spaniel named Yig and described by reporters as a "very good-natured dog," shared a bed with the boy in a private room in Charity Hospital on New York City's Blackwell Island. It was "natural," observed the editors of the *Boston Medical and Surgical Journal*, "that an attempt to temporarily unite a human being and a dog in a union as close as that of the Siamese twins should have excited the interest of a newspaper reporter and also of the lay mind." Daily press reports about the bone graft procedure prompted a series of letters critical of the "wanton brutality" of encasing the dog in plaster and emphasizing the "pitiful moaning" of the animal, the result of the devocalizing procedure performed to prevent the dog from disturbing the boy and other hospital patients.[76] The boy's plight, however, generated no similar outcry; his surgeon reported that, during his convalescence, John received "postal cards from persons praying that the effort to save his leg might be a failure." In an effort to refute what he described as "absurd rumors," the surgeon explained that both the dog and the boy had received careful medical attention and nursing care in the postoperative period. The surgeon noted how the dog and the boy "became friends, administering to each other's comfort," and moreover, how he, in "a prospective act of humanity," severed the bone graft between the boy and the dog, stitched the stump of the dog's leg, and allowed both of his "patients" to recover despite the apparent failure of the operation.[77]

Not all stories about grafting involved local doctors, hospitals, and patients. Newspapers published stories about unusual occurrences, including the 1903 lawsuit brought by Vera Anderson against a Philadelphia hospital and doctor for taking her skin for grafting another patient without her permission, and the case of Bertha Reed, a badly burned "Negro girl 8 years old" who received skin from white patients when the child's mother and other "volunteers of her race" refused to provide the needed tissue.[78] Newspapers around the country gave extensive coverage to the extraordinary gift of Willie "Crippled Newsie" Rugh. In September 1912, Rugh read about 22-year-old Ethel Smith, seriously burned when the gasoline tank on her motorcycle exploded. Learning that "skin-grafting alone could save her life," Newsie appeared at the Gary, Indiana office of Dr. J. A. Craig and offered to donate his "withered" leg for the grafting operation. When informed that so much skin was required that an amputation would be needed, Rugh reportedly hesitated only a moment before giving his consent to the operation.[79] Donor and recipient met on adjoining tables in the operating room before undergoing chloroform anesthesia. After 150 square inches of skin were removed from the man's leg and grafted onto the girl's body, Rugh received an additional dose of chloroform before his leg was amputated at the hip. Although Smith was discharged from the hospital after several days, Rugh developed pneumonia (news reports noted the anesthetic given for the amputation was too much for his weak lungs) and he died.

The extensive press coverage of Newsie's death emphasized his unselfish sacrifice. The special report to the *New York Times* noted: "when his foster mother knelt beside the bed and hid her face in the edge of the boy's pillow, he reached out a weak hand and stroked her hair. 'Don't cry, Mammy,' he begged. 'I never 'mounted to nothin' before, and now you know I done sompin' fer somebody.'"[80] The report in the *Los Angeles Times* similarly assumed that Newsie was a child, rather than a grown man, and speculated about the "thousands of atoms in the boy's dead body" that lived on in the woman patient who received the graft.[81] The idea that a mere boy and even the "crippled" could make a contribution to the social welfare was a favorite of the popular press. During the 1916 polio epidemic in New York City, newspapers reported the offer by a man left with a twisted leg and limp arm from an earlier bout of polio. Answering the call for blood donation to make polio serum, the man explained: "I am happy because you tell me that I may be able to save some other human being from my fate. If I can do that I shall feel that I have not been wasted in this life."[82]

Reports of Rugh's heroism moved the citizens of Gary to raise funds to erect a memorial in his name. Several people recommended that Rugh be awarded a medal from the Carnegie Hero Fund, established in 1904 with a $5 million grant from Andrew Carnegie in order that "the heroes and those dependent upon them should be free from pecuniary cares resulting from their heroism."[83] As one of Rugh's supporters noted,

> . . . it wasn't, indeed, a very good leg that Willie sacrificed, and possibly he is better off without than with it, but there seems to be no reason for supposing that he would have parted with the limb, poor specimen as it was, had he not heard that unless a very considerable amount of living cuticle could be secured the victim of the accident would not recover.[84]

Although the Fund did eventually recognize some "medical heroes," Rugh received no posthumous recognition from the commission.[85]

After World War I, a growing number of surgeons viewed the heroism of skin donors and the media coverage of donation as more of a hindrance than a help. "Every few months one picks up a paper describing a case of skin-grafting in which the relatives of the patient or the friends or fellow employees of the patient very generously and heroically contributed a certain amount of their own skin to cover the extensive area which had been destroyed by burn or injury," noted surgeon Arthur Dean Bevan in 1918.[86] His own experience with *isografts*, skin from individuals other than the patient, convinced him that such donations were of little use. More scathing of the practice was surgeon Emile Holman. "Iso- or homo-skin grafting," he complained in 1924, "is frequently employed by the profession to the wondering delight of a credulous laity, who enjoy contributing small squares of skin as sacrificial offerings on the altar of self-inflicted martyrdom."[87] Results from experiments with animals increasingly suggested the failure of using skin from other humans and animals, although the convincing demonstration came in Peter Medawar's work in the 1940s.[88]

By the 1920s, the self-sacrifice associated with giving one's own skin had become a Hollywood plot device. In two Hollywood films, the willingness to "go under the knife" established the nobility of the character. In the 1920 Robertson-Cole release, *A Woman Who Understood*, a sculptress agrees to undergo skin grafting to save the hands of her adulterous husband, a violinist. (Tellingly, the "other woman" refuses to undergo the procedure to save her lover.) In the 1923 film, *The Hero*, a returned war hero steals money from his church. On his way out of town, he passes a school fire, rescues several children, and requires skin grafting for his own serious burns.[89]

The Surgeon as Wizard

On the island of Doctor Moreau, the surgeon is no hero. In the early twentieth century, however, the American press often cast the surgeon in heroic terms. In part, this reflected the changing cultural status of surgery and surgeons.[90] One of the surgeons lionized by the press was Rockefeller Institute researcher Alexis Carrel. Born in France in 1873, Carrel came to North America in 1904. Even before he joined the staff of the Rockefeller Institute for Medical Research as head of the Department of Experimental Surgery, Carrel's surgical exploits had attracted public attention. During the summer of 1906, reports in Chicago and New York newspapers of his work on the transplantation of veins and arteries raised the possibility of organ transplantation in human beings.[91] Carrel conducted much of this early work with University of Chicago colleague Charles Guthrie, co-author of many of his early papers on transplantation of the kidney, ovary, thyroid gland, and limbs in animals. Although Guthrie achieved some notoriety with the report that he had grafted the head of one dog onto another (the two-headed animal "lived" for 26 minutes), he never received the attention accorded the French surgeon.[92] The Rockefeller connection and Carrel's Nobel Prize made him a popular focus of magazines and newspapers, where he was hailed as a magician, a "mender of men," and New York's version of the Wizard of Oz.

L. Frank Baum's memorable story of a young girl, scarecrow, tinman, and lion was only 12 years old when science journalist Carl Snyder invoked Baum's title character to represent the French surgeon. Contrary to popular belief, observed Snyder, the Wizard of Oz was alive and well and living in New York City, where he was performing "almost unbelievable things." These feats included developing a technique for joining together arteries and veins, work which enabled Carrel "to play with the animal machine as if it were made of tubes and rods of brass and iron." His exploits in this popular account in *Colliers'* included "transporting kidneys" from one animal to another, grafting the leg of one dog onto the body of another dog, and "introducing" the heart of a little dog into the neck of a larger animal, thereby having done "probably what has never been done before, all poetry and fancy to the contrary— made two hearts to beat as one!"[93]

Carrel cultivated the image of the surgeon as a miracle-worker. With his flair for publicity, he compared his work with the medieval miracle of the black leg. "The idea of removing a diseased member and replacing it with a sound one is by no means new," echoed *Scientific American*. "An old painting in Florence represents a miraculous operation of this kind in which the sacristan of the Church of St. Como and St. Damian is the patient, the saints are the surgeons, and the leg substituted for the sacristan's cancerous limb is taken, without regard to color, from a dead Moor."[94] This story of the brothers Cosmas and Damian, readers learned, was quoted by Carrel, who claimed the honor of converting the legend of the medieval saints into fact. The French surgeon did not perform the "miracle of the black leg" on human beings but on dogs, successfully grafting the black leg of a dog onto a white animal of the same height.[95] A popular subject of Renaissance painters, the miracle of the black leg has been frequently reproduced in medical journals and books that discuss transplantation.[96] Carrel may have been among the first to invoke the miracle when he talked to the press about his transplantation experiments, emphasizing its unusual, miraculous character.

Carrel's image as a surgical wizard was enhanced by his dramatic operation to save the life of the infant daughter of a New York surgeon. In 1908, the baby had lost a considerable amount of blood before the French surgeon surgically linked an exposed vein in her father's arm with an exposed vein in her leg. John D. Rockefeller claimed that this operation convinced him that he had invested wisely in medical research. In addition to his surgical feats, Carrel's personality enhanced his appeal, as did his preference for operating in black, rather than white, surgical garb. Although this preference was linked to maintaining a germ-free operating theater, the image of the "man in black" added to his mystique. In the French press, a 1913 illustration of Carrel as magician included the usual props of the magician, the pointed hat, the wand, dice, and cups. An image of horticultural grafts is supplemented by the tray the surgeon holds. This platter includes strange animal hybrids—a chicken with a fish head, a lizard with a rooster's head, and so on—suggesting the unnatural character of the surgeon's skill and perhaps the violation of traditional species boundaries. American references to Carrel's surgical wizardry seemed less freighted by the ominous character of the magician; instead, they emphasized the practical consequences of his operative exploits. In the *Woman's Home Companion*, Arthur Guiterman profiled Carrel in the magazine's section about "interesting people." Labeling Carrel a surgical wizard, Guiterman emphasized the man's "scientific needlework" that made his grafting possible, together with the work on a "stimulating tissue medium" that would repair broken bones in a week, a flesh wound or burn in a day, and make the practice of skin grafting obsolete.[97] The press coverage of Carrel and his surgical exploits encouraged speculation that clinical transplantation would soon be a reality. "The inference is inevitable," noted one reporter in 1908, "that hereafter, in cases of fatal accidents, the sound members and organs of victims may find resurrection by implantation into the frames of living patients."[98] Some reports went further. "We May Live 200 Years" read the headline of a 1912 article, which described experiments at the Rockefeller Institute in which "the brain of a child that had just died was put in pieces in a portion of an elderly millionaire's brain which had atrophied." This article described kidney transplants from one living person to another and, from a cadaver to a patient, the grafting of a human ear, culminating in the assertion that it was possible to take the healthy heart from a person dead from an accident and safely place it in another person's body. "Let a healthy young woman meet accidental and instantaneous death. It would be possible to use no inconsiderable part of her body for grafting or other justifiable procedures."[99]

Such speculation also prompted people across American to write to Carrel, seeking his assistance. As a visiting French surgeon noted in 1909, "those extraordinary Americans" with "typical American audacity" begged Carrel to experiment on them.[100] These letters, preserved in the Carrel archives, speak poignantly of loss and desperation, and illustrate a range of responses to the potential for interchanging body parts. They demonstrate that many Americans had already considered the possibility of human transplantation and what it might entail. Popular articles on Carrel produced a predictable crop of letters from people either seeking transplants or offering to serve as a donor in return for financial compensation. In 1908, for example, a 14-year-old boy, after reading an account of Carrel's dogleg transplants in the *Chicago Examiner*, wrote to Carrel about the loss of his foot in a streetcar accident. "Thinking that you would like to carry on the wonderful grafting discovery which astonished the medical world," the boy volunteered, "I will let you try to graft a new foot on my stump anytime you please, if you are inclined to do so."[101] In 1913, shortly after his fame reached dizzying heights when he became only the first American inhabitant to receive the Nobel Prize in Medicine or Surgery, Carrel received letters from people seeking transplantation of arms, hands, fingers, legs, breasts, feet, eyes, clitoris, ovaries, hearts, and kidneys. A physician from Warren, Ohio wrote to Carrel asking why a kidney could not be transplanted in a human subject, and described a 45-year-old man willing to take one chance in a hundred for relief. An Idaho woman who had undergone removal of her ovaries pled with Carrel to take her case: "If it is possible to replace or transplant a kidney, why would it not be possible to replace such an organ [ovary] as I mentioned. I would be perfectly willing to try even though it were death, to help my own condition and perhaps a good many others if such a thing can be done." A Massachusetts man with a weak heart from a bout of rheumatic fever expressed his willingness to "try the experiment of transplanting a heart or anything else." Some of these desperate letter writers acknowledged the issue of the organ source, mentioning both retrieval of organs from the newly dead or accidentally killed, as well as the possibility that criminals about to be executed could be persuaded to donate their body parts for transplantation.[102] Carrel's secretary issued a standard reply to these requests; she explained that the law did not permit such surgeries to take place.

Reports in the popular press accentuated the wonders and promise of the new surgery. Reporters were often graphic in their depictions of some realities of "spare parts" surgery. When he reported Carrel's experimental work in *Colliers'* magazine, Carl Snyder wrote vividly about the violence of American life—railway accidents, factory disasters, homicide, and suicide—that created "valuable material" for saving lives. "Depending upon the degree of mutilation—whether the bodies are blown to pieces, or chewed up, or merely punctured by a bullet, or killed electrically," he insisted, "here at a modest calculation are at least 50,000 good arms, as many legs, and perhaps a slightly less number of lungs, livers, hearts and other organs." Why shouldn't these limbs and organs, he asked, be placed in a cold storage facility from which surgeons could draw the materials to treat the injured and the maimed? Carrel had already investigated such cold storage. (Snyder did not mention that Carrel's work on the preservation of tissue included the skin and bone taken from an infant who died during childbirth.) It is possible that the response to the use of the dead reflected whose body was being used. When discussing Carrel's work on a tissue extract for the more rapid healing of broken bones and wounds, one reporter expressed enthusiasm, noting "if the tissues of the unidentified dead in the morgue may be used for the preparation of an 'optimum medium' for the healing of human wounds, we may hope to see a revolution in medical and surgical practice."[103] In this era, the bodies of the unclaimed dead were already being mobilized for medical education and research.

Snyder's article did not include kidneys for transplantation. When they reported the first transplant of a "corpse's kidney" in 1911, reporters did not shy away from the circumstances that made the organ available.[104] Instead, they emphasized the patient's "good luck" to have secured the kidney of a young, healthy man accidentally killed. Although most histories of kidney transplantation give 1936 as the date for the first human cadaveric kidney transplant., the New York press reported such a procedure 25 years earlier. [105] The transplant did not take place in Russia, but in Philadelphia, where surgeon Levi Jay Hammond transferred a kidney from a man newly dead in an automobile accident into a man with tuberculosis of the kidney. This "surgical feat," according to a *New York Times* journalist, "though unfortunate for the man who was killed by the motor car, was most fortunate for the subject of the operation, since the kidney of the man killed by accident was much better than that of a man dying of a malignant disease, of old age, or any illness."[106] The report describes in a matter-of-fact manner that, whereas Carrel had performed a transplant using a dog kidney in a human being, Hammond was the first to use a human kidney from a newly deceased person instead of using a kidney "kept in cold storage for the purpose."

The same day as this historic kidney transplant, Hammond also performed a human testicular transplant into a 19-year-old man, an elevator operator. This operation was apparently not reported in the popular press, but in the medical press. The patient, who had developed a painful swelling in the scrotal area, "finally gave his consent" to undergo an operative procedure to relieve the problem.[107] For "aesthetic reasons," the doctors explained, they hoped to substitute an "artificial testicle" after the removal of the diseased one, and made arrangement to acquire one from a live sheep: "but the thought came to us, if this transplantation can be successfully performed, why not substitute the human organ rather than the one from the lower animal?"[108] According to the case report Hammond and his fellow surgeon Howard Sutton published the following year, they explained to the patient the recent experimental work in animals and the success with blood vessel anastomosis: "the possibility of replacing his diseased organ by implanting a new one was left entirely to his own decision after assuring him of our willingness to undertake the experiment." Although initially averse to surgery, the patient reportedly accepted their proposal with enthusiasm, "and the details incident to the operative procedure were sources of entertainment to him."[109]

They located a healthy testicle in a 28-year-old man, newly dead from hemorrhage following the rupture of the liver. (Given the timing of the two transplants, it is likely this man—identified only as "killed by violence"—may have also furnished the cadaveric kidney to Hammond's other patient.) The organ, excised from the dead body, was placed in cold storage for 17 hours before it was transplanted into the injured elevator operator. The recipient spent 23 days in the hospital before being discharged. A month after the transplant, the doctors noted that the transplanted testicle had begun to atrophy. Still they considered their transplant not wholly a failure, for it demonstrated "that, under proper precautions, tissues, from subjects dying of injury and free from disease, can be removed, preserved and utilized in living tissues, without producing general systemic disturbances."[110]

Just which details of the operative procedure Hammond's patient found a source of entertainment is not specified in the doctors' account. It is hard to imagine what the patient would find amusing in these circumstances: the removal of the diseased organ? The use of sheep testicle? The transplant using cadaveric tissue? It is possible that the patient's seeming "entertainment" in the face of an operation he initially opposed masked anxiety about the procedure, and that his surgeons misinterpreted his behavior. But it is also possible that the notion of transplanting either a sheep testicle or a cadaveric organ did not trouble this particular patient, and that his physicians did not find his lack of concern remarkable.[111]

Certainly, the popular press found humor in the grafting cases. When a human ear graft was undertaken in 1903, such headlines as "lend me an ear" flourished. When the newspaper reported efforts to restore the sight of a boy blinded in a fireworks explosion, the reporter included a description of the substitution of the lens from a pig's eye for the boy's destroyed cornea, as well as the fact that the "porker" would spend its days "in peace and plenty on a Connecticut farm" if the operation succeeded. In the subsequent reports of the progress of the porcine eye (with headlines like "in a pig's eye") came the news that a museum had offered to purchase for $500 the one-eyed pig, an offer reportedly refused by the surgeon on the case.[112]

Physicians sometimes described how their patients found humor in undergoing the grafts. In the first two decades of the twentieth century, as many of the basic concepts of reproductive endocrinology were established, some surgeons transplanted ovaries—animal and human—in the hopes of restoring menstrual function to women. In 1906, Robert Tuttle Morris, an American pioneer in the field of ovarian transplantation, reported that one of his patients (a woman whose diseased ovaries were surgically removed) not only resumed menstruation following her transplant, but that she had conceived and given birth to a child. In his autobiography, Morris recalled how women responded to donating and receiving ovarian tissue. Whereas some women apparently balked at his request to donate their organs already scheduled for removal for therapeutic indications, other women, he noted, expressed the desire to give "a piece of themselves."[113] Morris found women much more likely than men willing to sacrifice a "solid organ." These women, he insisted, experienced so little dread of their upcoming surgeries that they often suggested the "self-sacrifice." The act of donation, of course, differs substantially from being a recipient. Morris had less to say about the recipients of ovarian tissue, except to note that one of his woman patients, "something of a wag," asked to know as she prepared to undergo the ovary transplant whether her donor was a Methodist or an Episcopalian.[114]

Morris's patients knew that their tissue was coming from another woman, either one who was having her ovaries removed for therapeutic reasons or from a dead woman. By his own account, he requested that his ovarian transplant patients to sign a paper with a "written expression of willingness to take risk" when the donated tissue came from the coroner's physician or from the medical examiner, because he feared liability for the transmission of syphilis. (The method used for preparing the ovaries for transplant did not permit the Wassermann test.)[115] He also asked that patients acknowledge that the grafting operation "would be wholly experimental" and that no outcome (especially a living child) could be guaranteed.[116] These conditions may have dissuaded some people, but Morris recognized desperation in these patients. Like Carrel, he received "pitiful letters" from women "willing to take almost any risk in order to have children." These desperate people seldom articulated concern about the retrieval of the tissue and other dark aspects of the practice.

Surgical Wizardry

In the late nineteenth and early twentieth century, American surgeons and the popular press expressed extraordinary interest in the possibility of restoring lost limbs, appendages, and other body parts. The transplantation of limbs, organs, and tissue was publicly embraced by Americans optimistic that human bodies, like machines, could be disassembled and reassembled with interchangeable parts. Like other industrial processes, surgery and the activities of surgeons were subjected to time and motion studies, and systematized. The human body became one more site for rationalization. The use of animal and human bodies—living and dead—as sources of skin, bone, corneas, nerves, and kidneys prompted wonder in the popular press. As the letters from individuals across the nation suggest, some Americans welcomed the opportunity to restore lost function and appearance, even if this entailed buying a pig, arranging to use tissue from an executed prisoner, or purchasing a human ear. Whereas in 1881, the use of skin from the dead repelled commentators, taking spare parts (kidneys, testicles, and others) after the turn of the century received little public censure; it had emerged as a feature of the "surgical wizardry" that remade bodies. Even the horrors of Doctor Moreau's island could be transformed into wonder by enthusiasts. French surgeon Alexis Carrel shared Wells' novel with his fellow surgeons. He then arranged meetings at which the doctors would have the opportunity to discuss what Carrel called a "quaint and curious" tale. No transcript of these discussions survives; just what the French surgeon considered either quaint or curious about Wells's story of a sadistic surgeon, a South Sea island, a puma-woman, and the revolt of the Beast Folk remains mysterious.

Notes

1. H.G. Wells, *The Island of Doctor Moreau*, ed. Robert M. Philmus (Athens: University of Georgia Press, 1993), 46.

2. See John Bertrand de Cusante Morant Saunders, "A Conceptual History of Transplantation," in *Transplantation*, eds. John S. Najarian and Richard L. Simmons (Philadelphia: Lea & Febiger, 1972), 3–25.

3. In *The Island of Dr. Moreau*, the "rhinoceros rats" are the work of Algerian soldiers.

4. Surgeons also used other materials (celluloid, paraffin, and petroleum jelly) for correcting deformity and massive loss of tissue. See John Staige Davis, *Plastic Surgery: Its Principles and Practice* (Philadelphia: P. Blakiston's Sons, 1919), 44–45.

5. W. W. Keen, "Address in Surgery," *Journal of the American Medical Association* 28 (1897): 1102–1110.

6. See C.O. Weller, "Report of a Case of Skin Grafting," *Texas Medical Journal* 12 (1897): 593–597. Also see Leland R. Chick, "Brief History and Biology of Skin Grafting," *Annals of Plastic Surgery* 21 (1988): 358–365.

7. See Herman Mynter, "Skin Grafting," *Medical Press Western New York* 2 (1887): 301–308. Hamilton used "pedunclated flaps," as opposed to free skin grafts, meaning the skin remained attached to part of the body.

8. Albert Ehrenfried, "Reverdin and Other Methods of Skin-grafting," *Boston Medical and Surgical Journal* 161 (1909): 911–927.

9. Arthur Dean Bevan, "Skin-Grafting: An Extensive Burn of the Chest Repaired by Thiersch Grafts," *Surgical Clinics of Chicago* 2 (1918): 717–725.

10. Gina C. Ang, "The History of Skin Transplantation,"*Clinics in Dermatology* 23 (2005): 320-324.

11. Rafael Morales, "A Successful Case of Transplantation," *Medical Record* 6 (1871): 80.

12. B. M. Cromwell, "A Case of Skin Grafting with Comments," *Atlanta Medical and Surgical Journal,* 13 (1876): 641–646.

13. M. Donelly, "St. Vincent's Hospital—Skin Grafting," *Medical Record* 7 (1872): 572–574.

14. Charles Leale, "The Use of Common Warts of the Hand in Skin-Grafting," *Medical Record* 14 (1878): 188.

15. Nicholas Senn, "Restitution of Skin by Plastic Operation in Cases of Extensive Traumatic Surface Defects of the Scrotum and Penis," *Philadelphia Medical Journal* 2 (1895): 964–966.

16. W. Symington Brown, "Skin Grafting," *Boston Medical Surgical Journal* 101 (1879): 829–833.

17. S. C. Bartlett and W. Lockwood Bradley, "Skin Grafting," *Proceedings of the Connecticut Medical Society* 4 (1874): 258. By 1924, 173 cases of total avulsion of the scalp were reported in the literature; see Clarence A. McWilliams, "Principles of Four Types of Skin Grafting," *Journal of the American Medical Association* 83 (1924): 183–189. See Claire Straith and Morrison D. Beers, "Scalp Avulsions: Report of Early Homo and Zoo-Grafting and Recent Split Scalp Grafting," *Plastic Reconstructive Surgery* 6 (1950): 319–326; and N.B. Aldrich, "Grafting with Pigeon Skin," *Boston Medical Surgical Journal* 128 (1893): 336.

18. The terminology for differentiating these grafts was not standardized.

19. This usage comes from H. Mynter, "Skin Grafting," p. 301. Surgeon John Staige Davis used autodermic, isodermic, and zoodermic to indicate donor. See his "Skin Grafting at the Johns Hopkins Hospital," *Annals of Surgery* 50 (1909): 545.

20. Thomas Bryant, Manual for the Practice of Surgery (Philadelphia: H.C.Lea's Son, 1881), p. 436.

21. Harold K. Shawan, "The Principle of Blood Grouping Applied to Skin Grafting," *American Journal of Medicine and Science* 157 (1919): 503–509.

22. T. Bryant, *The Practice of Surgery* (London: Churchill, 1872), p. 436.

23. Leonard Freeman, *Skin Grafting for Surgeons and General Practitioners* (St. Louis, C.V. Mosby, 1912), 9–10.

24. Lederer, *Subjected to Science*, pp. 11–12.

25. George Seeley Smith, "A Case of Frog-Skin Grafting," *Boston Medical Surgical Journal* 132 (1895): 79.

26. Paul A. Lombardo, "Phantom Tumors and Hysterical Women: Revising our View of the Schloendorff Case," *Journal of Law, Medicine & Ethics*, 33 (2005): 791-801; Susan E. Lederer, Ruth Faden, and Tom Beauchamp, *A History and Theory of Informed Consent* (New York: Oxford University Press, 1986).

27. M. Donelly, "St. Vincent's Hospital—Skin Grafting," *Medical Record* 7 (1872): 572. For difficulties with consent, see E.S. Howard, "A Case of Skin Grafting," *Pacific Medical Journal* 42 (1899): 70.

28. "Discussion," *Railway Surgeon* 1 (1894): 128.

29. L. Freeman, *Skin Grafting for Surgeons and General Practitioners*, pp. 26–27.

30. "Extraordinary Skin Grafting," *Scientific American* 75 (18 July 1896): 42.

31. George R. Fowler, "On the Transplantation of Large Strips of Skin for Covering Extensive Granulating Surfaces, with Report of a Case in which Human and Frog Skin Were Simultaneously Used for This Purpose," *Annals of Surgery* 9 (1889): 184.

32. Julius T. Rose, "Skin Grafting without Anesthesia," *Medical Record* 72 (1907): 809.

33. Leonard Freeman, "The Thiersch Method of Skin-Grafting," *Denver Medical Times* 14 (1895): 421–431.

34. J.T. Rose, "Skin Grafting without Anesthesia," p. 809.

35. Ibid.

36. Martin S. Pernick, *A Calculus of Suffering* (New York: Columbia University Press, 1985), 237.

37. For dispensing with anesthesia, see J. C. Masson, "Skin Grafting," *Journal of the American Medical Association* 70 (1918): 1581–1584. For colonic anesthesia, see Clarence A. McWilliams, "Principles of Four Types of Skin Grafting," *Journal of the American Medical Association* 83 (1924): 183–189.

38. G. R. Fowler, "On the Transplantation of Large Strips of Skin," p. 184.

39. John S. Davis, "Transplantation of Skin," *Surgery, Gynecology & Obstetrics* 44 (1927): 181–189. It would be interesting to compare concerns with scars left by blood transfusion and skin donation with the history of tattooing in this country. In the 1890s, tattooing apparently was quite fashionable among the rich and powerful in America; see Clinton R. Sanders, *Customizing the Body: The Art and Culture of Tattooing* (Philadelphia: Temple University Press, 1989), 16.

40. John M.T. Finney, "The Transportation of Skin Flaps from One Part of the Body to Another and from One Individual to Another," *Annals of Surgery* 50 (1909): 330.

41. See "Discussion," *Annals of Surgery* 50 (1909): 361.

42. F. Gregory Connell, "Removal of Skin from the Abomen during Laparotomy as a Source of Material for Grafting," *International Journal of Surgery* 22 (1909): 358–360.

43. David H. Agnew, "*Ulcers: Skin Grafting,*" *Medical and Surgical Reporter 31 (1874): 424-426.*

44. "Skin-grafting from Dead Bodies," *New York Times* 25 Aug. 1881, p. 4.

45. Jon H. Girdner, "Skin-grafting with Grafts Taken from the Dead Subject," *Medical Record* 20 (1881): 119–120.

46. E. P. Brewer, "The Limit of Skin Vitality," *Medical Record* 21 (1882): 483–484.

47. C. F. Timmerman, "Skin-Grafting on a Large Surface," *Medical Record* 55 (1899): 582. For use of an amputated foot, see Frank Overton, "Skin Grafting by Unusual Methods," *Medical Record* 54 (1898): 527.

48. F.G. Connell, "Removal of Skin from the Abomen during Laparotomy," p. 359.

49. R. Clement Lucas, "On Prepuce Grafting," *Lancet* II (1884): 586–587.

50. Frank Ashley, "Foreskins as Skin Grafts," *Annals of Surgery* 106 (1937): 252–256. See David Gollaher, "From Ritual to Science: The Medical Transformation of Circumcision in America," *Journal of Social History* 28 (1994): 5–36. Circumcision, of course, retained its religious meaning for Jews. For hospital childbirth, see Judith W. Leavitt, *Brought to Bed* (New York: Oxford University Press, 1986).

51. L.Freeman, "The Thiersch Method of Skin-Grafting," p. 19.

52. Charles A. Porter, "Massive Keloid of Face and Hands," *Annals of Surgery* 50 (1909): 332–335.

53. I.C. Eisenberg, "The Prepuce as Grafting Material," *Medical Record* 95 (1919): 514–515.

54. Stuart McGuire, "Methods to Hasten Epidermization, with Special Reference to Skin Grafting," *Virginia Medical Semi-Monthly* 8 (1903): 292–296.

55. N. Sabella, "Use of the Fetal Membranes in Skin Grafting,"*Medical Record* 83 (1913): 478–480. Two years earlier, surgeons at Johns Hopkins Hospital attempted grafts using amniotic membrane; see W. D. Gatch, "Report of a Case of Extensive Tiersch Skin Graft," *Johns Hopkins Hospital Bulletin* 22 (1911): 84–85.

56. Maximilian Stern, "The Grafting of Preserved Amniotic Membrane to Burned and Ulcerated Surfaces, Substituting Skin Grafts," *Journal of the American Medical Association* 60 (1913): 973.

57. N.B. Aldrich, "Grafting with Pigeon Skin," *Boston Medical and Surgical Journal* 128 (1893): 336.

58. Anthony Wallace, "The Early Development of Pedicle Flaps," *Journal of the Royal Society of Medicine.* 71 (1978): 834–838.

59. See Thomas Gibson, "Zoografting: A Curious Chapter in the History of Plastic Surgery," *British Journal of Plastic Surgery* 8 (1955): 234–242. See Straith and Beers, "Scalp Avulsions," p. 320. See "Discussion," *Annals of Surgery* 50 (1909): 361.

60. Samuel Lambert, "The Vagaries of a Vivisectionist Turned Clinical Surgeon and the Story of the Lady Who Lay with a Pig for Five Nights and Five Days on Professional Advice," *Proceedings of the Charaka Club* 9 (1938): 38–43.

61. M. E. Van Meter, "Note on the Use of Skin From Puppies in Skin-Grafting," *Annals of Surgery* 12 (1890): 136–137.

62. Alexander Miles, "Extensive Burn of Leg Treated by Grafting with Skin of Dog," *Lancet* I (1890): 594–595, noted that he was able to obtain a young greyhound as a skin donor for a badly burned schoolboy with "the co-operation of the friends of the child."

63. S. McGuire, "Method to Hasten Epidermization," p. 296.

64. G.R. Fowler, "On the Transplantation of Large Strips," p. 190.

65. In 1888, both British surgeon G.F.C. Masterman and Frenchman P. Redard explained that the idea of frog skin was so repulsive to their patient that they used the skin of young, wild rabbits and chickens. Why such sources were less repulsive is unknown; see Gibson, "Zoografting," p. 238.

66. "Skin Grafting with Pieces of Skin Obtained from Hens," *New York Medical Journal* 73 (1901): 37.

67. S. Lambert, "Vagaries of a Vivisectionist," p. 42.

68. "Bone from Chickens Ingrafted on a Man's Leg," *New York Times* 21 Apr. 1891, p. 2.

69. Horace Packard, "Skin Grafting," *Transactions of the American Institute of Homeopathy,* 1894; session 46–50: 1042–1053.

70. Hugh A. Baldwin, "Skin Grafting," *Medical Record* 97 (1920): 686–688.

71. "This Is Genuine Devotion," *New York Times,* 11 Jan. 1891, p. 10.

72. "A Surgeon's Sacrifice," *New York Times,* 5 Aug. 1891, p. 1–2.

73. "Six Square Feet of Skin," *New York Times,* 29 Dec. 1897, p. 4; "Man with a New Face," *Los Angeles Times,* 30 Mar. 1902, p. 2.

74. "Wreck Victim Made Over," *New York Times,* 27 Nov. 1903.

75. "A Human Crazy Quilt," *Los Angeles Times,* 14 Jul. 1896, p. 3.

76. "Dr. Phelps' Experiment," *New York Times,* 26 Nov. 1890, p.9; "The Boy and the Dog," *New York Times,* 9 Dec. 1890, p. 8; and "Grafting a Dog's Bone to a Boy," *Chicago Daily Tribune,* 22 Feb. 1891, p. 18.

77. "Transplantation of Tissue from Lower Animals to Man," *Medical and Surgical Reporter,* 2 May 1891, 64: 18; "The Bone Grafting Experiment," *Scientific American,* 7 Mar. 1891, 64: 15.

78. "Graft White Skin on Negro," *New York Times,* 21 May 1908, p. 1.

79. "Gives His Leg, Girl Saved," *New York Times,* 30 Sep. 1912, p. 8; and "By Real Heroism, Willie Rugh's Sacrifice Inspiring Others," *Boston Globe,* 4 Nov. 1912, p. 16.

80. "Newsie Died for Stranger," *New York Times,* 19 Oct. 1912, p.11.

81. "A Curious Incarnation," *Los Angeles Times,* 21 Oct. 1912, p. II6.

82. Naomi Rogers, *Dirt and Disease: Polio Before FDR* (New Brunswick: Rutgers University Press, 1992): 101. See Seth Koven, "Remembering and Dismemberment: Crippled Children, Wounded Soldiers, and the Great War in Great Britain," *American History Reviews* 99 (1994): 1167–1202, for an intriguing discussion of the social dynamics of sacrifice and disability.

83. Thomas S. Arbuthnot, *Heroes of Peace* (New York: Carnegie Hero Fund Commission, 1935).

84. "Certainly Earned a Medal," *New York Times,* 1 Oct. 1912.

85. The "kinds of peril" explicitly rewarded by the Carnegie Hero Commission included "drowning, suffocation in wells, railway trains, electric cars, burning, suffocation at fires, runaway teams, cave-in at mines, electric shock, attacks by enraged animals, attempted murder, falls, death by exposure, explosions, mad dogs, death by machinery, snake bites, contagious diseases, etc." One example of "medical heroism" was Leonard Williams, a 34-year-old tool-dresser who, in 1917, received a silver medal and $1,000 for attempting to rescue a fellow laborer from epidemic cerebrospinal meningitis. Williams stayed to nurse the stricken man after he was abandoned by everyone else in the community. *Annual Report,* Carnegie Hero Fund Commission (Pittsburgh, 1917): 35.

86. A.D. Bevan, "Skin-Grafting," p. 719.

87. Emile Holman, "Protein Sensitization in Isoskingrafting," *Surgery, Gynecology & Obstetrics* 38 (1924): 100.

88. Leslie Brent, *A History of Transplantation Immunology* (San Diego, CA: Academic Press, 1996).

89. See entries for both films in American Film Institute Catalog. In the play *The Hero,* on which the film was based, the war hero dies in the fire. So the film introduced the element of skin grafting. See Arthur Hobson Quinn, *Contemporary American Plays* (New York, Charles Scribner's Sons, 1923): 219–296.

90. Christopher Lawrence, ed. *Medical Theory, Surgical Practice: Studies in the History of Surgery* (Routledge: London and New York 1992).

91. Jon Turney. "Life in the Laboratory: Public Responses to Experimental Biology," *Public Understanding of Science* 4 (1995): 153–176.

92. "Startling Declaration: Surgeon Claims to Have Grafted Head onto Body of Living Dog." *Los Angeles Times,* 3 Jun. 1908; see also Samuel P. Harbison. "Origins of Vascular Surgery: The Carrel-Guthrie Letters." *Surgery* 52 (1962): 406–418, for tensions between the two collaborators.

93. Carl Snyder, "Carrel–Mender of Men," *Colliers* 50 (1912): 12–13; "Are the Parts of the Human Body Interchangeable?" *Current Opinion* 68 (1920): 358–359.

94. "The Transplantation of Members and Organs," *Scientific American* 72 (1911): 236–237.

95. Theodore I. Malinin. *Surgery and Life: The Extraordinary Career of Alexis Carrel* (New York: Harcourt Brace Jovanovich, 1979): 46–47. As most of Carrel's scientific publications describe the dog-limb transplants on animals of the same color, it raises the question whether he chose to repeat the miracle of the black limb for popular audiences. A drawing of the canine version of the black limb miracle appeared in "Assez Coupe Il Faut Recoudre," *Lectures pour tous,* 1913, reprinted in *Alexis Carrel 1873–1944,* Cahiers Medicaux Lyonnais Numero Special 1966: 74. The Cosmas and Damian miracle was reprised in "Are the Parts of the Human Body Interchangeable?" *Current Opinion* 68 (1920): 358–359.

96. See Thomas Schlich. "How Gods and Saints Became Transplant Surgeons: The Scientific Article as a Model for Writing History," *History of Science* 33 (1995): 311–331, for an explanation of the ubiquity of Cosmas and Damian in recent scientific discussions of organ transplantation, including the 1982 attempt by "humorous laboratory workers" to emulate the success of the saints by sewing the leg of a black rat onto a white rat.

97. Arthur Guiterman, "About People," *Woman's Home Companion* 40 (1913): 5.

98. "Transplanting Human Organs," *New York Times,* 8 Nov. 1908, p. 10.

99. "We May Live 200 Years," *Washington Post* 11 Aug. 1912, p. M2.

100. "New Organs for Old," *Washington Post,* 14 Jun. 1909, p. 5. The surgeon was Samuel Pozzi.

101. Roy Kemink to A. Carrel, 1 Dec. 1908, Alexis Carrel papers, box 45, sec. 15–1, f. 8, Georgetown University Library.

102. See letters in Carrel papers, box 45, sec. 15–1, f. 18. Carrel instructed his secretary to inform many of his correspondents that laws in the United States would not permit the donation of healthy organs.

103. "Tissue Extracts for Healing," *Los Angeles Times,* 6 Feb. 1913, p. II12.

104. "Transplant Corpse's Kidney," *Los Angeles Times* 14 Nov. 1911, p. I7.

105. The standard histories of transplantation assign priority to Russian surgeon Yu Yu Voronoy, who transplanted a human kidney in 1936. Hammond apparently did not publish an account of his transplant in the medical literature. For Voronoy, see L. H. Toledo-Pereyra and J.M. Palma-Vargas. "Searching for History in Transplantation: Early Modern Attempts at Surgical Kidney Grafting." *Transplantation Proceedings* 31 (1999): 2945–2948.

106. "Dr. Hammond Gives Patient New Kidney," *New York Times,* 14 Nov. 1911, p. 2; "Has Dead Man's Kidney," *Washington Post,* 15 Nov. 1911, p. 6 .

107. Levi J. Hammond and Howard A. Sutton. "An Abstract Report of a Case of Transplantation of a Testicle," *International Clinics* 22 (1912): 150–154. Hammond graduated from the University of Pennsylvania School of Medicine in 1886; see Thomas N. Haviland and Lawrence Charles Parish, "An Early 20th-Century Testicular Transplant," *Transactions and Studies of the College of Physicians of Philadelphia* 38 (1971): 231–234.

108. L.J. Hammond & H.A. Sutton, "An Abstract Report," p. 151.

109. Ibid.

110. L.J. Hammond & H.A. Sutton, "An Abstract Report," p. 154.

111. For a humorous account of a patient with a pig-skin graft, see Susan E. Lederer, "Animal Parts/Human Bodies: Organic Transplantation in Early Twentieth-Century America," in

The Animal/Human Boundary: Historical Perspectives, ed. Angela N. H. Creager and William C. Jordan (Rochester: University of Rochester Press, 2002).

112. See "Blind Boy May See through Eye of Pig," *New York Times,* 23 Jan. 1923, p. 14; "Says He Sees by Pig's Eye," 25 Jan. 1923, p. 9; "Believes Pig's Eye Works," 26 Jan. 1923, p. 12; and "Pig's Eye Tests Fail," 3 Feb. 1923, p. 2.

113. Robert T. Morris. *Fifty Years a Surgeon* (London: Geoffrey Bles, 1935), 166.

114. R.T. Morris, *Fifty Years a Surgeon,* p. 166.

115. R.T. Morris, *Fifty Years a Surgeon,* p. 166.

116. R.T. Morris, *Fifty Years a Surgeon,* p. 169. Elsewhere, Morris discussed how he kept blank forms in his office to be filled out by patients who may have forgotten what they were told about possible bad outcomes. He found these particularly valuable for fracture cases, enabling him to avert "many a lawsuit" (pp. 97–98).

2

Miracles of Resurrection

Reinventing Blood Transfusion in the Twentieth Century

In November 1906, a young Cleveland surgeon, George Washington Crile, published a preliminary clinical note about the direct transfusion of blood. Using a newly developed surgical technique, he sewed together the cut end of an exposed artery in a donor's arm with a similarly exposed vein in the arm of his patient. Crile's patient was a 23-year-old man who had lost a considerable amount of blood following the removal of several large kidney stones. "It was clear," the surgeon explained, "that the terminal stage was at hand with all the resources at command exhausted. It seemed therefore a suitable case for transfusion, and one which would afford a crucial test of its value."[1] With desperation as a justification, Crile performed the surgical cut-down to expose the artery in the arm of his patient's brother; he then joined this vessel with the exposed vein in patient's arm. The two brothers remained linked for 20 minutes, at which point the surgeon severed their connection. Crile described the direct transfusion as successful. Grace Crile, the surgeon's wife, who had witnessed the procedure, offered a more fanciful description; she called it a "miracle of resurrection."[2]

Such "miracles" offered physicians and surgeons a dramatic new method to save the lives of patients who had experienced severe blood loss and other medical emergencies. The so-called miracle required considerable technical dexterity to accomplish; imagine the technique required to sew the cut ends of delicate blood vessels (possessing the consistency of wet matchsticks) together so that blood flowed between them. And where could the surgeon find those donors willing and able to endure the physical and psychological rigors of donation, including the incision made on the arm or leg to expose a blood vessel and the surgical union with a dying recipient?

The technical demands of Crile's surgical transfusion were greatly reduced by the introduction of cannulas (small tubes placed within the blood vessels). The advent of indirect transfusion—the movement of blood mediated by needles, stopcocks, and bottles—in the second decade of the twentieth century further reduced the technical demands on the transfuser. Unlike previous episodes in the checkered history of blood transfusion—most of which ended in the procedure being abandoned—the early twentieth-century experience of the procedure and its dramatic potential as a life-saving measure established transfusion as a durable therapeutic measure of twentieth-century medicine. This success initiated a century-long search for individuals to supply blood for transfusion, as well as the quest for a blood substitute or artificial blood. Both searches continue today.

Moving blood between bodies was more than a surgical innovation. The vital fluid reeked with powerful cultural, ethnic, and religious associations. Blood represented identity and affiliation; it linked individuals and groups, parents and children, tribes, clans, and races. In the early twentieth century, blood transfusion was an invasive, dangerous, dramatic and, at times, successful undertaking. The sensational nature of blood transfusion, its physical intimacy and uncertain outcome, attracted enormous press attention. Hundreds of reports of transfusions appeared in the popular press, both reflecting and shaping expectations about the procedure, about participation as a donor or recipient, and about its place in modern medicine and surgery. In some ways, the advent of surgical transfusion, the physical union of two individuals mediated by surgeons, fostered a reconceptualization of the body, its fluids, and its parts. Just as the transport of skin, bone, and other tissues raised questions about the nature of the newly constituted individual, blood transfusion entailed incorporating the vital fluids of others, animal and human, living and dead, relatives and strangers.

Reporters capitalized on the new bond of blood by featuring stories of incongruous donors and recipients: the man who offered blood to save the life of the man he stabbed; the surgeon who offered his blood to his own patient; the seven Republican legislators in Utah who donated blood to their lone Democratic colleague (who died following the transfusion).[3] Reports of celebrities undergoing transfusion (tenor Enrico Caruso, silent film star Rudolf Valentino) or donating blood (shortstop Joe Tinker, batter Babe Ruth) appeared alongside descriptions of more ordinary individuals who participated in the transfusion process as either donor or recipient.[4] The press heralded the advent of a new profession—blood selling—and made much of those altruistic individuals who refused to accept payment for their vital fluids. This chapter considers those developments in surgery that advanced the science and practice of transfusion, as well as the cultural work that accompanied its integration into the body politic.

Transfusion before the Twentieth Century

Today, the idea of replacing blood lost through injury, childbirth, or surgery seems so straightforward as to require little explanation. But this seemingly simple notion represented a radical departure from the conventional therapies used to treat the sick before the twentieth century. Before 1900, most physicians and patients worried more about too much blood than too little; their efforts were directed at removing the excess blood rather than in replacing the lost fluid. In the centuries following Hippocrates and Galen, bloodletting—by lancet, cupping, or leech—was a sovereign therapy for treating illness and injury.

When the English physician William Harvey demonstrated that the blood in the body circulates, his book *De Motu Cordis* (1628) offered a new rationale for systemic therapy and interest in moving blood between bodies, between animals, and even between animals and human beings.[5] In undertaking these early experiments, in which animal blood was instilled into human recipients, the physicians took care to avoid overloading the circulatory system. In November 1667, as English physicians Richard Lower and Edmund King prepared to transfuse lamb's blood into the arm of a 32-year-old clergyman, they first drained some 7–8 ounces of blood from Arthur Coga. The young man described as possessing a "too warm brain" received some 8 ounces of lamb's blood. Why a lamb? The physicians hoped to transform "the frantic" Coga through cooling his blood with the vital fluid of an animal known for its mildness. The idea that the qualities of the animal would be transferred via its blood to the recipient was an ancient one. In the diary where he recorded his observations of Coga's transfusion, Samuel Pepys recalled the story of Dr. Caius, the founder of Keys College, a man "very old, and living only at that time upon woman's milk, he, while he fed upon the milk of an angry, fretful woman, was so himself; and then, being advised to take it of a good-natured, patient woman, he did become so, beyond the common temper of his age."[6] Observers noted how Coga happily received "the blood of the lamb," embracing its resonant Christian associations. The frantic clergyman appeared so benefited by his experience that he underwent a second lamb's blood transfusion and reported his improved condition to the members of the Royal Society.[7]

Earlier that same year in Paris, Jean-Baptiste Denys, physician to Louis XIV and professor of philosophy at Montpellier, similarly sought to infuse animal blood into individuals who had already undergone copious blood letting. Even though his first patient, a 15-year-old boy, had been bled some 20 times by physicians as treatment for a resistant fever, Denys first removed 3 ounces of blood before transfusing him with 9 ounces of blood from the carotid artery of a lamb. After the transfusion, in June 1667, his patient, Denis wrote, showed "a clear and smiling countenance," where once he had passed the time "in an incredible stupidity."[8] Denis performed several additional animal to human transfusions, including treating a madman who subsequently died after receiving three lamb's blood transfusions. In the wake of a trial about the circumstances of the man's death (he was actually poisoned with arsenic by his wife), transfusion became enmeshed in controversy. In 1668, the French court ordered that future transfusions be performed only with the authorization of the Faculty of Medicine of Paris; such authorization was not forthcoming.[9]

Even as the practice of transfusion largely disappeared in both France and England, medical and surgical writers in the late seventeenth and eighteenth centuries continued to include discussions and illustrations of animal to human transfusion in textbooks. Although the German surgeon Matthias Gottfried Purmann performed sheep to human transfusions on two soldiers and a leper, the engraving from his 1705 textbook on surgery suggested little practical experience with the procedure. In this idealized representation, the surgeon pointed his finger at a reclining lamb, whose artery has been opened to allow blood to flow into a tube in the patient's arm.[10] Whether this improbably placid depiction of what was surely a messier and more difficult undertaking encouraged transfusion remains unknown.[11]

Lamb's blood and the vitality that it reportedly possessed retained a reputation as a therapeutic agent among some late eighteenth-century American physicians, and was recommended as part of the efforts to reanimate General George Washington after his final illness. In December 1799, Washington, retired from the presidency and living at his Mount Vernon estate, developed fever and sore throat. Despite the care of three physicians (or as critics claimed, the malpractice of his three physicians, who ordered bloodletting of some 80 ounces of blood over a 12-hour period), the General succumbed to his disease. Shortly after his body had been removed to the dining room in preparation for his burial, a fourth physician arrived at the estate. William Thornton, who had trained at Edinburgh and was a longtime family friend, offered a radical suggestion to Martha Washington. To revive the dead Washington, he asked that the general's body be moved close to the fire, warmed with blankets, and vigorously rubbed. He insisted that doctors cut an opening in the General's throat in which to insert a bellows to put air into the lungs; this procedure, or tracheotomy, had been proposed while Washington remained alive, but it was not adopted. The final step to revive the dead man was an injection of lamb's blood, to supply a spark of vitality to his circulatory system. But Washington's widow did not agree to this radical plan, and it was abandoned.[12]

In the first two decades of the nineteenth century, the English physician James Blundell dramatically broke with past precedent in transfusion when he turned to human donors to rescue those patients close to death. Part of his rationale was based on medical science. Blundell had been impressed with the studies undertaken by John Leacock, a Barbados physician and fellow Edinburgh medical alumnus, who suggested that blood transfused from one animal would endanger an animal of another species. Following this lead, Blundell conducted extensive experiments on dogs. He removed as much blood as possible from the dogs, then transfused blood from such other animals as sheep and calves. His experiments supported Leacock's view about the danger of transfusion across species lines, but his rejection of animal blood was not absolute. In cases where human blood was not available, Blundell continued to accept lamb's blood as a substitute.[13] But Blundell was also a practical man. Transfusion using animal blood required "the presence of some animal in the bed-chamber." But as he astutely pointed out: "What then was to be done in an emergency? A dog, it is true, might have come when you whistled, but the animal is small; a calf, or sheep, might, to some, have appeared fitter for the purpose; but then, it could run not upstairs."[14] There were of course other difficulties in having animals bled in one's bedchamber.

Blundell's initial efforts at transfusing human beings with human blood were unsuccessful. In 1818, when he, in collaboration with surgeon Henry Cline, performed his first transfusion, he collected blood from several human donors and transfused it into a "poor fellow in Guy's Hospital" with "obstinate vomiting," apparently dying from stomach obstruction. The transfusion using a metal tube did not succeed, nor did his next five attempts. In at least two of these efforts, the patients had "ceased to respire" for some 4–6 minutes before the transfusion was undertaken, including the young man with a burst artery who received blood from one of Blundell's pupils.[15] Blundell's lack of success did not stop others. Inspired by Blundell's lectures and essays on transfusion, London physician Edward Doubleday successfully transfused a woman with blood from her husband ("who was willing to make this atonement"). After she received some 6 ounces of blood, the woman exclaimed "By Jasus! I feel strong as a bull."[16] In 1826, Blundell recommended to his fellow physicians that no more cases of transfusion be made public until a complete record of the procedure and its outcomes could be made, but physicians and journal editors continued to publish case reports and discussions over transfusion, which remained the subject of therapeutic controversy.

Who provided the blood for these early transfusions? As the cases above suggest, the doctor's pupils and the patient's relatives furnished blood. In 1827, 14 ounces of blood supplied by the medical assistant was used to revive a woman who had experienced severe postpartum blood loss. In 1829, when Blundell transfused a woman with severe blood loss, he took 8 ounces of blood from the arm of his assistant.[17] Male relatives of women who had experienced severe blood loss during childbirth were also tapped as a source of blood. Husbands were often close by during a woman's confinement, including the "hearty coal-heaver" who supplied blood to his wife when she hemorrhaged giving birth to their stillborn child in 1828.[18] In a few cases, female relatives also supplied blood for a female family member, but women were not Blundell's first choice for sources of blood. He preferred men to women, because men "bleed more freely and are less liable to faint."[19]

Transfusion remained controversial in Britain. Across the Atlantic, some American physicians demonstrated initial enthusiasm for blood transfusion. In 1828, the first volume of the *Boston Medical and Surgical Journal* reported Blundell's unsuccessful transfusion efforts; physician William Channing noted "Should the experiment be tried in the country, it will give the Editors of this Journal much pleasure to communicate the results in its pages."[20] By the 1840s, transfusion had lost much of its attraction for American physicians. Although American medical journals reported European efforts in transfusion, there continued to be only rare interest in attempting transfusion, a testament to the durable fear of plethora, or too much blood, and to the technical difficulties associated with transfusion. In the face of calamitous disease, like the terrible visitations of Asiatic cholera in 1849, physicians like William A. Hammond, then a young Army surgeon, turned to transfusion as a last-ditch effort. En route to Mexico, Hammond transfused as much as 20 ounces of blood from bulls into soldiers struck by cholera.[21] These therapeutic maneuvers reflected the physician's desperation, rather than confidence in transfusion.

In the 1850s, physicians at the Charity Hospital in New Orleans revived interest in transfusion. In 1854, the outbreak of cholera in the city prompted physician Samuel Choppin to attempt blood transfusion on a man dying of cholera. After receiving 2 ounces of blood in three separate attempts in an exposed vein in his arm, the patient weakened and died (perhaps as a result of air accidentally introduced into the vein by the syringe). Four years later, Dr. N. B. Benedict proved more successful when he attempted transfusion on "a person whose life is as dear to me as my own," his sister, afflicted with the dreaded yellow fever and suffering from prolonged bleeding by mouth. Although near death, she displayed immediate signs of recovery when she received blood from a young man who had suffered from yellow fever during an earlier epidemic. "There is no doubt," recorded one observer in his diary, "that death had begun its work before this took place." After receiving only 2.5 ounces of blood, "she was like a new creature, and was saved."[22] The New Orleans transfusions were undertaken in patients who had lost considerable body fluid. Both yellow fever and cholera produce prodigious vomiting, diarrhea, and blood loss in sufferers. But, for physicians at this time, transfusing blood had less to do with returning blood volume than in providing *vital blood*, blood that could restore the spark of life. Despite Benedict's successful resurrection of his sister, most American physicians remained much more comfortable with the idea of removing blood rather than moving blood into the body. In so doing, these orthodox physicians retained "the therapeutic perspective" of an earlier era, a perspective, as historian John Harley Warner has noted, that valorized blood letting in principle, even as the practice of letting blood declined.[23]

Despite the enormous toll in loss of life, limb, and blood, the war that racked America in the years 1861–1865 prompted little interest in moving blood from one body to another. Transfusion expert Paul J. Schmidt has written that surgeons in the Union Army recorded only four cases in which transfusion was performed during the conflict.[24] The transfusion recipients included a private from Massachusetts who suffered a deep wound that required the amputation of his leg, a private from Illinois who had suffered a musket ball in his thigh, and a young man with an aortic aneurysm. At least one Confederate surgeon, A. Clendinen, claimed that he had successfully performed transfusions during the war to treat cases of threatened collapse from hemorrhage.[25] This is hardly an impressive record considering the injury and bloodshed that marked those years.

In 1871, when physician W. B. Drinkard compiled the history and statistics of blood transfusion, he was able to locate only four American cases among a total of 170 published cases. "I can hardly think that all American cases are comprised in this list of four," Drinkard noted, "but these are all that a very patient investigation of published records has discovered."[26] His four American cases included one performed at the Quartermaster's Hospital in Washington during the Civil War, and three others performed in Philadelphia. Drinkard apparently overlooked the reports from New Orleans, as well as the successful 1866 attempt by W. W. Myers, who transfused 5-year-old Henry with blood taken from "a healthy male laboring under plethora." The physician saved the blood from this patient, taking care to keep it from "contact with atmospheric air," until he injected it into the anemic child, who made a rapid recovery.[27]

One thing that Drinkard's survey of the literature made clear was that loss of blood during childbirth remained the most common indication for blood transfusion in the nineteenth century. More than half of Drinkard's recorded cases (89 out of 170) were performed in cases of postpartum hemorrhage. After 1871, blood loss during childbirth continued to furnish opportunities for American experiments in transfusion. In 1872, physicians in Louisville, Kentucky attempted to transfuse a woman "sinking under anemia dating from the birth of her child." At her husband's insistence, her doctor dissected out a vein in her arm, placed a tube (cannula), and instilled 1 ounce of blood. The physician would have preferred to give her more blood, but the patient's relative who had agreed to supply the blood fainted after only 1 ounce was drawn. After one of the doctors agreed to furnish his blood, she received an additional 6 ounces but she died 20 minutes later.[28] Blood loss and profound anemia provided the indication for twice attempting transfusion on Mrs. B, the mother of four children. In April 1878, a Wisconsin medical student furnished 6 ounces of blood, which was injected through six punctures into the woman's arms, with good results. In January 1879, after she again lay close to death's door, physician C.F. King furnished 150 cc of blood, which was introduced into the opened veins of the sick woman, who recovered rapidly. Unfortunately for her physicians, "her ambition domineered over her judgment." After exposing herself to the cold, she drove a horse down an embankment, sending her into decline and the care of a practitioner from a competing medical sect; she fell "into the hands of homeopathy, and the grave, on the 16th of April, 1879."[29]

Over the next three decades, blood transfusion remained a little used, if sensational, technique. American physicians followed European developments in transfusion in the medical literature, debated the utility of transfusion, discussed different methods and instruments to accomplish it, and considered both the indications for undertaking the procedure and the uncertain outcomes. Many such discussions touched on various technical difficulties encountered in performing transfusion. Perhaps the most pressing issue was clotting. Blood exposed to air begins to clot very quickly, clogging the tubes and making the movement of blood from donor to recipient difficult. This was no trivial problem. That blood exposed to air clotted so readily may explain why some transfusion recipients apparently survived, even when they received multiple transfusions of lamb, calf, and dog blood; these transfusion recipients were unlikely to have received the number of ounces described by physicians. Even when patients received blood from other humans rather than animals, the survival of these patients when they received dissimilar human blood (the blood groups would not be identified until 1900) may have resulted from the small amounts of blood actually transfused.

The discovery that a substance in the blood, fibrin, could be separated from the serum or fluid portion offered one solution to the clotting problem. The work of the German physician Theodor Bischoff made it possible to create "de-fibrinated blood." After removing blood from a donor, the physician stirred it with an eggbeater, a whisk, or a neatly-tied bunch of broom, creating clots. These clots were then strained through clean linen or damask. The liquid that remained was rewarmed and then instilled into an opened vein in the patient. But some surgeons complained that the very process of defibrination robbed the blood of its vitality, because large quantities of the "red globules" were lost in the process. Others continued to find value in transfusing the fluid. In August 1870, a "German gentleman aged 45" at the Pennsylvania Hospital agreed to undergo transfusion as his condition worsened. His nephew, "a stout, vigorous young man," furnished blood, which was defibrinated and injected into the patient, who also received "champagne and broths by mouth." Although the transfusion of defibrinated blood gave him a temporary reprieve, the gentleman succumbed to cancer of the stomach 4 months later.[30]

A second solution to the clotting problem was to avoid using blood altogether, substituting some other fluid—usually milk or saline—that did not coagulate. Physicians noted that milk from a cow or a goat did not form clots. Moreover, milk was "more allied to chyle, the material of which nature makes blood, than any other fluid" known to medical practitioners. The injection of milk into the veins, physicians like T. Gaillard Thomas argued in 1878, was a safer and more efficient treatment not only for severe blood loss but also in such other disorders as Asiatic cholera and typhoid fever.

Before the twentieth century, reports of transfusion using blood, milk, or saline appeared occasionally in the popular press. In 1886, a Chicago policeman severely injured in the Haymarket Riot received blood from his brother-in-law in a last-ditch effort to save the man's life. Erich Egerlis reportedly "stripped to the waist, and his large muscular arms and deep, brawny chest, covered with hair, won the admiration of the onlookers." Egerlis emitted a "stifled groan" as his artery was opened and 4 ounces of blood taken. The physicians considered the transfusion a technical success; it was not sufficient, however, to save the policeman's life.[31] In 1887, the *Washington Post* described "a "peculiar effect" of transfusion in the case of Mrs. Hoyt Sherman, who received blood from the arm of her son, an inveterate smoker. After the transfusion, his mother described how she smelled and tasted tobacco.[32] In 1890, transfusion figured in the romantic triangle of a Wisconsin lumber merchant, the woman he loved, and her fiancée. When the young woman fell seriously ill and required a transfusion, her husband-to-be refused to donate. The lumber merchant supplied the blood for transfusion and won the lady's hand in marriage.[33]

The operation of transfusion remained sufficiently known that it could be adapted for use in political cartoons. During the election of 1880, William Rogers, a political cartoonist for *Harper's Weekly*, depicted an emaciated and skeletal "Democracy" receiving a transfusion from General Winfield Scott Hancock, the Democratic candidate for President, in the hotly contested political race. Rogers's caption read: "Transfusion of blood: is it too late?" Apparently yes—Garfield won the election.

Crile's Miracles

George W. Crile must have seemed an unlikely champion of the new method of surgical transfusion, for his medical career began inauspiciously. Trained as a schoolteacher, he worked his way up to elementary school principal, then decided to

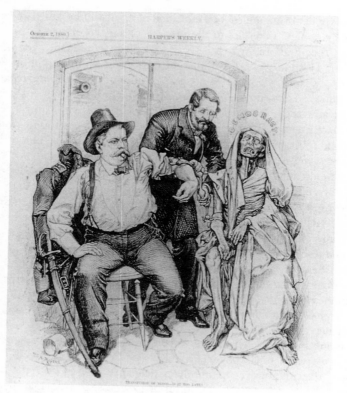

Figure 2.1 In this cartoon, William Allen Rogers depicted Hancock's efforts to revive democracy using blood transfusion, a risky and desperate measure only rarely undertaken in nineteenth-century America. (Source: *Harper's Weekly* [Oct. 1880]: 637.

pursue medical training at the Wooster Medical School in 1886. This institution offered three advantages of the late nineteenth-century medical education: the course of study was short, the tuition was low, and the school offered summer sessions, which enabled Crile to retain his day job as principal. When he graduated from medical school in 1887, he served as a house officer at University Hospital in Cleveland, where he impressed his superiors with his surgical skill, an avid interest in research, and a desire for improvement. Crile was ambitious and, like all ambitious late-nineteenth-century American doctors and surgeons, he went abroad to visit hospitals and laboratories in London, Paris, and Vienna, where he met such medical dignitaries as English physiologist Victor Horsley and the German surgeon Theodor Billroth.[34]

Crile focused his attention on the problem of shock, the body's often fatal response to trauma or surgery. During his hospital experiences in Cleveland, he often witnessed the complications that victims of railway and factory accidents developed in the face of severe blood loss and injury. Crile began experimenting with animals to study the nature, causes, and treatment of shock. In 1897, Crile's first important work "An Experimental Research into Surgical Shock," received the prestigious Cartwright Prize from Columbia University, even as the animal experiments he described made him notorious among animal protectionists. Along with Harvard neurosurgeon Harvey Cushing, Crile worked tirelessly to popularize the measurement of blood pressure with a sphygmomanometer (developed by Italian physician Scipione Riva-Rocci and introduced into America by Cushing in 1901). Crile's researches on blood pressure and its importance in shock prompted Cushing to monitor blood pressure during all surgical operations, leading, in the estimation of historian Peter English, "to the general acceptance of blood pressure measurements in clinical medicine."[35]

Crile's interest in blood transfusion developed from his investigations into surgical shock. In 138 experiments on animals (in shock induced by Crile through trauma or surgery), he systemically compared the therapies then recommended to treat shock, including intravenous saline infusion, strychnine, and the newly discovered extract from the adrenal glands (adrenaline). It was the failure of saline infusions to raise the blood pressure in cases of shock that persuaded Crile to consider blood as a potential therapeutic measure. Blood, he assumed, was safe to use in the body, carried oxygen, and was generally available. Here Crile drew on technical innovations in the suturing of blood vessels, especially Alexis Carrel's technique for surgically connecting arteries and veins. Crile studied with the French surgeon and practiced extensively on dogs in order to master the delicate task of sewing blood vessels end to end. With his colleagues at Western Reserve, he performed a series of experiments in its newly established Laboratory of Surgical Research.[36] Western Reserve was, along with the Hunterian Laboratory at Johns Hopkins, among a handful of schools that possessed such facilities in the early twentieth century.

Crile's first attempt at surgical transfusion in human beings took place in December 1905. To save the life of a delirious, 23-year old woman, he linked an exposed vessel in her arm with the exposed radial artery of her husband. Crile ended the transfusion process after only a few minutes in the face of the man's pre-existing heart condition and his evident nervousness. The patient, whose condition continued to worsen, died after several hours.[37] Crile's second attempt at clinical transfusion proved more successful. This was the "clinical test" undertaken in August 1906, in which he linked the blood vessels of two brothers and reported in the November 1906 *Journal of the American Medical Association*.[38]

Crile's brief report stressed the careful deliberation and experimentation that preceded his decision to attempt such a novel procedure. He described 74 "carefully conducted" animal experiments, which justified his decision to undertake the novel therapy of sewing the blood vessels of two people together: " . . . after having covered by experiments every conceivable phase that would have a clinical bearing," Crile performed the clinical test only when it became certain that the patient would "otherwise inevitably die." Although the young man required a second transfusion from a second brother, he survived. Crile reported additional successes: he described how a woman who had been bleeding from the bowel for more than 4 months experienced "extraordinary" benefit from a surgical transfusion. Two typhoid hemorrhage patients, the surgeon noted, were "wonderfully revived by the transfusions" even though they died. Another patient with a severe kidney hemorrhage received a transfusion but did not survive his ordeal.

Crile's reports on transfusion suggest that he believed that some justification for "clinical tests" was necessary. This may explain his repeated emphasis on the number of animal transfusions he had performed. This emphasis may also suggest a kind of overcompensation about the human transfusions. Like the French chemist Louis Pasteur, whose laboratory notebooks contradicted his claims about prior animal experiments before the human trial of the rabies vaccine, Crile's chronology of the transfusion indicates that the animal transfusion tests occurred after the start of human trials.[39] Although historian Peter English has argued that Crile began transfusing animals in 1904 and "cautiously began the procedure in humans in 1906," Crile's autobiographical account identified December 1905 as the time of his first, and unsuccessful, human transfusion. In his book, *Hemorrhage and Transfusion* (1909), the first American text on transfusion, the surgeon offered a somewhat different chronology. Here, Crile described the experimental studies on animal transfusion studies as beginning September 1906, 9 months following the first clinical attempt at surgical transfusion (the delirious young woman) and nearly 1 month after his successful transfusion of the two brothers. Crile's repeated justifications for his human trials may reflect the ambiguity over the animal trials preceding the human trials.

Hemorrrhage and Transfusion documented how Crile performed 61 transfusions on 55 patients (some patients required a second or third transfusion) between the years 1905–1909. The surgeon described how his technique developed as he accumulated clinical experience with transfusion. In the first 32 transfusions, Crile used sutures to join the cut ends of the vein in the donor and the artery in the recipient. This was a complex procedure requiring exquisite dexterity and special thread and needles, which discouraged its use in emergencies. Prompted to refine the procedure and the instruments, Crile introduced, in December 1906, a cannula (available in various sizes), which served as a tube to unite the inner surfaces of the donor's artery and recipient's vein. These cannulas, similar to miniature napkin rings, reduced the time necessary to perform the surgery, although the procedure remained technically challenging.[40]

What kinds of patients received these transfusions and for what indications? Twenty of Crile's patients received blood, like the young Russian man, because they had lost a great deal of blood. But Crile also attempted transfusion for other medical conditions, including blood disorders (pernicious anemia, leukemia) cancer, goiter, and tuberculosis. Amid concern that American cancer rates were on the increase, Crile pursued the possibility of a cancer vaccine. Assuming that immunity to cancer would result from implanting small bits of cancerous tissue, Crile collaborated with S. P. Beebe at Cornell University Medical College to study dogs who were transplanted with a type of cancer (lymphosarcomata) and then transfused with blood from dogs considered "immune" to the tumors.[41] Crile and Beebe reported that transfusions of large quantities of blood reduced the size, in some cases dramatically, of the tumors but they offered no explanation. Following a series of studies of cancer in dogs, Crile attempted transfusions in six of his patients who had been diagnosed with sarcoma of the neck, jaw, testicle, forearm, and thigh. He described the clinical value of transfusion for sarcoma as encouraging, if not yet conclusive. Crile performed only one transfusion on a small child, an 18-month-old boy with a tumor in his kidney.

However, one of the most dramatic illustrations of the therapeutic potential of surgical transfusion came from Alexis Carrel, who developed the technique for joining together blood vessels. In March 1908, Mary Lambert, the 5-day-old daughter of a New York surgeon, developed life-threatening hemorrhages from her mouth, nose, stomach, and bowels. Her doctors diagnosed melena neonatorum, or hemorrhage of the newborn, a disastrous condition lacking any effective treatment (and now treated with Vitamin K, a factor needed for clotting). In a last-ditch effort to save his daughter's life, surgeon Adrian Lambert appeared on Carrel's doorstep and begged him to attempt a transfusion. Although Carrel reportedly protested that he had not performed the procedure on humans (and lacked a medical license to practice in New York), he was persuaded to travel to the Lambert home. There he sewed the arterial vessel in her father's left arm to the exposed vein in the right leg of his daughter, who was tethered to an ironing board in the family dining room. "His blood rushed from his big, healthy body into that of the child with such good effect that the baby rallied almost immediately and is not only out of danger, but fast gaining flesh and the rosy look a healthy baby ought to have."[42]

Carrel did not perform subsequent transfusions, but other American physicians adopted transfusion as a means to treat infants with bleeding problems. In Chicago, physician V. D. Lespinasse credited the direct transfusion of blood with a cure in virtually all of his 14 patients. These infants were sutured to the blood vessel of a parent for 5 to 15 minutes (15 minutes in one case, because the father fainted). The babies experienced an immediate improvement in their color and their ability to make "a great protest every time the needle is passed" to sew up the incision. When the infants were returned to their mothers for nursing, they weighed 8 to 14 ounces more than they had before the transfusion. In addition to his 14 cases, Lespinasse pointed to 23 other cases in the medical literature that demonstrated the therapeutic power of transfusion "so long as there is a spark of life."[43]

Uniting the inner surfaces of the donor vein and recipient artery allowed transfusers to avert the difficulties associated with blood clotting.[44] But surgical transfusion offered no panacea. Success with the procedure required a skilled operator and a trained corps of assistants; Crile recommended a first and second assistant, a nurse for the two patients, an instrument nurse, and an orderly. He also advised that the procedure worked best when performed in an operating room where donor and recipient occupied adjoining operating tables. There were other difficulties as well.

Determining just how much blood moved between giver and receiver during such a transfusion required guesswork. Some transfusers used time and blood pressure readings to estimate the amount of blood moved, and the length of time a donor and recipient remained linked varied considerably. In his transfusions, Crile joined blood vessels of givers and receivers for anywhere from 8 to 58 minutes. At Johns Hopkins Hospital, vascular surgeon Stephen Watts reported allowing

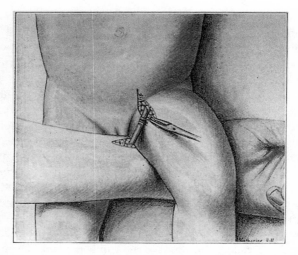

Figure 2.2 Image showing the placement of donor vessel and the infant's vessel. Some preferred to transfuse babies through a vein in the head (Source: *Journal of the American Medical Association* 62 [1914]: 1868)

direct transfusions to continue for 80–110 minutes.[45] More cumbersome than these time/flow calculations was attempting to weigh patients to determine how much blood had been transferred.

Knowing how much blood was transfused was no trivial issue. Too much blood in the recipient could place extreme demands on the heart and lead to death. When Johns Hopkins surgeon Bertram Bernheim performed his third surgical transfusion, the blood from a large male donor "swelled the patient's veins almost to bursting," and "literally knocked that women's heart out the same as if it had been hit with a sledge-hammer."[46] Too much blood also compromised the welfare of the donor. Many accounts of transfusion described how the waxy pallor of the recipient gave way to pink and rosy skin. But some transfusions ended only when the physician noticed the unhealthy pastiness and apparent distress of the donor. Crile advised physicians to watch closely for physical manifestations of distress in donors, including loss of color in the donor's mucous membranes, pallor of the skin, quickening of the pulse or respiration, lowering of blood tension, and shrinkage of the face. In 1912, Doctor Burton Lee described to his fellow members of the New York Surgical Society how one 26-year-old man collapsed after serving as a blood donor to a patient with gastric bleeding. The young man was linked via a cannula to the patient for 40 minutes, when he began to look pale. During the last 10 minutes of the transfusion, his blood pressure dropped, he broke out in cold perspiration, his extremities became cold, and he collapsed. Four days later, he was sufficiently recovered to leave the hospital. What caused his collapse? Perhaps it was the cocaine anesthesia he received when the cut-down was performed. Perhaps, another surgeon speculated, the transfusion should have been stopped at the first indication of paleness, and the donor treated with coffee and whiskey per rectum. The legal liability of the surgeon also occupied the assembled physicians, but perhaps they were reassured by advice from a surgeon at Mt. Sinai Hospital, where "they had a printed release which the patient was requested to sign before operation. While such a release had no legal value, patients who signed it were not so apt to sue as might otherwise be the case."[47]

Participation in surgical transfusion required the donor to sacrifice an artery or, when some surgeons advocated transfusing vein-to-vein, a vein. With either a vein or an artery, the cut-down produced a scar on the skin. In addition, the procedure demanded that the donor possess the emotional stamina to be cut into and directly linked to an obviously dying patient. Crile acknowledged the "psychic factor" in his transfusions. In an effort to minimize the stress on the donor, he administered morphine or cocaine (the donor experienced the prick of the needle); the surgeon also recommended that the faces of both the donor and recipient be covered with a damp towel, thereby avoiding "too much bright light and headache."[48] Despite the physical and emotional demands of the procedure and the attendant risks, Crile reported that family members and friends readily agreed to serve as donors. The surgeon's account also suggests the enormous pressure put on family members and friends to provide blood for the operation: "The gravity of the patient's condition and the reason for wishing to transfuse are carefully explained in detail, and the painlessness of the operation to both donor and recipient is assured. Almost always," he noted, "the offer to serve is made voluntarily." If family members and friends did not always immediately come forward to donate blood, Crile found that their initial objections to the procedure could be overcome in many cases. "Ignorant people," he conceded, with a "certain amount of distrust of both surgeons and hospitals" sometimes refused when asked to donate blood. He described how the parents of one of his patients, a 9-year-old child whose legs had been crushed in an accident, refused to donate blood "because the child was so much mutilated by the injury that it was not worth saving."[49]

In these early transfusions, Crile did not distinguish between the bloods of individuals. "It has been found," he noted in 1909, 9 years after Karl Landsteiner's discovery of human blood groups, "that contrary to common belief, normal blood of one individual does quite as well as that of another. Kinship apparently is of no special advantage."[50] (Blood types are considered in Chapter 5.) Crile's clinical experiences contradict this claim. Kinship conferred a distinct advantage in recruiting donors. More than two-thirds of Crile's 55 patients received blood either from a husband or close family member. Despite the case of the child described above, children were especially likely to receive blood from a relative. Crile's initial series involved transfusing six children. Five of these children received blood from a father, brother, or mother. Only one child—a 17-year-old boy—received blood from an unrelated male donor. Women were also more likely to receive blood from a husband or a male relative. Sixteen of the 29 women who underwent direct transfusion received blood from a husband; nine received blood from either a male (a brother

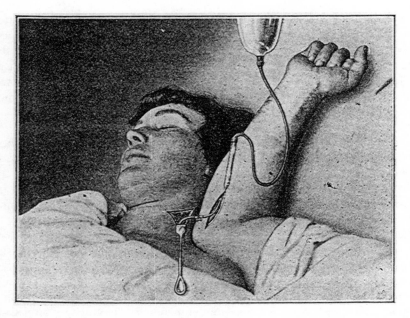

Figure 2.3 Position of donor and recipient; irrigator containing warm sterile saline solution for continuous flushing of the blood vessels (Source: A.L. Soresi, "Clinical Indications for Direct Transfusion of Blood," *Medical Record* 81 [1912]: 839).

or son) or female relative (a sister or daughter). Only three of his female patients received blood from an unrelated male donor. (In one case, the donor was not identified.) In transfusing male patients, Crile also relied heavily on family members to serve as donors. Ten of his 20 male patients received blood from a brother (six cases), a son (three cases), or a nephew (one case). Only one of Crile's male patients received blood from a female relation, a 40-year-old American man suffering from carcinoma, who underwent direct transfusion with his sister-in-law. Men, however, were more likely to receive blood from an unrelated donor. In nine cases, unrelated male donors supplied the blood necessary for transfusion.

Kinship encouraged some individuals to provide blood, and physicians believed that it might also have served to limit transfusion reactions that occurred when the donor and recipient bloods were not compatible. When the Medical Superintendent of the Hebrew Hospital in Baltimore reported two cases of transfusions, he explained that the selection of the mother as a blood donor for her 7-year-old daughter made sense as "the sentiment of a member of a family being of great assistance in the management of both patients." But the physician also assumed that their close family tie promised a smoother transition. Using the parent was "beneficial on account of the close similarity of the blood, although any human blood may be used."[51] In Brooklyn, physician William Francis Campbell echoed these sentiments when he identified the closeness of blood relationship (because it lessened the risk of hemolysis or cell rupture) as one of the three key factors in selecting a blood donor (he also recommended that donors be young, healthy, and thin adults, as fat people as a rule possessed small arteries).[52]

Crile was familiar with Landsteiner's work on the different types of human blood. He acknowledged that the state of knowledge about the blood was in transition. "At the present time," Crile noted in 1909, "we are probably only on the boundary line of knowledge concerning the different constituents of the blood and their reaction. Moreover, what is apparently true to-day may be contradicted to-morrow, so that we cannot feel very sure of our ground until more research work has been undertaken and the results tested by time."[53] Although blood types did not figure into Crile's selection of the donors for his transfusions, he did recommend some tests to ensure that the donor's blood did not react badly with that of the recipient. This could be tested by both suspending the red cells from the patient in the recipient's serum and the reverse (suspending the recipient's red cells in the serum of the donor) and watching to see whether the red cells would rupture or lyse (hemolysis). These laboratory tests did not guarantee that what took place in vitro would necessarily occur in the body (in vivo). The cumbersome nature of these tests and the imprecision of the results made Crile less interested in matching blood.

Some physicians challenged Crile's sanguine assumptions about the near-interchangeability of human blood. In 1907, doctors William Pepper and Verner Nisbet reported a transfusion in which a 33-year-old man received blood from his wife and his brother-in-law. Following the second transfusion, the patient experienced distress, his urine became bloody, and he developed "jaundice, oppression, and other evidences of hemolysis." The patient's death 2 days later prompted Pepper and Nisbet to challenge the "innocuousness of introducing blood from normal individuals into other normal persons, or those suffering from hemorrhage or disease."[54] But routine blood typing did not take hold in clinical practice until the end of World War I.

Despite concerns about safety, American interest in blood transfusion did not wane. Physicians and surgeons offered a host of new techniques and equipment for transferring blood, including a cannula shaped like a Y with a syringe (Curtis and David, 1911), a glass storage tube coated with paraffin (the Kimpton-Brown tube, 1913), and several variations on syringe-needle-stopcock devices (Bernheim, Lindemann, and Unger).[55] These technical improvements made transfusion easier to perform.

Other physicians recommended different positions and elevations of operating room tables to improve the flow of blood from donor to recipient. When he performed a transfusion at the home of a young woman hemorrhaging from a stomach ulcer, Brooklyn physician J. E. Jennings had the family take down a 7-foot door so that he could place the blood donor (the young woman's fiancé) at a 45-degree angle from her bed. Using the saphenous vein in the leg to move blood into her body, he described how the patient's ears which were "white and waxy became pink." The transfusion was stopped when the donor became pale and weak.[56]

In 1915, the independent discovery that the addition of sodium citrate to the blood would retard clotting furthered stimulated interest in blood transfusion. Physicians Luis Agote (Argentina), Richard Weil (Belgium), and Richard Lewisohn (United States) each described successful transfusions using citrated blood. In the leading newspaper of Buenos Aires, Agote explained that he had received a large quantity of citrated blood intravenously without adverse consequences. Not only was the transfusion of citrated blood well tolerated by the recipient, but the procedure using citrated blood could be performed by a single physician. This innovation made transfusion accessible to even "the untrained physician" and greatly increased the popularity of the practice.[57]

Not everyone accepted the safety and efficacy of blood modified by the addition of sodium citrate. The controversy over fresh blood versus modified blood ensured that the practice of direct transfusion did not wholly disappear from American surgical practice. At some hospitals, the procedure of direct transfusion continued to be performed well into the 1920s. Despite the aversion of professional donors to the inch-long incision over the radial artery and the technical demands of the surgery, some physicians continued to champion direct transfusion.[58] By 1921, many of the numerous blood transfusion techniques allowed practitioners to obtain blood from donors by needle "thus avoiding the destruction of a useful vein" and making the process of donation less onerous.[59]

Blood transfusion did not remain risk-free. Long before the twentieth century, physicians had recognized the potential for disease transmission through the transfusion of blood. Indeed, this was one of the reasons for longstanding suspicion about the safety of vaccination (that the process of moving serum from body to body transferred more than immunity to smallpox, possibly also allowing the infection of people with syphilis and other serious diseases).[60] Physicians acknowledged that surgical transfusion could result in disease transmission between donor and recipient. When he selected a donor for his typhoid fever patients experiencing hemorrhages, Crile, for example, deliberately chose individuals who already had typhoid fever in an effort to minimize risks from infection. By 1915, reports of transfusion-transmitted diseases—measles, malaria, and syphilis—began to appear. After a 9-month-old infant received a blood transfusion from her mother, she developed fever and rash, and physicians confirmed that she had measles. Her mother, who had no visible signs of measles before the transfusion, developed the disease 2 days after the transfusion. Although she survived, her infant daughter did not; she died 3 weeks after the transfusion.[61] Reports about patients developing malaria following transfusion also appeared. Although measles and malaria posed dangers, the disease most dreaded by patients and physicians was syphilis (so stigmatized that, before 1913, the New York Times avoided the word altogether; the paper referred to it as a "loathsome blood disease.")

In 1917, Johns Hopkins surgeon Bertram Bernheim described an early case of the transmission of syphilis from donor to recipient in blood transfusion. When he was asked to donate blood to his father, suffering from pernicious anemia, the son of Bernheim's patient refused to take the Wassermann test for syphilis. When his father took a turn for the worse, the son donated blood. His father subsequently developed a virulent form of syphilis.[62] Establishing transfusion as the source of infection was not a simple matter. In order to prove that syphilis was transmitted in a given case from donor to recipient, it was necessary to establish that the donor had the disease before the transmission and the recipient did not. This was easier to establish in some cases than others. In Bernheim's case, the son's refusal to take a Wassermann test was taken as an indication that he was aware that he had the disease. When a 17-month-old boy developed syphilis in 1927, following a blood transfusion at the Jewish Hospital of Brooklyn, both the physicians and parents were able to rule out "exposure though sexual contact because the patient was an infant." In this case, the age of the child and the fact that his parents were free of the disease encouraged the Brooklyn physicians to consider the professional donor who supplied the blood as the source of the infection. (The donor could no longer be located through the commercial agency.) "In this country, where transfusions are so popular," warned the physicians, "there must have occurred many more similar cases which have not been reported, probably because it is an unpleasant subject for publication."[63] At this time, physicians assumed that syphilis was prevalent in America. The Public Health Service estimated that 10% of all Americans had the disease. In a survey of prospective donors in New York City, Dr. Herman Goodman found that .68% of the white applicants were positive for syphilis, but among Negro applicants, 25% of the men tested positive for the disease. Given this prevalence, the transmission of syphilis by transfusion was no trivial matter. "The transmission of syphilis to an adult," noted one physician, "even in an attempt to save life, is a disaster than which no other could be worse but the transmission of syphilis to an infant." By 1931, ten cases in the medical literature prompted warnings that physicians should exercise extreme caution when transfusing. Six years later, there were 59 cases of transfusion syphilis in the medical literature, which did not include 11 cases recorded by the Department of Health of New York City but not publicly reported. Physicians assumed that the actual number was much greater. [64]

Physicians had little problem asking professional blood donors to undergo blood tests to rule out syphilis; they were willing to take much more on faith when it came to the family members of their patients who offered blood. For that reason, the cases of transmission of syphilis via transfusion from family members may have been more common than transmission from professional donors. (A similar issue developed during the early days of the AIDS epidemic, when some patients insisted on directed donation by family members, who felt compelled to give blood even though they had an infectious disease.) In some cases, donors who knew or suspected that they had syphilis provided blood for a family member. When Mrs. M.J., "an undernourished Negress," needed blood following a miscarriage, her sister provided the blood. When Mrs. M.J. developed syphilis and had a positive Wassermann test 2 weeks later, the doctors tested her husband who was negative. The sister had not undergone a Wassermann test before the transfusion; only after "considerable difficulty" did the doctors induce the "obviously reluctant donor" to submit to a blood test that showed her infection.[65] But, in some cases, family members remained unaware of their infections or uncertain of their status as donors.

When his sister developed syphilis after he donated blood for a transfusion for birth-related hemorrhage, one man "admitted that he was exposed to syphilis" 4 years earlier. He had not volunteered this information earlier because he had failed to develop any symptoms and because an earlier Wassermann test had been negative.[66]

Performing the blood test did not resolve all problems. Some donors tested negative for syphilis and only later developed the disease. One such case occurred at Johns Hopkins, where a 6-year-old child, being treated for sickle cell anemia and undernutrition, developed syphilis after several injections of blood from her mother. The mother initially tested negative for syphilis but, by the end of the injections, she tested positive for the disease.[67] In other cases, laboratory errors resulted in the use of donors with syphilis. To prevent the transmission of syphilis not yet detectable by laboratory methods, some physicians opted to add antisyphilitic drugs to the blood being transfused. At Georgetown University Hospital, three patients—two "colored females" and a "white male"—received one-tenth of a gram of Mapharsen (a drug to combat syphilis) in the sodium citrate added to the blood they received. They apparently did not develop syphilis.[68]

By 1935, patients who had developed syphilis from transfusion began suing physicians and hospitals. Some physicians insisted that transfusion-related syphilis could no longer be upheld as an "accident" but rather negligence. Physician R. Straus, who worked at the laboratory of Cleveland's Mount Sinai Hospital, criticized the laxity of donor examination not only in the United States but in the "naively conducted" organization of blood donors in Germany, in which "only donors of pure Aryan ancestry are accepted—as a rule only students or members of the National Socialist Party." Straus suggested that the German reliance on the donor's "word of honor" that neither he nor any member of his family had become infected with syphilis was entirely unsatisfactory as a means of ensuring safe transfusions and insisted that all who provided blood had to undergo syphilis testing.[69] Bemoaning the poor supervision of blood donors and the failure to adequately test for syphilis, Philadelphia physician John Stokes explained that the damage suit would be a fine educator. "Nothing will serve better (and with the howling popularity of syphilis at this time the figures will rise) than a judgment for a hundred thousand dollars against a careless medical man or surgeon who transmits syphilis by transfusion."[70] Although it could locate no case law relating to the transmission of syphilis by transfusion as of 1938, the Medical Protective Company of Fort Wayne, Indiana warned physicians: "from a medicolegal standpoint, our experience in defending such cases has not been good. The Courts have allowed the cases to go to a jury and the juries have returned verdicts against doctors who made a transfusion without a Wassermann test."[71] In some cases, physicians were able to avoid liability by obtaining "a denial of venereal infection." When his sister-in-law needed blood in an emergency, one man offered such a denial to her physician. Because time was short, the physician did not perform the Wassermann test. When the patient later developed syphilis, this denial from the donor insulated the physician from liability.

Covered in Blood

In the early twentieth century, transfusion was more than a surgical procedure. It was a dramatic spectacle. The sensational features of blood transfusion—near-death, sacrifice, and danger—quickly attracted newspaper reporters; in the first three decades of the twentieth century, hundreds of articles describing blood transfusions appeared in American newspapers. This was especially true in New York City, where newspapers published frequent reports of blood transfusion, often with a local angle. If George W. Crile was the motive force in advancing surgical transfusion, it was the flamboyant Alexis Carrel who received the lion's share of credit for the innovation. Crile was at Western Reserve in Cleveland, but Carrel was a senior member of the Rockefeller Institute for Medical Research in New York City, an institution funded by the largesse of John D. Rockefeller and one seeking to cement its status as a leading institution through publicity about its breakthrough investigators. In March 1908, when Carrel's surgical expertise saved the life of a 5-day-old baby, newspapers made much of his surgical feat. The transfusion persuaded John D. Rockefeller, whose financial gifts funded Carrel's research at the Rockefeller Institute, that his money had been well spent. Moreover, the stories played a role in the Institute's ongoing battles with opponents of animal experimentation.[72]

Rockefeller was not the only one impressed by transfusion. The spectacle of surgical transfusion suffused medical accounts of the procedure. Physician Samuel Lambert described how his brother Adrian's blood "was allowed to flow into the baby to change her skin from a pale transparent whiteness to a brilliant red color." Reporting his own case of a successful direct transfusion, Spokane physician Arthur

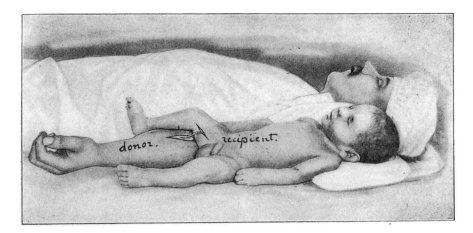

Figure 2.4 This transfusion of a child and adult was similar to that performed by Alexis Carrel, and it persuaded J.D. Rockefeller that his investment in medical research was worthwhile (Source: A.L. Soresi, "Clinical Indications for Direct Transfusion of Blood," *Medical Record*, 81 [1912]: 839).

Cunningham vividly recalled the scene: "The clinical picture of a patient, across whose features the shadow of death is rapidly appearing, being suddenly changed into an animated being, red blood coursing through the previously pulseless vessels, the flush of life suffusing the pale cheek, the awakened interest in surrounding scenes; such a transformation is comparable only with the miraculous biblical accounts of the raising of the dead."[73]

Newspaper editors similarly welcomed vivid reports of the dramatic and colorful story of moving blood between bodies. The popular press carried hundreds of reports of transfusions during the first three decades of the twentieth century. Some of these stories reflected the celebrity of the donors and recipients. When Tennessee senator Luke Lea gave a quart of blood to his wife in 1911, his "story of sacrifice" earned him "universal admiration."[74] Newspapers reported how suffragist Inez (Milholland) Boissevain received six blood transfusions as treatment for pernicious anemia, and the story about the Standard Oil magnate John D. Archbold, who received blood from his chauffeur after suffering complications from an appendectomy, appeared on the front page. Popular singer Anna Held, the common-law wife of impresario Florenz Ziegfeld, underwent transfusion for myeloma, but succumbed to her illness. Admiral Robert E. Peary appeared to be gaining after he received a blood transfusion, but died as a result of pernicious anemia 10 days after the procedure.[75]

The majority of newspaper stories about transfusion involved more ordinary people. In 1913, Samuel Bernberg was on the road to recovery "through the self-sacrifice of his 14-year-old sister Annie."[76] Like many such stories, the report of the 12-year-old's transfusion was brief. In addition to the names of donor and recipient and the outcome of the transfusion, the report identified his illness—pernicious anemia—and the physicians who performed the procedure. Often these stories served to illustrate the power of kinship; husbands donating to wives, sisters to brothers, uncles to nieces, and parents to their children.

Stories of transfusion similarly demonstrated the importance of affiliation. In 1914, blood from a "brother physician" gave hope for the recovery of Otto Ramsay, the chair of obstetrics and gynecology at Yale Medical School; a private in the Salvation Army received blood from Charles Wiseman, commander of the Salvation Army Corps.[77] In 1915, Mrs. Leslie Lynch, the wife of a White Plains businessman, received blood donated by her maid, Miss Mary Ryan.[78] Patrolman Frank Smith gave a pint of his blood to an "old chum" and fellow policeman; a school teacher "sacrificed" her blood for a pupil afflicted with scarlet fever; and the coach of Howard McNamara, the captain of the Brunswick School football team, gave his blood in an effort to treat the teenager's leukemia.[79] In one strange case, a New York man, Julian Dick, received a blood transfusion from the brother of the man who had shot him.[80] These stories celebrated sacrifice, but in many cases, illustrated that transfusion did not save all recipients. The "blood gift" of his brother failed to save Paul Knight, a Cornell University law student diagnosed with leukemia; John Gilmurray "vainly sacrificed" a quart of blood for his brother, and the principal of Jamaica High School (New York City) "vainly gave his blood" to save his wife.[81] "Life fluids" from his father, brother, wife, cousin, and chum, failed to save Leight Bourne Middleton, afflicted with "poverty of blood" (aplastic anemia).[82] By the 1920s, it often seemed that the large number of transfusions was the story. Despite operations over the course of 2 years and 27 transfusions, Adelaide Jones died of pernicious anemia in 1922. A veteran of the world war received 107 transfusions before he succumbed. [83] Finally, many of the stories about transfusion featured descriptions of interns, medical students, and college students who sold their blood to pay for a wedding or new baby, or to fund college studies.[84]

What impulse prompted more than a thousand such stories of transfusion—about donors and recipients—in the first four decades of the twentieth century? What made transfusion newsworthy? Perhaps, rather than news, these transfusion stories represented a new form—a medicalized form—of the human-interest story. Such stories became popular with the rise of the penny press in the middle decades of the nineteenth century; at mid-century the phrase "human interest" was explicitly invoked in the office of the *New York Sun* to refer to those "chatty little reports of tragic or comic incidents in the lives of the people."[85] By the late nineteenth century, even more serious newspapers included what James Gordon Bennett, editor of the *New York Herald*, had called "a correct picture of the world—in Wall Street—in the Exchange—in the Post Office—at the Theaters—in the Opera—in short, wherever human nature or real life best displays its freaks and vagaries."[86] To the exchange and the post office, editors added the sick room, the operating theater, and the hospital, with their real life dramas, comedies, and tragedies.

This medical form of the human interest story, like other narratives of its kind, reflected public curiosity about the social worlds of "others": the interest of the poor in the rich, the rich in the poor, the sick in the well, and the well in the sick—what newspaper magnate William Randolph Hearst called "the interesting" rather than "the important." In so doing, the popular newspaper offered informal education in the world of science, nature, medicine, and health. This was not limited to stories of transfusion. When the *New York Sun* covered the Sanitary Conference of American Republics, the "human interest" angle developed around the discovery by Charles W. Stiles of the role of hookworm disease, in what the paper called "the Germ of Laziness." The cartoons, jokes, and comments had the effect, according to Mark Sullivan, of "making Stiles the target for newspaper and stage humorists the world over; next, the object of scorn and vituperation in all the region south of the Potomac River and east of the Mississippi; and finally, years later, one of the heroes of medical science in his generation."[87]

Such medical human interest narratives also resonated with early twentieth-century newspaper interest in developments in medical science and medical research. As historian Bert Hansen has demonstrated, the popular press first began to accord medical discoveries high visibility in the late nineteenth century.[88] The *New York Times* covered such developments in depth, with a particular eye to local events and local luminaries, including John D. Rockefeller (whose failure to attend church services on a Sunday because of a snow storm was front page news) and surgeon Alexis Carrel. Transfusion represented an innovation, an American innovation, at a time when Americans were eager to take their place in the larger world. Although Carrel was not an American (and never accepted American citizenship), his surgical research at the Rockefeller Institute—transplantation, transfusion, and the "glass heart"—made him an object of American admiration. When Carrel received the Nobel Prize in 1912, Americans embraced him as the first worker in America to receive the prize in medicine or physiology.

Transfusion also attracted attention because of the dramatic spectacle it presented: a patient on the brink of death, the self-sacrifice of a relative or friend, and the possibility of restoring vitality to a bloodless body. This was especially true of surgical transfusion, which required much more from donors and recipients than transfusion mediated by syringes and stopcocks. The movement of blood between bodies called into question the conventional boundaries of the self in American society. Moving blood from men into women, Gentiles into Jews, Negroes into whites (and vice-versa) elicited speculation about the dissolution of the boundaries and the implications for the reintegrated person. It afforded the opportunity to speculate about whether someone would take on the character or nature of the donor, whether such dissolution transgressed sexual or species boundaries. Even more, transfusion stories offered a platform for moral contemplation of the limits of human responsibility. Few questioned whether a son should donate blood to his father, a mother to her child, a husband to a wife. But what were your obligations to more distant relatives, to your brother-in-law or your neighbor? How far did the obligations extend even to the closest relatives? Did it require you to lay on a bed adjacent to your loved one, to be cut open, to have your artery or vein exposed and then sewn to the vessel of the patient? Did it require you to incur these risks and the general unpleasantness of the experience, particularly when the outcome was likely to be failure? Transfusion stories facilitated speculation about the hero and the enigma of the altruist, about the bonds of human community, and the intimacy of blood relations.

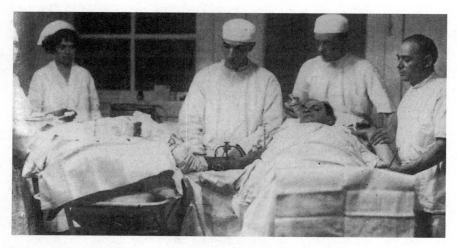

Figure 2.5 This photograph of a transfusion in action illustrates that transfusion was a complex procedure requiring trained doctors and nurses (Source: H. Harlan, "This Business of Selling Blood," *Hygeia*, 7 [1929]: 471).

Given the press's interest in transfusion, it is perhaps not surprising that transfusions were incorporated into American mass culture, especially in Hollywood films. Between 1916 and 1940, more than 32 American films included blood transfusion as a specific subject. In such silent films as *Doctor Neighbor* (1916), the willingness of the individual to give blood represented extreme self-sacrifice and forgiveness. Dr. Neighbor, for example, dies after donating blood to the man who misused his niece. In the 1916 film *Her Surrender*, the transfusion of a man's blood into a woman's veins signals their romantic relationship (in the film it is called "transfusion of love").[89] In the 1920s and 1930s, such films as *Night Nurse* (1931) and *And Sudden Death* (1936) featured the transfusion of blood in hospital and operating room scenes. In the popular 1934 film *Little Miss Marker*, when the character played by child star Shirley Temple is thrown by a horse, she undergoes an emergency transfusion. "Anybody who saw Little Miss Marker, way back when Shirley Temple was a new discovery, probably has a pretty fixed idea about how transfusions are given. Remember the poor little kid and the big bad man lying in the operating side by side with their arms joined together by a lot of tubes? And you just knew the blood was pouring into the kiddie's arms to save her life—and it did."[90] Perhaps, then as now, such scenes on the big or small screen (think of the cardiac resuscitation scenes in such television programs as *E.R.*) encouraged viewers to believe that these procedures seldom failed.

American mass culture also capitalized on some of the fears excited by the transfer of blood, especially the blood of animals. In the 1925 silent melodrama *Wolf Blood*, a logger in a remote forest is seriously injured and requires a blood transfusion. The only blood source available is a wolf, which is placed on a table and then surgically connected to the logger. As his anxiety over the effects of the animal blood coursing in his veins grows, the logger begins to behave in strange ways until he is saved by a young woman.[91] This film, and others that included the transfer of ape and monkey blood and serum into human beings with tragic consequences, expressed some of the disquiet about strange blood and its effects on the body, even as the transfusion of blood from animals made a comeback in the 1920s. Beginning in 1921, Rene Cruchet, a professor of pathology at the University of Bordeaux, revived animal to human transfusions. Cruchet first attempted the transfusion of sheep, ox, and horse blood into dogs. He explained that the promising results of these trials encouraged him to undertake injections of sheep's blood into eight patients, horse blood into 12 patients (nine tuberculous patients, one "insane," and two others). Despite the fact that one of the recipients died suddenly from the introduction of horse blood, Cruchet insisted that the conditions of his other patients improved and that his patients "even asked urgently for repeated transfusions" with animal blood.[92]

Blood in the Bank

In the 1930s, a major innovation in transfusion took place. This involved using stored blood rather than fresh blood administered immediately after being taken from a donor. The idea of using "canned blood" was not new. In World War I, physician Oswald Hope Robertson had used such preserved blood to treat battlefield casualties. Trained at the Rockefeller Institute, Robertson gained familiarity with the method of preserving blood with sodium citrate and dextrose developed by Rockefeller researchers Francis Peyton Rous and J.R. Turner. In November 1917, Robertson collected blood from soldiers with blood type O, preserved it with the Rous solution, and stored it on ice. After waiting 5 days for the red cells settled at the bottom of the blood bottle, he drew off the fluid, and returned the red blood cells to an ice container. When fighting took place, he placed the preserved blood cells on ice using a converted ammunition case and took it to the Casualty Clearing Station, where he reconstituted the cells with distilled water, warmed it up, and administering it to badly wounded Canadian soldiers. His blood work, historian Kim Pelis notes, not only earned him an enduring place in historical memory, but persuaded "an international coalition of young medical officers, including the Canadian Norman Guiou, the British Kenneth Walker, and the Australian A. W. Holmes-á-Court, to experiment further with transfusion close to the front lines."[93]

After the Great War, when physicians and surgeons returned to civilian practice, few saw any need to use preserved blood. They preferred to use blood that was "fresh" and still warm from the donor's body. In the United States, surgeons and physicians helped organize donors so that they could be called quickly when needed. In the 1920s, Soviet physicians at the Central Institute of Hematology and Transfusions in Moscow introduced "blood conservation"; they removed blood and stored it for later use in transfusions. Between 1931 and 1934, two physicians from the Leningrad Blood Transfusion Station reported 1529 transfusions using "canned" blood. In 1930, Russian surgeon Serge Judin retrieved blood from a corpse (dead 6 hours from a fractured skull), mixed it with saline, and injected it into the body of a young engineer whose suicide attempt had resulted in enormous blood loss. As the engineer received the blood, "consciousness returned, and by the end of the transfusion the patient had a good pulse and his colour had improved." Judin's successful use of corpse blood continued; by 1937, he reported the results of his first 1000 cases. Cadaver blood, like the blood of live donors, could be preserved with sodium citrate, dextrose, and glucose. Although some surgeons flirted briefly with cadaveric blood, it proved unattractive to most American physicians.

In 1937, the Cook County Hospital opened the first "blood bank." When physician Bernard Fantus introduced the term "blood bank" to refer to the system of blood collection and distribution that he had organized at the Chicago hospital, he acknowledged the Russian lead in the preservation and storage of cadaveric blood. But blood taken from the dead, Fantus explained, proved "revolting to Anglo-Saxon susceptibilities." For this reason, he advanced what he described as "the blood bank proposition," based on simple rules and policies for obtaining and dispensing blood in the hospital setting. "Just as one cannot draw money from a bank unless one has deposited some, so the blood preservation department cannot supply blood unless as much comes in as goes out."[94]

Fantus's concept of the blood bank spread rapidly. Hospitals and communities around the country adopted similar methods for making blood available when needed.

In 1938, the surgical staff at Philadelphia General Hospital opened a blood bank. Physicians at Memphis's John Gaston Hospital opened a blood bank the same year. In 1939, surgeons at Johns Hopkins Hospital in Baltimore, physicians at the Presbyterian Hospital in New York City, doctors at Jefferson Davis Hospital in Houston, and surgeons at Children's Hospital in Washington, D.C. organized blood banks. In 1941, the Irwin Blood Bank opened in San Francisco.

Availability of blood was one factor in the growing popularity of blood transfusion in clinical practice. One index of this recognition was the number of transfusions reported by the Blood Transfusion Betterment Association (BTBA), which began monitoring blood transfusion in New York City in 1929. In 1930, the BTBA recorded 3125 blood donations. By 1934, the number of donations climbed to 5216. Three years later, the BTBA reported 9820 blood donations. Other medical centers reported similar increases in blood transfusion. At the Mayo Clinic in Rochester, Minnesota, doctors performed 841 transfusions in 1933; in 1935, they performed 1289 transfusions.[95] In 1937, when physicians Philip Levine and Eugene Katzin surveyed 700 American hospitals about their transfusion practices, 77% of the institutions reported a "decided increase" in the number of transfusions in 1936 over the number performed in 1935. By the end of 1939, transfusion expert Alexander Wiener had collected reports of at least 15,000 transfusions in American hospitals.[96]

The major indication for transfusion on the eve of America's entry into World War II remained the replacement of lost blood. Transfusing blood into someone who had experienced severe blood loss immediately expanded the number of red blood cells that carried oxygen to the tissues and increased blood volume—both essential in the management of shock. Physicians acknowledged that patients who experienced hemorrhage enjoyed "the most spectacular results from blood transfusion." As Alexander Weiner noted in 1943, most emergencies in civilian practice resulted from automobile accidents or attempted homicide. He cited one analysis of 292 cases of gunshot wounds to the abdomen, in which hemorrhage was the single most important cause of mortality, and one in which "a significant reduction in the mortality rate was observed among patients receiving blood transfusions."[97]

Transfusion was also regarded as significant in the treatment of other kinds of hemorrhages, including the profound loss of blood that occurred in typhoid fever, peptic ulcer, and pulmonary tuberculosis. Women who experienced blood loss in pregnancy and childbirth (ruptured uterus, postpartum hemorrhage) also benefited from transfusion; in some cases of ectopic pregnancy rupture, surgeons used blood recovered from inside the patient's own body to perform "auto-transfusion" when fresh blood was not readily available.

Surgeons recommended the use of blood transfusion as preparation for surgical procedures. Undertaken to prevent shock, these transfusions were viewed as a means to convert poor surgical risks into better surgical risks. At the Jewish Hospital of Brooklyn, transfuser Richard Lewisohn explained that transfusion preceded "every brain operation and before other operations in which much bleeding was anticipated."[98] Physicians also found transfusion valuable in treating a variety of blood disorders, including hemophilia, sickle cell anemia, purpura, and hemorrhagic disease of the newborn. Although the biochemical mechanism in hemophilia was not yet understood, surgeons recognized that transfusion decreased the time needed for clotting, and that as little as 100 cc of blood was sufficient to stop bleeding. In 1946, Harvard biochemist Edwin Cohn and his colleagues demonstrated that the "anti-hemophilic factor," now called factor VIII, could be isolated (fractionated) in plasma. In cases of sickle cell anemia, physicians used transfusions to increase the number of oxygen-carrying red blood cells. Some sickle cell patients received hundreds of transfusions to aid their recoveries from episodes of severe anemia. (Transfusion, which reduces the risk of stroke, remains an important therapy for the treatment of sickle cell anemia.) In hemorrhagic disease of the newborn, transfusion was once the only available life-saving measure. Even with better understanding of the role of blood clotting and the importance of vitamin K, transfusion remains an important adjuvant treatment in managing this disease of early infancy.[99]

Indeed, the popularity of blood transfusion prompted some physicians to caution their colleagues about the willingness to see transfusion as a panacea. Some surgeons warned about caving in to the demands of the patient's family. "Transfusion has acquired such popularity among the laity," Richard Lewisohn observed, "that we are often forced to resort to it against our better judgment, in order to ease the mind of the sorrow-stricken family."[100] But physicians also turned to transfusion despite the slim chance of success. The desire of physicians "to leave no stone unturned in the general care of patients" encouraged them to undertake transfusions where benefit was unlikely. Boston physician Arlie Bock warned that cases of acute leukemia encouraged consideration of transfusion despite the lack of adequate justification. "Once the diagnosis [of acute leukemia] is made, the family should be informed of the inevitable outcome, and, if the subject of transfusion is brought up, they should be advised against it. If transfusions are attempted, one of two things generally happens, either a severe fatal transfusion reaction occurs or life may be miserably prolonged for a few weeks." Bock warned that transfusion did not benefit patients with Hodgkin's disease, malignant hypertension, or chronic kidney infections.[101] Physicians needed to exercise good judgment in deciding when, where, and for what indications transfusions should be undertaken.

Blood for Battlefields

The outbreak of war in Europe brought fresh demands for blood. In the spring of 1940, Alexis Carrel returned from France to describe the dramatic need for blood plasma to treat battlefield casualties. The BTBA considered the possibility of shipping plasma to France and England. In June 1940, members of the Association's Board of Trustees met with representatives from the American Army, Navy, National Research Council, Rockefeller Institute, and major pharmaceutical firms to discuss the idea in earnest. Although plasma production and shipment was in its early stages, those gathered supported the idea of trying to mount a large-scale effort in the collection, processing, and transportation of blood plasma. With the aid of the New York chapter of the American Red Cross, physicians at Presbyterian Hospital in New York City began collecting blood in August 1940.

Between August and January 1941, Americans made some 14,556 donations to the Blood for Britain Program. Although originally distributed to France as well, Britain became the sole beneficiary of these products once France fell to the Nazis.[102] The medical director of the project was surgeon Charles Drew, who had organized the blood bank at Presbyterian Hospital in New York City and who had written a dissertation on banked blood at Columbia. Drew set up criteria for the mass collection of the blood, participated in the protracted debates over the best types of collecting bottles and stoppers, and made recommendations about the criteria for the blood donors.[103] Once blood was collected, technicians diluted the blood with saline solution and separated the red blood cells from the plasma portion using a centrifuge or by sedimentation. The liquid plasma was stored in Baxter 1000-cc bottles, which could be shipped in Clipper planes to the British.

The success of the Blood for Britain program created optimism about the large-scale collection of blood plasma as Americans prepared for war. In January 1941, the Surgeons General of the Army and the Navy asked the American Red Cross "to secure voluntary donors in a number of the larger cities of this country, to provide the necessary equipment, to transport the drawn blood rapidly to a processing center, to arrange for separating the plasma and for storing the resulting product in refrigerated rooms." The plasma amassed by the Red Cross would be "of greatest service if a military emergency arises, but also of ultimate use in any national catastrophe."[104] The Red Cross opened its first blood donor center in New York City in February 1941, and eventually operated some 35 centers between 1941 and December 1945.

The Red Cross's initial decision to exclude African Americans as blood donors created problems for the organization (see Chapter 5). Although this policy was rescinded and African Americans accepted as donors, the organization's decision to apply racial labels to the blood and to process plasma from black donors separately from "white" blood further antagonized potential supporters. Despite these missteps, the Red Cross appealed to Americans to donate blood, capitalizing on "the enormous emotional advantage that donations of blood could save the lives of wounded men."[105] Perhaps not surprisingly, the number of blood donors peaked at particular points during the war. After the invasion of Normandy, Americans poured into the Red Cross centers; during the week of June 10, 1944, the Red Cross collected some 123,284 pints of blood. Between 1941 and 1945, the organization collected more than 13 million pints of blood from some 14.6 million Americans (10.3% were rejected for various reasons, including anemia, high blood pressure, or disease).[106]

Most of the donated blood (10 million pints) was processed into plasma, which was shipped to both the European and Pacific theaters. But whole blood was also used for American soldiers. American military physicians used some 600,000 pints of whole blood collected by the Red Cross. The Army shipped over 200,000 pints of type O blood to Europe; the Naval Air Transport delivered more than 181,000 pints of type O blood to the Pacific. The massive deployment of blood and blood plasma for British and American forces was hailed as one of the great success stories of World War II. The mortality rate in combat, according to Brigadier General Douglas Kendrick, who supervised the American Army's blood program, was reduced by

50% in World War II because of the availability of "prompt and adequate resuscitation, in the routine of which whole blood and plasma play major roles."[107] Along with penicillin, the transfusion of blood and the system for mobilizing blood and blood components validated both American medical and military interests.

When American surgeons returned from military service, they expected blood and blood components to be readily available for their civilian practices. New surgical procedures increased the need for blood. The advent of open-heart surgery, for example, greatly magnified the demand for blood. The introduction of the heart-lung machine in 1953 made possible for the first time surgical repairs of ventricular septal defects; these machines, however, required as much as 60 pints of donated blood for each operation. In addition to cardiovascular surgery, the use of the "artificial kidney" or kidney dialysis machines boosted the demands for blood. The success of kidney transplantation at the Massachusetts General Hospital in 1954 further stimulated increased clinical demands for donated blood. To meet the growing demand for blood in post-war America, the American National Red Cross announced, in 1947, plans to develop regional blood centers to help supply the need for blood and blood products. Between 1948 and 1963, the Red Cross opened 56 regional centers. By 1962, Americans donated blood to some 4400 hospital blood banks and 123 community or medical-society blood banks.[108]

The Red Cross supplied only part of the solution to America's need for blood. In 1947, a coalition of independent and community-based blood organizations met in Dallas and formed the American Association of Blood Banks (AABB).[109] The AABB and the Red Cross differed in their approach to the operation and function of blood banks. Among the salient differences were the role of physician governance, the responsibility for paying for blood, and individual versus community responsibility for blood supplies. Almost from the start, these differences created considerable friction. In 1948, surgeon John Scudder, director of the Presbyterian Hospital Blood Bank in New York City and a member of the AABB, criticized the operation of a newly established Red Cross blood center in Rochester, New York. The Red Cross, Scudder insisted, should not be permitted to collect blood because they lacked appropriate medical supervision; they did not require, for example, a physical examination before blood donation. Moreover, Scudder maintained that the steps taken by Red Cross personnel were not adequate to prevent contamination of the donated blood.[110] In the 1950s, several organizations attempted to create a more unified system for supplying America's blood needs. The Red Cross and the AABB, together with the American Medical Association and the American Hospital Association, established a National Blood Council in 1954. Despite these efforts at coordination, the attempt foundered.

In 1971, a British professor of social policy compared British and American blood programs and offered a scathing condemnation of American policies. In *The Gift Relationship*, Richard Titmuss caustically described the American reliance on paid (rather than voluntary) donors and the threat to the safety of the blood supply this fostered. Moreover, Titmuss argued that the commercialization of blood and donor relationships repressed the expression of altruism, erodes the sense of community, lowers scientific standards, limits both personal and professional freedoms, legalizes hostility between doctor and patient, subjects critical areas of medicine to the laws of the marketplace, places immense social costs on those least able to bear them (the poor, the sick, and the inept), and increases the danger of unethical behavior in various sectors of medical science and practice.[111]

In the face of this stark censure, the Department of Health, Education, and Welfare appointed a special task force to review blood policies. Like Titmuss, the members of the task force found that American blood was of uneven quality, that it contributed to high rates of post-transfusion hepatitis, that its distribution was inefficient and inadequate, and that its provision created economic burdens on many Americans. To address these shortcomings, the federal government created a National Blood Policy. This new national policy did not alter the landscape of the American blood suppliers, nor did it influence the collection of blood for blood components. As Ronald Bayer has noted, this "bifurcated system of blood collection, regulated by the Food and Drug Administration (FDA) in close collaboration with the industry that it was charged with overseeing" fell under the silent shadow of human immunodeficiency virus (HIV) in the 1980s.[112]

In 1982, the Centers for Disease Control Morbidity and Mortality Weekly Report described three patients with hemophilia who had developed symptoms very similar to those found in some homosexual men and Haitians. Some blood bankers initially downplayed the threat that acquired immune deficiency syndrome (AIDS) could be transmitted in blood and blood products (especially the factor VIII that enabled hemophiliacs to live more normal lives), but it became clear that there were a growing number of cases of transfusion-associated AIDS cases. In 1985, the FDA licensed a new test to detect exposure to the virus in donated blood, which proved very effective in eliminating HIV-infected blood from the blood supply. However, some 29,000 Americans had become infected with HIV when they received blood transfusions between 1978 and 1984.[113]

The AIDS epidemic stigmatized transfusion, transforming the procedure from a life-saving measure to a potential death sentence. The threat of transfusion-associated AIDS elicited bizarre proposals (including a blood bank containing only blood donated by certified virgins) and misconceptions about the ways in which the virus was transmitted. Many Americans erroneously assumed that HIV could be transmitted not only if they received a transfusion but even if they donated blood for transfusion. Apparently, a significant number of Americans continue to believe that donating or giving blood can transmit the HIV virus. For a study of HIV-related stigma and knowledge, researchers surveyed approximately 2000 American adults about HIV transmission. In 1991, 32.2% of those polled indicated that donating blood could transmit the HIV virus. By 1999, this percentage had increased slightly (32.9%) rather than decreased, despite the educational efforts of organizations like the Red Cross and the AABB.[114] In 2005, the AABB's website, for example, continued to post the frequently asked question "Can you get AIDS or hepatitis from donating blood?" and the response "No. Sterile procedures and new disposable equipment are used by all blood donor centers. All items used—the finger lancet, the needle, the cotton balls, swabs, and solutions—are discarded after a single use."[115] Nonetheless, the association of AIDS with transfusion and blood donation persists.

Other, newer dangers are associated with blood transfusion. In the 1990s, reports that the agent responsible for bovine spongiform encephalopathy (mad cow disease; a variant form of Creutzfeldt-Jakob disease, a rare, fatal neurologic disease) in Europe could be transmitted through the blood supply raised questions about the safety of blood transfusion. In 2002, when the United States experienced an unprecedented outbreak of infections by West Nile virus, a mosquito-borne agent, American researchers discovered that the virus was transmissible by both blood transfusion and organ transplantation. Fortunately, researchers had rapid access to a screening test for the virus, the nucleic acid test (NAT).[116] Still, the threat to the blood supply from emerging infectious diseases remains.

Miracles of Resurrection

In the early twentieth century, a Cleveland surgeon revived medical interest in moving blood between bodies when he successfully sutured the cut end of a blood vessel in a donor to that of recipient. Grace Crile recorded her impressions of the "midnight resurrection" in 1906, when she accompanied her husband to St. Alexis Hospital in the middle of the night. She described the donor's "contracted features, the deep orbital spaces, the greenish pallor of the patient," all signs of impending death. Once George Crile had sutured the vessels of the patient and his brother, she recorded how the pallor receded, how "his cheeks, his lips, even his ears, took on a rosy glow."[117] The spectacular nature of using blood to bring patients back from the brink of death excited physicians and surgeons, as well as the interest of the popular press and members of the public. Who would not be affected by the sight of two individuals united in flesh and blood?

Notes

1. George Crile, "Direct Transfusion of Blood in Treatment of Hemorrhage," *Journal of the American Medical Association* 47 (1906): 1482–1484.

2. Grace Crile, ed. *George Crile: An Autobiography* (Philadelphia: J.B. Lippincott, 1947), vol. 1, 166.

3. "Offers Blood to Save Life of Man He Stabbed," *Chicago Tribune*, 27 Dec. 1914, p. A7; "Seven Republicans Give Blood to Democrat," *New York Times*, 25 Mar. 1921, p. 9; "Six Offer Blood to Save Negro," *New York Times*, 25 Oct. 1928, p. 24.

4. "Tinker's Blood for Wife," *New York Times*, 15 Jul. 1913, p. 1; "Blood of Babe Ruth Is Given to Daughter," *New York Times*, 6 Aug. 1938, p. 15.

5. See Douglas Starr, *Blood: An Epic History of Medicine and Commerce* (New York: Alfred A. Knopf, 1998).

6. Samuel Pepys. *Diary*. Accessed on line at http://www.pepys.info/1667/1667nov.html on July 8, 2005.

7. Thomas Birch, *The History of the Royal Society of London* (London: A. Millar, 1756–1757), 216.

8. Geoffrey Keynes, ed. *Blood Transfusion* (London: Simpkin Marshall, 1949), 15.

9. Pete Moore, *Blood and Justice* (West Sussex, England: John Wiley & Sons, 2003).

10. M. G. Purmann, *Lorbeer Krantz, oder Wund Artznei* (Frankfurt, 1705).

11. N.S.R. Maluf, "History of Blood Transfusion," *Journal of the History of Medicine and Allied Sciences* 9 (1954): 59–107.

12. David M. Morens, "Death of a President," *New England Journal of Medicine* 341 (1999): 1845–1849.

13. Kim Pelis, "Transfusion, with Teeth," in Robert Bud, Bernard Finn, and Helmuth Trischler, eds. *Manifesting Medicine: Bodies and Machines*, (Amsterdam, The Netherlands: Harwood Academic Publishers, 1999), 1–29.

14. James Blundell, *The Principles and Practice of Obstetricy, As At Present Taught, by James Blundell* (Washington, D.C.: D. Green, 1834), 264.

15. James Blundell, *Researches Physiological and Pathological: Instituted Principally with a View to the Improvement of Medical and Surgical Practice* (London: E. Cox, 1825), 136–137.

16. "Another Successful Case of Transfusion," *The Lancet* 5 (1825): 111–112.

17. "Successful Case of Transfusion," *Lancet* 11 (1829): 431–432.

18. J. Howell, "Successful Case of Transfusion," *Lancet* 9 (1828): 698–699.

19. J. Blundell, *Researches Physiological and Pathological,* p. 123.

20. W. Channing, "On the Transfusion of Blood," *Boston Medical and Surgical Journal* 1 (1828): 97–102.

21. Paul J. Schmidt, "Transfusion in America in the Eighteenth and Nineteenth Centuries," *New England Journal of Medicine* 279 (1968): 1319–1320.

22. James Polk Morris, III. *Blood, Bleeding, and Blood Transfusion in Mid Nineteenth-Century Medicine* (Ph.D. dissertation, Tulane University, 1973.) See pages 156–157.

23. John Harley Warner, *The Therapeutic Perspective: Medical Practice, Knowledge, and Identity in America, 1820–1885* (Cambridge: Harvard University Press, 1986).

24. Paul J. Schmidt, "Blood Transfusion in the South Before the War between the States," *Southern Medical Journal* 72 (1979): 1587–1589.

25. "Transfusion of Blood," *New York Times*, 19 Jun. 1880, p. 2.

26. W.B. Drinkard, "History and Statistics of the Operation and Transfusion of Blood," *National Medical Journal* 2 (1871–1872): 181–194.

27. W. W. Myers, "Transfusion in Anemia," *Medical and Surgical Reporter* 15 (1866): 255–256.

28. "Transfusion," *American Practitioner* 6 (1872): 58–60.

29. F. H. Epley, "A Case of Transfusion." *Chicago Medical Journal and Examiner* (1879): 234–240.

30. Thomas G. Morton, "On Transfusion of Blood, with a Report of Eight Cases, and a Description of a Convenient Apparatus for Performing the Mediate Method," *American Journal of the Medical Sciences* 18 (1874): 110–118.

31. "He Gave His Life Blood," *National Police Gazette*, 3 Jul. 1886, 48(459), p.6.

32. "The Peculiar Effects of Blood Transfusion," *Washington Post*, 4 Mar. 1887, p.1.

33. "His Life for Hers," *Washington Post*, 9 Feb. 1890, p. 16.

34. Robert G. Frank, Jr. "The Telltale Heart: Physiological Instruments, Graphic Methods, and Clinical Hopes 1854–1914," in William Coleman and Frederic L. Holmes, eds., *The Investigative Enterprise: Experimental Physiology in Nineteenth Century Medicine* (Berkeley: University of California Press, 1988), 211–290.

35. For American opposition to animal experimentation, see Susan E. Lederer, "The Controversy over Animal Experimentation in America, 1880–1914," in *Vivisection in Historical Perspective*, ed. Nicolaas A. Rupke (London: Croom Helm, 1987), 236–258. Peter C. English, *Shock, Physiological Surgery, and George Washington Crile* (Westport, CT: Greenwood Press, 1980), 98.

36. G. Crile, *George Crile*, p. 162.

37. George W. Crile, *Hemorrhage and Transfusion: An Experimental and Clinical Research* (New York: D. Appleton, 1909), 381–382. The patient suffered from an exophthalmic goiter.

38. See William Schneider, "Blood Transfusion in Peace and War, 1900–1918," *Social History of Medicine* 10 (1997): 105–126.

39. Gerald L. Geison, *The Private Science of Louis Pasteur* (Princeton: Princeton University Press, 1995).

40. George W. Crile, "The Technique of Direct Transfusion of Blood," *Annals of Surgery* 46 (1907), 329–332.

41. G. W. Crile, *Hemorrhage and Transfusion*, p. 242.

42. "Father's Blood Saves Baby," *Washington Post*, 21 Mar. 1908, p. 3. For the medical report, see Samuel W. Lambert, "Melaena Neonatorum with Report of a Case Cured by Transfusion," *Medical Record* 73 (1908): 885–887.

43. V. D. Lespinasse, "The Treatment of Hemorrhagic Disease of the New-Born by the Direct Transfusion of Blood," *Journal of the American Medical Association* 62 (1914): 1866–1869.

44. Kim Pelis, "Blood Clots: The Nineteenth-Century British Debate over the Substance and Means of Transfusion," *Annals of Science* 54 (1997): 331–360.

45. Stephen H. Watts, "The Suture of Blood Vessels: Implantation and Transplantation of Vessels and Organs. An Historical and Experimental Study," *Bulletin of the Johns Hopkins Hospital* 18 (1907): 153–179.

46. Bertram M. Bernheim, *Adventure in Blood Transfusion* (New York: Smith & Durrell, 1942), 15.

47. "Collapse of a Transfusion Donor," *Annals of Surgery* 55 (1912): 892–894.

48. George Crile, "The Technique of Direct Transfusion," pp. 329–332.

49. G.W. Crile, *Hemorrhage and Transfusion*, pp. 300–301.

50. George W. Crile, "Further Observations on Transfusion with a Note on Haemolysis," *Surgery, Gynecology & Obstetrics.* 9 (1909): 16–18.

51. Charles Bagley, Jr., "Report of Two Cases of Transfusion of Blood, Occurring at the Hebrew Hospital," *The Hospital Bulletin* 6 (1910–1911): 7–10.

52. William Francis Campbell, "Blood Transfusion as Therapeutic Measure," *New York State Journal of Medicine* 9 (1909): 232–237.

53. G.W. Crile, *Hemorrhage and Transfusion*, pp. 319–20.

54. William Pepper and Verner Nisbet, "A Case of Fatal Hemolysis Following Direct Transfusion of Blood by Arteriovenous Anastomosis," *Journal of the American Medical Association* 49 (1907): 385–389.

55. William H. Schneider, "Blood Transfusion in Peace and War, 1900–1918," *Social History of Medicine* (1997): 105–126.

56. J.E. Jennings, "A Contribution to the Surgery of Blood Transfusion," *Long Island Medical Journal* 4 (1910): 153–157.

57. P.L. Mollison, "The Introduction of Citrate as an Anticoagulant for Transfusion and of Glucose as a Red Cell Preservative," *British Journal of Haematology* 108 (2000): 13–18; Henry M. Feinblatt, *Transfusion of Blood* (New York: Macmillan, 1926), p. 96.

58. J. Shelton Horsley, Warren T. Vaughan, and A. I. Dodson, "Direct Transfusion of Blood," *Archives of Surgery* 5 (1922): 301–313. See J. Shelton Horsley, "Blood Transfusion: A Study of Two Hundred and Forty-Five Cases," *Archives of Surgery* 7 (1923): 466–468.

59. I. S. Ravdin and Elizabeth Glenn, "The Transfusion of Blood with Report of 186 Transfusions," *American Journal of the Medical Sciences* 161 (1921): 705–722.

60. Silik H. Polayes and Max Lederer, "Transmission of Syphilis by Blood Transfusion," *American Journal of Syphilis* 15 (1931): 72–80.

61. Harry Bauguess, "Measles Transmitted by Blood Transfusion," *American Journal of Diseases of Children* 27 (1924): 256–259.

62. B. M. Bernheim, *Adventure in Blood Transfusion*, p. 62.

63. Silik H. Polayes and Max Lederer, "Transmission of Syphilis by Blood Transfusion," *American Journal of Syphilis* 15 (1931): 72–80.

64. "Transmission of Syphilis by Blood Transfusion," *Journal of the American Medical Association* 97 (1931): 106–107; R. Straus, "Kline Exclusion Test in Prevention of Transfusion Syphilis," *Archives of Dermatology and Syphilology* 36 (1937): 1039–1043.

65. Clyde L. Cummer, "Transfusion Syphilis," *American Journal of the Medical Sciences* 185 (1933): 787–789.

66. Harry Mandelbaum and A. N. Saperstein, "Transmission of Syphilis by Blood Transfusion," *Journal of the American Medical Association* 106 (1936): 1061–1063.

67. H. B. Taussig and H. E. Oppenheimer, "Severe Myocarditis of Unknown Etiology," *Bulletin of the Johns Hopkins Hospital* 59 (1936): 155–170.

68. Frank J. Eichenlaub and Robert Stolar, "Syphilis Acquired from Transfusion and Its Control," *Pennsylvania Medical Journal* 42 (1939): 1437–1443.

69. R. Straus, "Kline Exclusion Test in Prevention of Transfusion Syphilis," *Archives of Dermatology and Syphilology* 36 (1937): 1039–1043.

70. "Discussion," *Journal of the American Medical Association* 110 (1938): 19.

71. Joseph V. Klauder and Thomas Butterworth, "Accidental Transmission of Syphilis by Blood Transfusion," *American Journal of Syphilis* 21 (1937): 652–666. For out-of-court settlements involving transfusion-related syphilis, see Clyde L. Cummer, "Transfusion Syphilis," *American Journal of the Medical Sciences* 185 (1933): 787–789. See also "Malpractice: Syphilis Transmitted by Blood Transfusion," *Journal of the American Medical Association* 117 (1941): 2192.

72. See George W. Corner, *A History of the Rockefeller Institute* (New York: Rockefeller Institute Press, 1964), 77; and Susan E. Lederer, "Political Animals: The Shaping of Biomedical Research Literature in Twentieth-Century America," *Isis* 83 (1992): 61–79.

73. Arthur T.R. Cunningham, "Some Observations on Direct Blood Transfusion with Report of a Case," *Northwest Medicine* 3 (1911): 42–43.

74. "Story of Sacrifice," *Washington Post*, 25 Jun. 1911, p. 1.

75. "Mrs. Boissevain Better: A Sixth Blood Transfusion Is Made to Suffragist," *New York Times*, 17 Nov. 1916, p. 4; "Chauffeur Gives Blood to Save Mr. Archbold," *Los Angeles Times*, 1 Dec. 1916, p. 1. "Blood Transfusion for Anna Held," *New York Times*, 4 May 1918, p. 15; "Admiral R.E. Peary, Pole Discovered; Dies at Capital," *New York Times*, 21 Feb. 1920, p. 1.

76. "Saved by Sister's Blood," *New York Times*, 19 Sep. 1913, p. 2.

77. "Fight for a Doctor's Life," *New York Times*, 8 Jun. 1914, p. 1; "Gave His Blood to Woman," *New York Times*, 14 May 1914, p. 7.

78. "Maid Saves Mistress's Life," *New York Times*, 13 Jun. 1915, p. 1.

79. "Policeman Gives His Blood," *New York Times*, 8 Jul. 1921, p.9; "Gives Blood to Save Pupil," *New York Times*, 25 Mar. 1923, p. E2; "Fail to Save Athlete," *New York Times*, 30 Apr. 1927, p. 24.

80. "Julian Dick Dies, Despite Blood Transfusion from the Brother of the Man Who Shot Him," *New York Times*, 3 Jan. 1921, p. 1.

81. "Blood Gift Fails to Save," *New York Times*, 2 Dec. 1913, p. 2; "Brother's Sacrifice Vain," *New York Times*, 1 Mar. 1914, p. C4; "Vainly Gave His Blood to Save Wife," *New York Times*, 8 Apr. 1914, p. 13.

82. "5 Blood Transfusions Fail," *Washington Post*, 1 Aug. 1913, p. 5.

83. "27 Blood Transfusions Fail," *New York Times*, 1 Dec. 1922, p. 6.

84. These stories are discussed in Chapter 3, Banking on the Body.

85. Gary A. Fine and Ryan D. White, "Creating Collective Attention in the Public Domain: Human Interest Narratives and the Rescue of Floyd Collins," *Social Forces* 81 (2002): 57–85.

86. Helen MacGill Hughes, "Human Interest Stories and Democracy," *Public Opinion Quarterly* 1 (1937): 73–83.

87. Hughes, "Human Interest Stories," p. 80. Stiles also earned the label "Privy Counselor" for insisting that building sanitary privies (outhouses) would limit the spread of hookworm.

88. Bert Hansen, "New Images of a New Medicine: Visual Evidence for the Widespread Popularity of Therapeutic Discoveries in America after 1885," *Bulletin of the History of Medicine* 73 (1999): 629–678.

89. The number 32 comes from a keyword search of the American Film Institute's On-Line Catalog. See "Her Surrender," *Moving Picture World* 30 Sep. 1916, p. 2101.

90. Hannah Lees, "Life by the Pint," *Colliers* 100 (25 Sep. 1937): 18, 69–71.

91. See entry for "Wolf Blood" in the *AFI On-line Catalog*.

92. Rene Cruchet, "Transfusion of Blood from Animal to Man," *British Medical Journal* 2 (1926): 975–978.

93. Kim Pelis, "Taking Credit: The Canadian Army Medical Corps and the British Conversion to Blood Transfusion in WWI," *Journal of the History of Medicine and Allied Sciences* 56 (2001): 238–277.

94. Bernard Fantus, "Cook County's Blood Bank," *Modern Hospital* 50 (1938): 57–58.

95. De Witt Stetten, "The Blood Transfusion Betterment Association of New York City," *Journal of the American Medical Association* 110 (1938): 1248–1252, p. 1251; "Annual Report for 1935 of the Section on Anesthesia: Including Data on Blood Transfusion," *Proceedings of the Staff Meetings of the Mayo Clinic* 11 (1936): 421–432.

96. Philip Levine and Eugene M. Katzin, "A Survey of Blood Transfusion in America," *Journal of the American Medical Association* 110 (1938): 1243–1248; Thomas Hale Ham, "Transfusion Therapy," *New England Journal of Medicine* 223 (1940): 332–339.

97. Alexander Weiner, *Blood Groups and Transfusion* (Springfield, IL: Charles C. Thomas, 1943): 78.

98. Richard Lewisohn, "Clinical Results in Two Hundred Transfusions of Citrated Blood," *American Journal of the Medical Sciences* 157 (1919): 253–272.

99. A. Weiner, *Blood Groups and Transfusion*, pp. 84–91.

100. R. Lewisohn, "Clinical Results," p. 269.

101. Arlie Bock, "The Use and Abuse of Blood Transfusions," *New England Journal of Medicine* 215 (1936): 421–425.

102. Douglas B. Kendrick, *Blood Program in World War II* (Medical Department of U.S. Army, 1964), 13. Kendrick's account is silent about the decisions to exclude African Americans as donors and the subsequent difficulties and criticism that this policy produced.

103. Spencie Love, *One Blood: The Death and Resurrection of Charles Drew* (Chapel Hill: University of North Carolina, 1997).

104. G. Canby Robinson, *Adventures in Medical Education: A Personal Narrative of the Great Advance of American Medicine* (Cambridge, Harvard University Press, 1957), 284.

105. D.B. Kendrick, *Blood Program in World War II*, p. 119.

106. D.B. Kendrick, *Blood Program in World War II*, p. 140.

107. Douglas B. Kendrick, *Memoirs of a Twentieth-Century Army Surgeon* (Sunflower University Press, 1992), 90.

108. Louis K. Diamond, "A History of Blood Transfusion," in Maxwell M. Wintrobe, ed. *Blood Pure and Eloquent* (New York: McGraw Hill, 1980), 681.

109. Louanne Kennedy, "Community Blood Banking in the United States from 1937 to 1975: Organizational Formation, Transformation and Reform in a Climate of Competing Ideologies" (Ph.D. dissertation, NYU, 1978), 94–112.

110. John Scudder, "The Blood Bank Controversy," *New York Times*, 23 Feb. 1948, p. 24.

111. Richard M. Titmuss, *The Gift Relationship: From Human Blood to Social Policy* (New York: Vintage Books, 1971), 138.

112. Ronald Bayer, "Blood and AIDS in America: The Making of a Catastrophe," in Eric Feldman and Ronald Bayer, ed. *Blood Feuds: AIDS, Blood, and the Politics of Medical Disaster* (New York: Oxford University Press, 1999), 20–58.

113. R. Bayer, "Blood and AIDS," pp. 33–34.

114. Gregory M. Herek, John P. Capitano, and Keith F. Widaman, "HIV-related Stigma and Knowledge in the United States: Prevalence and Trends, 1991–1999," *American Journal of Public Health* 92 (2002): 371–377.

115. http://www.aabb.org/All_About_Blood/Donating_Blood/donate.htm; Accessed Aug. 1, 2005.

116. Jay S. Epstein, "Insights on Donor Screening for West Nile Virus," *Transfusion* 45 (2005): 460.

117. G. Crile, *George Crile*, p. 166.

3

Banking on the Body

We are hardly accustomed to thinking of our body parts and fluids as commodities. Yet the American practice of selling blood, skin, and other body parts to be used in or on other people's bodies is more than a century old. Over the course of the twentieth century, so-called "professional blood sellers" and even "professional skin sellers" advertised their availability, the quality of their product, and their services. In New York City, in 1938, a group of professional blood sellers actually unionized, joining the American Federation of Labor (AFL) and promising not to strike. Until the 1970s, much of the blood used in this country for transfusions and the manufacture of blood products came from individuals who were paid for supplying this vital fluid.

This commodification of the body, its fluids, and its parts was never complete nor was it uncontested. Long before the creation of a National Blood Policy (by the U.S. Department of Health, Education, and Welfare in 1974), which sought to promote "voluntary" blood donation, some Americans had expressed reservations about "making money from human misery" by selling blood.[1] And as early as the 1920s, some observers cautioned about "the despicable traffic in organs." That people would worry about the economic exploitation of the indigent, forced to sell part of his body to survive, may not be as surprising as the body part that excited this concern—namely the human testicle, harvested for transplantation into the bodies of aged men in an effort to restore lost vitality and strength. Forty years later, the success of renal transplantation in the 1950s and heart transplantation in the 1960s raised the specter of a market in human kidneys and human hearts. Concern about commodifying the human body prompted the United States Congress, in 1984, to enact the National Organ Transplant Act, which included provisions that expressly forbade the sale of human tissue.

Despite such regulatory efforts and apparent distaste for commercializing the sale of body fluids and tissues, the market in human tissue continues to operate. Sometimes the market in what some have called "renewable body assets" is open, if largely unregulated. College newspapers routinely carry advertisements seeking young women to donate (sell) their eggs to infertile couples for in vitro fertilization. Sperm banks have long paid healthy young men a fee for their deposits. Other individuals sell their plasma (blood is taken, centrifuged, and the red cells separated from the liquid portion are mixed with a saline solution and returned to the individual's blood stream). Some plasma, not surprisingly, is more valuable than others, and the pay scales reflect this. Given the prohibition on the sale of organs like kidneys, it was perhaps predictable that a clandestine trade in kidneys would arise. Critics have attacked so-called "transplant tourism," wherein wealthy Westerners travel to developing countries to avoid the long waiting time for a cadaveric organ and receive organs purchased from desperate, indigent individuals. These organ sellers generally receive only a trifling sum (the big money goes to the broker) and they experience substantial risk in the surgery and after-care they receive.[2]

In popular culture, the corrupting power of money in the organ trade is a favorite trope. Films, television programs, and the Internet play on such urban legends as the businessman who wakes up in a hotel room minus a kidney, or how the young and ethical doctor discovers that the mysterious "brain deaths" of healthy young people are linked to a network that supplies organs for ailing millionaires.[3] Perhaps even more surprising is the fact that such tales about unscrupulous surgeons and nefarious schemes to induce vulnerable individuals to sell their body parts are not a recent development. Stories about the tragic consequences of selling hands and hearts date from the early twentieth century. Then, as now, film companies transformed these stories into cinematic treatments about the perils of the trade in human bodies.

How did blood and tissue acquire economic value in American society? What role did physicians play in these transactions? Who sold their blood and tissue, and under what circumstances? What lessons, if any, can be drawn from this durable effort at commodifying the body?

The commodification of the human body has a long history. Women and men have long bought and sold their own bodies and those of other people for sexual purposes. (Today, so-called "sex tourism" in countries like Thailand, where children and adults are coerced into selling sexual services, coexists alongside transplant tourism.) The legally sanctioned enslavement of human beings and the attendant purchase and sale of slaves, for example, only ended in the United States by government fiat in 1865; in other parts of the Western hemisphere, slavery remained legal until the 1880s.[4] Physicians had never been wholly absent from the large-scale enslavement of Africans, who were captured, transported, and then bought, sold, and bred like livestock. As the evaluators of a slave's "soundness" for labor and production, physicians inspected slave bodies before sale.[5] After sale, physicians offered advice and services to keep slave bodies working. In some cases, doctors purchased slaves or made other financial arrangements to have access to slave bodies, which could then be used to attempt novel therapies or procedures. In perhaps the most notorious case, the Alabama physician James Marion Sims entered contractual arrangements with the owners of enslaved women who suffered from childbirth injuries. In the 1840s, Sims agreed to house and feed these women in exchange for the opportunity to attempt to surgically repair their defect (vesicovaginal fistula). By his own account, some of these women participated in as many as 30 surgical operations before he successfully developed an effective method using silver sutures to repair their bodies.[6]

In the nineteenth and twentieth century, American physicians participated in a clandestine market involving the bodies of the dead. As in Britain, the acquisition of sufficient "material" for anatomic dissection prompted the theft of newly dead bodies for delivery to medical schools and private dissectors. Some medical educators and anatomists chose to purchase the bodies of the newly dead from so-called "resurrection men," professional grave robbers. In the late nineteenth century, American "traffic in corpses" included shipping bodies in zinc-lined trunks by train to medical schools. In 1899, the city undertaker of Memphis, Tennessee was arrested when he confessed that he received up to $200 per body when he arranged for the bodies of three black males and one white female to be shipped to Iowa.[7] By 1902, some claimed that dead bodies had become a "drug on the market," a glut because the newly passed anatomy laws gave medical schools access to the bodies of the unclaimed dead. Still, reports of traffic in dead bodies continued to appear, even after the development of willed-body programs.[8]

The medical market for the living body was less developed than the underground economy based on the dead body. Physicians sometimes paid individuals to undergo discomfort and/or risk to test theories or study biologic processes. In 1667, at the Royal Society, English physicians Richard Lower and Edmund King paid Arthur Coga, the young man with the "too warm brain" the sum of 20 shillings for his willingness to undergo the "experiment" of transfusion. In *Zoonomia* (1794), English physician Erasmus Darwin, one of the inspirations for Mary Shelley's *Frankenstein*, advocated blood transfusion as a therapy for malnutrition and putrid fevers. He advised one elderly patient to imbibe daily a few ounces of blood from an ass, "or from the human animal, who is still more patient and tractable."[9] The human animal, in Darwin's scheme, would permit for a fee the opening of a vein and placement of a tube to allow blood to flow to the recipient. Darwin's elderly patient preferred to meet his death without such an intervention. When English physician James Blundell became the first to transfuse humans with human blood, he too suggested that money could make blood available. In 1825, as he acknowledged the difficulty in obtaining arterial (rather than venous) blood for his transfusions, Blundell explained "persons may be induced occasionally, sometimes from motives of affection, and sometimes for hire, to submit to the opening of the artery."[10]

Indeed, physicians paid some individuals for the privilege of performing medical examinations or unusual anatomic feats. In 1796, the eminent Philadelphia physician Benjamin Rush was among those who paid a substantial fee (one-quarter of a dollar) for entrance to Mr. Leech's Tavern to observe Henry Moss, a 38-year-old man born "entirely black" but who had inexplicably "become as white and fair as any white person."[11] Moss earned his freedom and his living demonstrating the apparent instability of black skin; in a special meeting of the American Philosophical

Society, Rush reported his theory that black skin represented a form of leprosy and that Moss was undergoing a spontaneous cure.

In the 1820s, when the gunshot wound to his abdomen left a permanent opening to his stomach, the French-Canadian voyageur Alexis St. Martin agreed to permit Army surgeon William Beaumont to perform 1 year of "reasonable experiments" in exchange for $150, plus food, clothing, and lodging. St. Martin found many of these experiments unpleasant: the studies included removing gastric fluid or inserting into the abdominal opening a piece of food tied with string that was removed at various points in the digestive process. After St. Martin returned to Canada, Beaumont expressed resentment that he had been "obliged to pay high wages to induce [St. Martin] to return and submit to the necessary examination and experiments upon his stomach and its fluids." He paid the wages because he recognized that the trapper's anatomic irregularity was essential to his work.[12]

Physicians and dentists also participated in transactions in which money was exchanged for pieces and parts taken from living bodies. In the late eighteenth century, one of the by-products of English surgeon John Hunter's investigations into human teeth was a vogue for live-tooth transplantation. This practice entailed removing healthy teeth from the mouths of impoverished young people and securing them into the mouths of wealthy individuals with damaged or rotting teeth. (The young possessed healthier and more attractive teeth.) By 1800, fear of transmitting disease, especially syphilis, and the numerous cases of failure of tooth transplantation damped enthusiasm for using teeth from live donors. Some British dentists did continue the use of teeth taken from the bodies of the dead; in the early nineteenth century, some called these "Waterloo teeth," because it was assumed that they had been obtained from battlefield corpses.[13]

Human hair and human milk continued to be bought and sold in the nineteenth and twentieth centuries. Human hair was used for making wigs and hairpieces. In 1904, "real white hair" from an American woman reportedly sold in New Jersey for $25 an ounce. According to one trader in human hair, most of the hair used to make wigs came from Russia, Scandinavia, Italy, Germany, Spain, and France, and "the cheaper sorts from Japan, China, and South America." American hair was a scarcer commodity because "Americans as a people are more prosperous and don't have to sell their locks."[14] For centuries, middle-class families had employed wet-nurses to suckle newborn infants. In Progressive Era America, female milk sellers replaced wet nurses as breast milk was transformed into what one physician called "therapeutic merchandise." In the 1910s, physicians set up milk bureaus at hospitals such as the Boston Floating Hospital, which paid lactating women about $4 a week (for a quart a day) for their breast milk. Some enterprising women were able to parlay their biologic products into considerable earnings; one Italian American woman reportedly earned $987.98 during a single year of milk selling.[15]

In the late nineteenth and early twentieth centuries, developments in medicine and surgery opened up new possibilities for commodifying body parts and fluids. Fueled by patient demand, this new commerce was largely managed by physicians and surgeons who often brokered the sale of parts and services between patients and suppliers. In the 1930s, American physicians and surgeons appropriated the language and concepts of financial institutions—deposits, withdrawals, and banking—for the storage of bodily fluids and tissues. More than a metaphor, banking captured the transactional nature of commerce in the body. Originally adopted to refer to stored blood, banking became the organizing principle for making available a variety of tissues, including eyes, bones, skin, nerves, organs, and sperm.

Traffic in Organs

In 1900, Charles Mixer published a short story that drew on the surgical imaginary of possible organ transplantation made possible by nineteenth-century surgical advances. "The Transposition of Stomachs" offered more than surgical switching of the digestive organs of two individuals; it also involved a financial arrangement between a retired steamship company president and one of his former employees, "a strapping, robust, rosy-cheeked fellow" with a strong appetite. For the sum of $25,000, the longshoreman agreed to allow an eminent surgeon to surgically transpose his healthy Irish stomach with the dyspeptic organ of the aging gourmand. After the operation (with its acknowledged risks) goes well, the rich man is amused to learn that his supplier has driven "the identical bargain" with another longshoreman. But instead of the sum of $25,000, this transaction is for $5000. "So if all goes well, Jerry will have a better stomach than he ever had, and twenty thousand in the bank."[16]

This little story, and others like it, illustrates how the potential surgical alteration of the body through replacing worn out organs with new ones or revitalizing the blood became available for both speculation and speculative fiction. As Mixer's story makes clear, some of the conjectures prompted by these surgical developments were financial. The "transposition of stomachs," for example, involved not only commodifying the body and its parts, but also its recommodification—the resale of used body parts. Who knows, the rich man muses, where his old stomach will end up and in whom? Yet, the most fantastic part of Mixer's tale was not the switching of stomachs or that a rich man would purchase a body part from a working-class man willing to sell one. Instead, it was the enormous sum initially offered and accepted. $25,000 was a great deal of money (in 2006 terms, the comparable sum would be more than $583,000). The working-class man was far more likely to receive much less for the sale of his body parts or fluids.

Just 3 years later, in November 1903, the *New York Times* published a front-page article about an advertisement that had appeared in metropolitan newspapers:

> $5000 will be paid for right ear, $2^{1}/_{2}$ inches long, $1^{1}/_{4}$ inches wide, with
> perfect curves and full lobe; the ear may be from either male or female,
> and must be from a person in perfect health; offers by mail considered.[17]

With a thirst for the sensational, reporters contacted Dr. Andrew Linn Nelden, who explained that the ear was intended for a "Western millionaire," who had lost his own in an accident and was seeking a replacement on the eve of his marriage. The millionaire was willing to accept a female ear of the appropriate size, Nelden told reporters, because a woman would be able to more readily disguise her surgical disfigurement by altering her hairstyle.

Nelden had apparently first made the rounds of hospitals seeking a prospective donor. "It is necessary to get some one whose blood is absolutely pure," he informed reporters. "Such persons are not so numerous among those who would be likely to part with an ear."[18] Nelden sought to ensure that the recipient would not develop syphilis as a result of the graft; because newspapers at the time did not print the word "syphilis," the reference was made to "pure" blood. After locating two possible donors, Nelden asked each to sign a written contract indemnifying the surgeon and the recipient from legal liability in case of a bad outcome. This legal formality apparently dissuaded the prospective donors, and Nelden chose to advertise. The advertisement brought 150 persons to the physician's home and hundreds of letters from people seeking to sell an ear. Once he narrowed the pool to six candidates, he selected a German man as the donor and required him to sign a written agreement reproduced at length in a metropolitan newspaper:

> This agreement, made this ___ day of November 1903 between _____ party of the first part and _____ party of the second part, and Dr. Andrew L. Nelden, party of the third part, witnesseth that for and in consideration of $1 by each party to the others in hand paid, the receipt of which is hereby acknowledged.
>
> The party of the second part hereby sells, transfers and sets over to the party of the first part all his right, title and interest in and to his ear now on the right side of his head and hereby consents to allow his said right ear to be removed and grafted on the head of the party of the first part by Dr. Andrew L. Nelden, party of the third part, in such manner and form and at such time and places as the said Dr. Nelden shall specify, and the said party of the second part hereby agrees to release and hold harmless the said party of the first part and said party of the third party from any and all damages, injury or detriment that may result to him from the said transfer, removal or grafting.
>
> And the party of the first part, in consideration of such transfer, consent and agreement hereby agrees to pay to the party of the second part $5000 at the completion of said operation, and the said party of the third part agrees to use his best ability as a surgeon to accomplish the said removal and grafting of said ear with the least possible pain or injury to the parties of the first and second part, and does promise and agree not to reveal the name or address of the party of the first or second part. [19]

The physician was reportedly disturbed when newspapers resurrected an old New York law making the severing of someone's ear a criminal offense (the crime of mayhem). Although the Manhattan District Attorney promised not to intervene in the case, Nelden decided to perform the operation in Philadelphia. According to a report in the *Philadelphia Inquirer*, the Philadelphia district attorney promised there was nothing in Pennsylvania law that would make it a criminal offense to cut off a man's ear unless it was done without consulting him about the price.[20] The operation, performed in a private hospital on November 19, 1903, required that the donor and recipient be physically linked for 12 days to ensure that blood circulation could be achieved in the grafted ear. In December, F. E. Sturdevant informed newspaper reporters that he visited the "celebrated patient" and saw his new ear. Despite the scars of the stitches which held the ear to his head and large amounts of congealed blood and pus about the area, the ear was reportedly "without blemish of any description except for the high coloring and fullness." Nelden pronounced the operation a complete success.[21]

This unusual transaction involving the sale of a body part in which a surgeon essentially mutilated a donor for the benefit of a third party provoked hilarity among newspaper writers ("Lend me your ear!" was but one of the puns the incident produced). There was little, if any, public criticism. The transaction, observed one editorialist in the *New York Times*, suggested the prevailing lack of financial security even at a time of national prosperity in the United States. The writer also noted how little cultural baggage was associated with the ear; he made reference to the absence of an American national superstition about the loss of an ear ("akin to a Chinaman's pigtail"). He also speculated about the potential of such surgeries to alter humanity. "This kind of graft is in its infancy, and that not only ears, but hands and arms and legs, bid fair in the future to be attached in like manner to alien bodies, making possible the building up of composite human frames (useful for the purposes of life, but hard to identify in the tumult of the resurrection)."[22] Given the penchant for humor, the editorial concluded with a plea that the surgeon be given a "fair hearing" (in yet another pun occasioned by the episode). Physicians offered little public comment about the sale of a human ear for surgical attachment to another man's body. Editors of the *New York Medical Journal* did publish one moral objection to the surgery. As the $5000 payment required the donor and recipient to spend 2 weeks in bed physically linked head to head (in an effort to ensure that the graft would "take"), the editors criticized the prospect of intimate physical contact between an unrelated female donor and the male recipient.[23] No one mentioned that the sale of a body part offended public morality, nor did anyone publicly object to the mutilation of a healthy body for the benefit of another.

Paying someone $5000 for the physical intimacy of being surgically joined for 12 days and then losing an ear seems bizarre. For some British and French observers, it offered one illustration of the ways in which surgical developments redrew American boundaries of corporeal commerce. In 1902, the *British Medical Journal* joked about the advertisement placed by a Chicago surgeon, seeking two individuals willing to undergo an ear "amputation" for $300. Although two willing subjects presented themselves, the surgeon received conflicting reports about the legality of such a transaction and did not perform the operation.[24] In his 1908 scientific romance, French writer Maurice Renard extended the theme of erasing the boundaries of the body explored in *The Island of Doctor Moreau*. (Indeed, Renard dedicated the book to H.G. Wells.) As a prelude to transplanting human minds into animal bodies, Renard's fictional French surgeon begins with such feats as performing an ear graft on "X, the Pickle-King, the American millionaire [who] had only one ear, and desired to have a pair. A poor devil sold him one of his for five thousand dollars."[25] By 1927, however, American newspapers reported that a French pianist paid 20,000 francs to replace his deformed finger with the healthy finger of a needy Parisian.[26]

American authors did not neglect the dramatic potential of buying and selling body parts. In 1906, the *Saturday Evening Post* featured a short story about the unfortunate outcome of a hand transplant. Written by popular attorney-author Arthur Train, "Mortmain" described surgeon Penniston Crisp, whose technical agility allows him to transgress the bounds of flesh, blood, and sinew in both animals and human beings. The surgeon could do "more things to a cat in 20 minutes than would naturally occur in the combined history of a thousand felines"; he could also "handle the hidden arteries and vessels of the body as confidently and accurately as you or I would tie a shoe string."[27] Through extensive experimentation on animals, Crisp perfects the technique for replacing lost limbs through grafting. He undertakes the case of a young aristocrat, Sir Richard Mortmain, whose hand has been badly mangled in an accident. Mortmain pays a young clerk for one of his hands; but, following the surgery, Mortmain struggles with the hand that is not his own. It is, for one thing, the hand of a lower-class man rather than an aristocrat; instead of long, sensitive, tapered fingers, the hand is thick, hairy, and blunt. Worse, the hand Mortmain receives turns out to be the hand of a murderer. The struggle with this murderous flesh is played out in the story. (In French, Mortmain is literally "dead hand.")

Train's short story was fiction, but the inspiration for the story developed out of the writer's friendship with a prominent New York surgeon, Robert Abbe. A specialist in hand surgery and other reconstructive procedures, Abbe recalled a visitor in 1893, "a well-to-do man from the West," who had lost both hands below the wrists in a fishing accident involving dynamite cartridges. "With Western energy, he had come East to see if there was not someone who could graft a new hand upon his arm." Abbe recounted that the man expressed confidence that he would be able to persuade a Territorial Governor to release a convict willing to sacrifice one of his hands. Although he declined to perform the surgery, Abbe conceded, "In view of the fact that surgeons have replaced a finger, an end of a nose, and small parts of flesh under favorable conditions, I asked myself why not a major part, such as a hand or a leg?"[28] Abbe's subsequent experiments with grafting limbs on dogs and cats helped furnish the premise for Train's short story.[29]

In 1915, "Mortmain" became the basis for a "grewsome [sic]," if well-received film in which a musician observes a researcher successfully graft the paw of one cat to another. After he loses his hand following an injury, the musician believes that this same doctor has grafted the hand of a murder suspect onto his stump. In this version, the hand surgery turns out to be a hallucination; the musician successfully discovers the true murderer.[30] In his autobiography, Train described the surreal experience of seeing a version of the film with Turkish captions in a theater in Constantinople. He was even more astonished when he realized that his story had been first plagiarized by a French novelist and then "highjacked in turn from him by a German film company" that released the movie in 1928.[31]

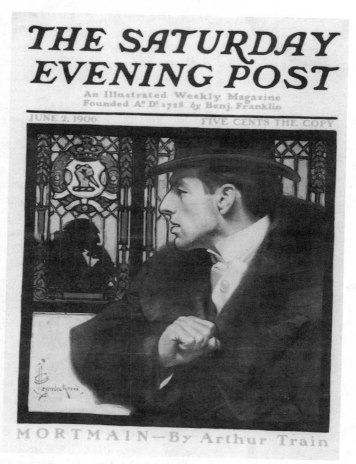

Figure 3.1 The June 1906 issue of *Saturday Evening Post* featured one of the earliest popular stories about the awful consequences of transplanting a "murderous hand" to one's body (© 1906 SEPS: Licensed by Curtis Publishing Co., Indianapolis, IN. All rights reserved. www.curtispublishing.com).

Nor was the film the only early release to use buying organs as a plot device. In the film *After His Own Heart* (1919), a young man desperate to obtain money to marry agrees to an offer of $250,000 from Dr. Spleen (!), who plans to exchange the young man's healthy heart with the aging organ that belongs to his fiancée's elderly uncle. The younger man backs out of this unholy bargain when he learns that the previous heart transplant recipients—two dogs in the surgeon's island sanitarium—died shortly after the surgery. Spleen's heart attack prevents him from carrying out this scheme. In the 1922 melodrama, *The Blind Bargain*, the surgeon, played by Lon Chaney, persuades a young man to participate in gland transplant experiments by offering him money for the surgical operation his mother needs to survive. A talented actor, Chaney also played the apish, misshapen laboratory assistant, the outcome of one of the surgeon's earlier grafting efforts.[32]

In these fictions and films, the "dark side" of transplantation refracts the corrosive power of money. It is wealth that enables Mortmain to purchase the hand of the murderer; it is money that compels a young man to undergo ape-gland grafting in order to get the funds that will save his mother's life. If his money buys Mortmain a hand, it remains an organ that comes from an individual outside his socioeconomic class (and a killer to boot!). Money makes the hand available, but class difference makes it impossible for the offending tissue to be successfully incorporated into the aristocratic body. In the other two films, the need for money leads young men to make "unholy arrangements" with surgeons corrupted by their thirst for power over nature. Despite the potent threat, each film—in true Hollywood fashion—ends with virtue triumphant. The young men are able respectively to marry a sweetheart and to procure a life-saving operation for a mother.

In fact and fiction, Americans avidly discussed the purchase of skin, flesh, bone, and organs. In the late nineteenth century, skin grafting created a new, if limited, market for individuals willing (or desperate) to sell their skin. In 1889, a Los Angeles physician placed an advertisement for eight to 10 healthy boys. Needing skin to treat a badly burned man, the doctor paid several boys 5 cents a cut for the 10 cuts he made to their arms. In 1891, Mrs. Lucy Pratt, a trained nurse at a San Francisco children's hospital and recently widowed, received $100 when she allowed surgeons to remove 45 square inches of skin to treat a badly burned railway clerk.[33] In 1903, the emergence of human skin as an "article of commerce" in New York and Philadelphia prompted one reporter, describing a case in which a surgeon paid $5 for skin to place on a badly burned child, to remark: "there is no reason why healthy men and women should not sell the article."[34]

Some enterprising individuals began to appear at clinics and hospitals, offering their skin for sale. In 1906, Thomas Morris appeared at the Department of Agriculture's Bureau of Chemistry in Washington, D.C. seeking to sell blood, skin, or a limb to Harvey Wiley—the head of the bureau and well-known in the press for his creation of the "Poison Squad," a group of young men subjected to tests of the safety of food additives. After he made a similar appeal to President Theodore Roosevelt, the unsuccessful seller was taken to the Washington Asylum Hospital. In 1907, Mrs. Mary Pasquan received a different reception when she approached surgeons at New York's Bellevue Hospital. The hospital superintendent declined her offer to purchase skin, but he advised her to try the Cornell Medical College, where such procedures were more common.[35]

Some American surgeons advised that patients undergoing surgery might be approached as potential skin donors. When F. Gregory Connell performed laparotomy (a surgery that involves opening the abdomen), he asked the patient's permission to use the skin removed during their surgery. He advised his fellow surgeons to do the same. Consent should always be secured, Connell argued, "otherwise misunderstandings with more or less annoying consequences might arise." Perhaps Connell had been influenced by the occasional reports of nonvoluntary skin donation.

In 1899, the National Society for the Prevention of Cruelty to Children intervened in a British case when a physician removed skin from the foot of an orphan in order to treat the ulcerated leg of a woman in the workhouse.[36] This may explain why physicians believed that compensation could serve a useful purpose. As Connell noted, "In case the donee be affluent and the donor the opposite, financial recompense might not be unreasonable."[37]

A small cohort of dedicated skin sellers also participated in the skin trade. In Chicago, the press reported a new industry in the treatment of burned patients. When they needed skin to treat the badly scalded abdomen of a Joliet businessman, surgeons at the city's Presbyterian Hospital called in a "professional skin seller." The seller was a young German man named John Baumann, who expressed only enthusiasm about the money he made allowing skin to be stripped from his forearms. "I like the work," he told reporters, "if you can call it work, and I intend to follow it as a regular profession as long as there is demand for good healthy skin." The pay scale was apparently better in Chicago than in New York; instead of 50 cents a square inch, Baumann received from $3 to $5 a square inch. His compensation for the skin for the Joliet man was $60 ($1230 in 2005 terms), "not so bad for 15 minutes work."[38]

Selling skin prompted little critical comment in the popular press. If anything, it struck some observers as easier to understand how money motivated donation rather than less lucrative incentives. When a young man gave up 32 square inches of skin from his thigh to aid a severely burned 7-year-old boy and refused financial compensation, "the identity and motives" of the young donor roused great curiosity among the citizens of Nutley, New Jersey. The child's doctor strove to emphasize the seriousness and extent of the donation, some 32 inches of skin, "as thick as my coat here, cutting right down to the fat."[39] The donor explained that his only motive was to save the child's life. Just why someone would be willing to undergo such rigors for a stranger puzzled not only the physician but the child's parents and neighbors.

Skin was not the only body part that could be marketed. Some of the people who wrote to Rockefeller surgeon Alexis Carrel volunteered to sacrifice body parts to other patients for financial compensation. Popular articles about Carrel's exploits led some to offer specific organs for sale. One Montana woman offered an eye to any patient "who has $25,000 and no eyes."[40] She expressed the willingness to part with an arm or hand if payment was made. Maurice Harris of Jersey City, New Jersey wrote in August, 1913 of his willingness to undergo any operation that Carrel devised for remuneration. Carrel responded to these offers, as he did to all such correspondence, by saying that such transactions were not legal.

Like Carrel, the Russian physician Serge Voronoff received offers to sell him similarly precious organs. In the 1920s, the notorious gland-grafting surgeon described how men had contacted him offering to sell their testicular material for the right price. Voronoff rejected these offers on the grounds that the amount of money required by these sellers would restrict the grafting operation to millionaires. In the United States, the Chicago surgeon Max Thorek was one of Voronoff's most committed followers. Like his mentor, he acknowledged the difficulty in getting healthy, live human donors of testicular tissue. Thorek worried that the "stress of poverty" might lead a young man to part with one or part of his sex glands in exchange for money. He was more comfortable with donations from near relatives, who wished to provide "therapeutic help," for example, a son to a father. According to his clinical cases reports, Thorek permitted one unrelated donor to supply part of his testis to a 64-year-old musician. "Evidently there was some close relationship existing between the two, the nature of which I could not ascertain," Thorek noted, "but the donor was most cheerful after having matters explained to him." [41]

The sale of testicular tissue prompted the most emphatic denunciation of a market in body parts. In 1923, the vogue of human testicular transplants prompted biologist Paul Kammerer to denounce the "despicable traffic in organs." Pointing to the corrupting power of money, the biologist also cited cases in which legal contracts were drawn up to formalize the sale of organs, as well as the reports of "gland theft" in the popular press. In 1922, for example, a young man in Chicago was "knocked unconscious and then robbed of the long-sought-for organ." [42] Amid press speculation about a wealthy man who had paid medical students to obtain the gland for his rejuvenation, a University of Chicago medical student was held in police custody. But the truth seemed even more bizarre. The young man's attackers were alleged to be Nathan Leopold and Richard Loeb, the notorious perpetrators of the "crime of the century," the less-than-perfect murder of 14-year-old Bobby Franks in 1924. In his defense of the two young men, eminent attorney Clarence Darrow argued that a disturbance in glandular secretions (and suspicions of homosexuality) mitigated their responsibility for the crime, saving them from execution. Amid the flurry of intense interest in the gland operations, including the gland surgery that tycoon Harold McCormick reluctantly conceded that he had undergone, two Illinois state representatives proposed legislation to make it a felony "to purchase, sell, give or take any gland from any living person for the purchase of transplanting such gland into any other living person." [43] Thomas C. O'Grady and Laurence C. O'Brien expressed particular concern that glands might be obtained from ex-soldiers, hungry and desperate for money, for the benefit of "a wealthy old steer." [43] This legislation lacked popular support; Chicago ministers opposed the measure as unnecessary, as did the disabled veterans of Chicago. Not only was it wrong for the rich to purchase such material from those in need, but the poor also benefited. "There are many instances," noted one reporter, "in which the bodies of the very rich have been used for experiments which turned out to the advantage of many." [44] Offers from those willing to sell their glands appeared in newspapers around the country.

The sale of skin, testicular material, and other tissue largely subsided by the 1930s. One enterprising New York plastic surgeon announced the opening of a "grafting donors' bureau," which registered 15 people willing to sell cartilage from their ears or ribs for money. These tissues would be used to reconstruct "bashed-in noses," and the surgeon held out the possibility of selling and transplanting whole ears or sections of skin. [45] The isolation of testosterone and estrogen by endocrinologists in the 1930s rendered testicular transplantation unnecessary (the procedure had also lost its medical currency among surgeons). The market in human blood, however, continued its vitality.

Easy Money

Before the twentieth century, human blood had only limited monetary value. In a handful of cases, doctors who needed blood to perform transfusions arranged to pay those proximate to the emergency and willing to supply blood. In February 1883, when physicians were called in to treat an unconscious man in a New York hotel, they ordered a blood transfusion. The only person apparently willing to give the 8–10 ounces of blood was Edward Banks, a "colored porter" at the hotel, who was persuaded to participate at a rate of 10 cents a drop. After the transfusion, the patient recovered with the porter's assistance. At the end of his stay, the man gave Banks only $5 to discharge his debt. The porter brought a lawsuit against the blood recipient, arguing that the blood he provided was worth $192 (at 10 cents a drop). Blood, as one physician argued at the trial, "had no commercial value, but in this case, as given to save life" that it should be considered valuable.[46] Banks prevailed in his lawsuit; the judge awarded him $197.90 and $12 in court costs.[47] Reports of blood sales appeared in the press. In 1899, when a young man in San Francisco "made desperate by hunger" advertised his willingness to sell his body to a physician for scientific purposes, a physician reportedly offered him $200 "to submit to the operation of transfusion."[48]

The advent of surgical transfusion in the early twentieth century increased the need for and the demands on the blood donor. George W. Crile was not only among the first to perform direct surgical transfusion, but he was also among the first to introduce the practice of hiring donors as sources of blood. Crile found "the commercial attitude" difficult; his two "hired donors" proved to be "not as tractable as those who responded to the appeal of sentiment."[49] As surgeons in other American cities adopted Crile's technique for direct transfusion, they followed Crile's lead in engaging blood sellers when they too experienced difficulties in recruiting friends, family members, and other volunteers to serve as blood donors. "Securing a donor is perhaps the most frequent obstacle to the performance of transfusion," F. D. Gray, a New York surgeon complained in 1910. "Not even members of the patient's family are always willing to submit to what they fear is a painful and possibly dangerous procedure."[50]

When one of Gray's patients, an 11-year old boy with hemophilia, required a transfusion, the surgeon found no family members willing to donate. Although one of the nurses at the hospital, presumably a young, unmarried woman, volunteered to give blood, the hospital superintendent refused to permit it because her parents lived at a distance and could not be consulted. In the end, the boy received blood from the ambulance driver, who agreed to donate his blood for an undisclosed "financial consideration." When New York newspapers described in 1909 how one Bellevue Hospital physician offered $10 to a young transient at the Mills Hotel to furnish blood, the Hospital was "besieged by people who implored them to buy a pint or so of blood." Whenever a similar story appeared in the newspaper, "hundreds go thither in the course of the year for that grewsome purpose [of selling blood]." At another New York hospital, the surgeon reported a direct transfusion using "a healthy girl of twenty-three years, who was paid by the patient's friends" as the blood supplier.[51] By 1915, the *New York Sun* hailed "a new profession"—men who make a business out of selling their blood.

The financial compensation for this service varied tremendously. Some sold 15 ounces of blood for $10. In 1909, nearly 100 New York City men responded to an advertisement seeking "Healthy man, 20 to 30 years old, over 150 pounds, to give blood transfusion; reward." Some of the advertisements were placed by physicians, others by family members, like Henry Friedman, who sought blood for his ailing brother-in-law. Some "sixty men of many kinds" appeared at his doorstep offering "Irish blood, Jewish blood, German blood, native-born American blood, and several other kinds" for no less than $25 a quart. Responding to a 1913 advertisement for a "transfusion hero" to provide blood for the 16-year-old son of a Park Avenue lawyer, Joseph Wiley, a healthy 23-year-old man, provided 4 quarts of blood and received $120. The "easy money" led Wiley to offer his services as "Transfusion Expert." Worried about the dangers of his new job, his mother exclaimed: "why the next thing I know some one will be advertising for a new head and Joe'll sell his."[52]

Blood selling was not confined to New York. In Baltimore, Johns Hopkins surgeon Bertram Bernheim initially offered $100 to his earliest donors for surgical transfusion. Recruiting the mostly "homeless men from the Friendly Inn," Bernheim later halved this $50, because "most people could not afford the larger sum and anything less than $50 seemed too little."[53] Other Baltimore surgeons offered the "derelicts" from the Friendly Inn $25 for submitting to transfusions, plus $1 a day to keep themselves in good condition until they were needed.[54] In Washington, D.C., the transfusers at Emergency Hospital, Georgetown University Hospital, and Providence Hospital had many Washingtonians "on a string" who would part with a pint of blood for $25. Many of these donors were medical students or hospital staff, including one woman who sold blood for 60 transfusions, worth an estimated $3000 "including gratuities and the thank offerings dating over a period of 3 years."[55]

Paid donors offered a number of advantages. Because these men and women "were not troubled with the heroic attitude which naturally accompanies the unpaid giving of blood," their participation in the practice streamlined the procedure. Without a personal investment in the patient undergoing transfusion, they were less emotional and more experienced with what was required. This was also an advantage when relying on medical students and interns to provide blood for a fee. Already present at the scene of the medical emergency, young doctors and medical students added blood selling to participation in medical experiments as a means of earning needed cash.[56] In 1920, students and interns at the Johns Hopkins Hospital routinely sold their blood for $50–$100 a pint. One third-year medical student reportedly earned $600 for 11 transfusions, all without missing a day of class.[57] Another Hopkins intern informed a reporter that he would have preferred to donate blood free of charge to the hospital patients, but "he needed all the money he could get for his approaching wedding."[58] As an intern at the Boston City Hospital, physician Lewis Thomas recalled how he received $25 a pint for his donations, as well as the pint of whiskey stipulated by a 1937 Massachusetts law.[59] (Whiskey, of course, was essential (!) to restoring the lost blood.)

In the 1910s and 1920s, college students around the country joined medical students in selling their blood for use in patients who lacked friends and family members as donors. In 1915, when the price of 8 ounces of blood jumped from $25 to $75 in New York City, Columbia University students competed for the right to sell blood at area hospitals.[60] In 1925, Yale University posted blood selling as an occupation for students applying for jobs.[61] For many of these sellers, selling blood was a short-term occupation, an opportunity to obtain cash to tide them over until their circumstances changed, the chance to become a hero, or both. "It is the easiest way I know of making $30," explained University of Southern California student Monte Harrington in 1927, "and it gives me the feeling that not only have I earned my money, but that I have actually done a good deed."[62]

The need for a dependable stream of blood donors prompted some physicians to look to professionals to supply blood. At first physicians and hospitals placed newspaper advertisements for blood donors. Advertising proved impractical because blood was generally needed on short notice, the demand was unpredictable, and reliable methods of storage were lacking. Physicians and hospitals responded by setting up their own networks of paid donors who could be called on short notice for blood donation. By the 1920s, professional donors began to organize their services, especially in New York City, with its large concentration of hospitals and surgeons. Enterprising individuals opened agencies or bureaus that supplied donors to participating hospitals in exchange for a percentage of the compensation received by the donor. In 1930, for example, the Mixon Blood-Donor Agency in New York City maintained a roster of over 300 donors. The agency maintained a minimum of 12 men on call at its office at all times, "some of whom eat and sleep there, having no other home since the depression."[63] Some professional donors even specialized; Thomas Kane, a one-time sailor and "champion blood donor," received $40 to $100 per quart for providing blood solely to women and children.[64]

The majority of blood sellers were men, preferably in robust physical condition and seemingly free of infectious disease. In the case of direct transfusion, American surgeons preferred to perform the cut down and exposure of an artery on men, because as one transfuser remarked, "one disliked the idea of making an incision in the wrist of a woman."[65] Preference for male donors continued with the advent of indirect transfusion. The physical differences between men and women, some transfusers noted, made it easier to use men as donors. Even though women were considered more likely to volunteer as donors, the larger and more accessible veins of men, as well as lesser amounts of subcutaneous fat, decreased the technical demands on the physician.[66] Moreover, research into the health effects of blood donation on the donor suggested that women donors were slower to recover cell volume and hemoglobin levels after donations and more likely to develop anemia after serving as a donor. At the Mayo Clinic, which employed some professional women donors, physicians speculated that more than biology was involved in the tendency of women to develop anemia from transfusion: "the diet of men, including as it does a larger amount of meat, is more effective in blood regeneration, and the work and habits of women are not conducive to blood regeneration."[67] Some physicians complained that using women as donors was less efficient, as the women couldn't get dressed and on their way as fast as men, nor were they as steady in the operating room, where squeamishness hindered both the procedure and the donor's recovery.

Many of these blood sellers no doubt lived in hope of generous gifts from grateful recipients and their families. Even doctors reaped the benefits of appreciation from wealthy patients. When the ambulance surgeon from Mary Immaculate Hospital in Ridgewood, New Jersey supplied blood to a man suffering from acute anemia, the physician received an automobile from the grateful man.[68] In 1923, the press reported the largesse of the Italian tenor Enrico Caruso to his professional blood seller. Three years earlier, Caruso was performing the role of Elazar at the Metropolitan Opera House in New York City, when he collapsed. The press issued daily reports of the tenor's medical care in the penthouse suite of New York's Vanderbilt Hotel. Caruso received two blood transfusions from Harry Fenstad, who received $500 for his services. When Caruso recovered from the transfusion, the tenor was reportedly outraged to learn that his "professional benefactor" had received such a trifling sum. "Only $500 for two pints of blood! The blood of a man is worth more than that. It is worth $750 a pint at least." Caruso instructed his business manager to pay his surprised donor an additional $1000, the most generous compensation he had ever received.[69] Fenstad's story of Caruso's generosity (or self-valuation) appeared in the newspapers when the apartment house superintendent was arrested for being drunk and disorderly in a New York tavern.[70] At his arraignment, Fenstad claimed that alcohol was essential to his blood regeneration. This report, in turn, provoked criticism from his professional brethren, who charged that Fenstad was no professional. "True professionals" were the men who devoted themselves to producing a quality product for sale. Fenstad was released, as was another blood donor, Vito Panarella, in 1929, whose "weakness due to having given a quart of blood in a transfusion caused him to lose his temper." Despite upbraiding a policeman and resisting arrest, Panarella received a suspended sentence.[71]

Harry Fenstad was happy to benefit from Caruso's generosity. Other blood sellers were less than pleased with the compensation they received. In 1911, one Chicago woman sued the estate of her late employer for $20,000, when she became "greatly enfeebled" after supplying blood to a rich widow; she settled for $1000.[72] After the death of Ethelbert W. Peck in Chicago in 1916, blood supplier E. B. Fisher pursued a claim against his estate in Probate court. Fisher claimed that he had supplied some 16 ounces of blood to the dying man, for which he received no payment. Claiming injury and discomfort as a result of this supply, Fisher presented an itemized list of charges for the blood:

For painful suffering and injuries $5000

Loss of time from business 600

Services rendered 200

Total $5800

The *Chicago Daily Tribune* labeled this haggling over blood money "repulsive." Dispute over a similar deathbed donation ended up in a San Francisco courtroom when Mrs. G. P. Hilliard died after receiving blood from Leona Standiford. Although she was assured that she would be well paid, she sued when the woman's husband paid her only $35 for her services. Like Fisher, Standiford claimed that she experienced shock and illness from the transfusion process. In 1923, she successfully sued the Hilliard estate for $2500.[73]

Feeling Like Shylock

How did the exchange of money influence transfusion? It seems clear that for some Americans, trading in blood seemed problematic. In a 1911 editorial, the *Los Angeles Times* noted the success of transfusion in modern medicine and the willingness of near relatives and friends to serve as blood donors, but expressed reservations about the prospect of buying blood. "If, however, the selling of one's blood for such a purpose shall ever become a business matter of bargain and sale, a new and uncertain factor may enter into the question." Little more than a decade later, another reporter noted that blood selling had its dark side: "A donor must feel pretty much like a Shylock the first time he sells his blood. It would be heroic to give it—that would be sacrifice—but selling it—how could that ever be?"[74] If the allusion to Shylock, Shakespeare's Jewish merchant who demands a pound of flesh from his debtor, offered blood selling a classic pedigree, it also colored the practice as sordid, ruthless, and un-Christian. The shame that some people associated with blood selling may have encouraged others to conceal their participation. Science writer Herbert Harlan described the dilemma for college and medical students who served as frequent blood retailers: "How will they explain that little scar on the arm to their parents? Perhaps it will not be noticed. If it is, it may be interpreted as the result of an accident. Some may even be brave enough to tell just where they got it."[75]

Some Americans worried that putting a price on human blood would make it unavailable to the poor and working class. Concern about "profiteering in blood" led women medical students at New York's Flower Hospital to furnish blood to patients free of charge when prices for blood rose too high in 1920. When some blood sellers demanded more money, the press offered harsh criticism in the press: "Even in dire extremity, however, there are limits to the extent to which the public allows itself to be stung, and an impasse was reached, the patients refusing to comply with what they considered to be an exorbitant demand and the life savers declining to be tapped for less consideration."[76] At the University of California Hospital in San Francisco, the hospital director noted the urgent need for funds to provide blood for indigent patients. Although the professional donors received $50, it was often left to the physicians to find money to cover these expenses.[77] One response to the concern for the poor was to form blood benevolent societies to ensure that no one would go untransfused if they lacked the money to pay a donor. In St. Louis, for example, a window washer organized the Blood Donors Benevolent Association;

by 1935, the organization boasted 110 members—housewives, janitors, truck drivers, clerks, shoemakers, and mechanics. The association, according to one newspaper report, was especially "proud because few of its members are from the white-collar class."[78] Thus, working-class Americans could participate in the philanthropy of the body.

Altruistic blood donation prompted media attention. Reporters praised the "everyday heroism" of those who gave skin or blood without compensation to save the health of an injured or dying person: "splendid proof that the world is full of kindness and unselfish affection, and that no sacrifice stands in the way of duty to those in distress."[79] This everyday heroism was sometimes rewarded; after he had given blood without compensation to a dying Colorado man, "Blind Charley," a San Diego newspaper seller, learned that he had received $15,000 from the dead man's estate.[80]

Some people regarded the willingness to donate blood without compensation as a sign of moral worthiness. When the man who donated blood to her husband and "afterward refused to accept any remuneration for the sacrifice" was indicted for theft, Mrs. Norbert Gunsberger appeared before the magistrate to make a plea for leniency. "I cannot believe that this young man can be guilty of burglary," she insisted, "after doing such a thing [as giving blood]."[81] Some donors were lionized in the American press for their refusals to accept money for their frequent, life-giving donations. The former vaudeville showman Edward "Spike" Howard of Philadelphia appeared in the popular press for his extravagant blood donation. Once able to break iron chains with his chest, editors of the new photo-weekly *Life* noted, "his greater claim to fame" was his status as the world's most generous donor. In February 1938, Howard made his 871st donation of blood: "Because he thinks there is something sacred about blood," *Life* noted, "Howard has never accepted payment, and has passed up more than $22,000 in fees."[82]

The female equivalent of Spike Howard was Rose McMullin, a Philadelphia woman variously hailed as the "champion woman blood donor in the United States" and the "lady with the golden blood." McMullin began appearing in newspapers in 1940, as the number of donations she gave increased. McMullin's blood was called "golden" because it had been modified when she received a preparation of *Staphylococcus aureus*, made from the infected blood of her 3-year-old niece. In September 1935, as her niece's grave condition worsened, physicians at Hahnemann Hospital in Philadelphia suggested using a heat-killed preparation of the child's blood as a last-ditch measure. McMullin and her brother-in-law, the child's father, received four subcutaneous injections of the preparation. Each later provided this now-modified blood for transfusion to the child, who made a complete recovery.[83]

McMullin credited Rose Marie's recovery to her "golden" (from *aureus*) blood, and she began to respond to appeals from the families of sick children and adults for more of her therapeutic blood. In 1937, she traveled to the home of a child dying of a similar staph infection in Pennsylvania, and she provided blood for a Chicago dentist and a young Manhattan mother. By April 1940, she had reportedly given blood for more than 300 transfusions. At first, her donations were limited to

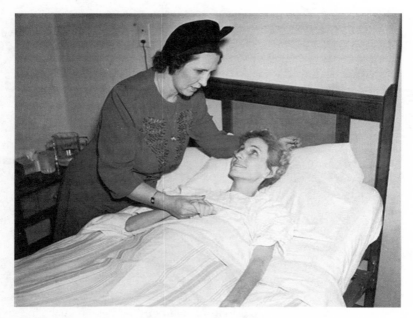

Figure 3.2 "The Lady of the Golden Blood," Mrs. Rose McMullin comforts Mrs. Hazel Farmer at the American Hospital in Chicago, Dec. 4, 1940, shortly before she gives the ailing woman a half-pint of her blood (AP Images).

individuals with the same condition as her niece. But when she received appeals from families of children with leukemia, she also responded to these and to other requests. Some of the recipients were famous, including the son of Brigadier General William (Billy) Mitchell, who succumbed to leukemia despite having received two transfusions from McMullin.[84] Although many of the recipients were less well known, her arrivals and departures made newspaper headlines across the country. She appeared several times on the radio program *We the People*, where she also received gold medals from the American Legion for her life-giving services. Throughout her career as a blood donor, Mrs. McMullin claimed that she never accepted money for her blood. Although she did accept (and require) money for travel expenses, she explained "I don't want to make money out of human misery." [85]

The American Medical Association (AMA) grew increasingly skeptical about the "golden lady's" altruism when they began receiving inquiries from physicians. These doctors sought information about the qualities of her blood and the nature of her services. In October 1940, Max Wintrobe, then a junior physician at the Johns Hopkins Hospital in Baltimore, complained to the AMA about the "Golden Girl's" claim that her blood could cure leukemia. (Parents of children with leukemia wrote to the AMA and to the American College of Surgeons asking for information about

McMullin's blood as a treatment for leukemia.) Wintrobe challenged her claims about refusing money for her blood. Although the mother of his patient was informed that there were would be no charge for blood for her child, McMulllin asked the woman for $500 for travel expenses to Baltimore. In another case, she asked for $300 for the trip from Philadelphia to Newark, New Jersey. Other physicians similarly complained about the travel expenses requested by the Lady with the Golden Blood. As one Alabama physician noted, her expenses "would make our national debt pale into pauper figures."[86] Several physicians also expressed concern about McMullin's practice of using the names of the physicians, whose patients received her blood, as testimonials to the value of her blood. In February 1941, Morris Fishbein, the powerful editor of the AMA's journal, published a column critical of her claims and billing practices. When McMullin came to Chicago in March, she refuted the accusations that her blood was not effective in treating staph, strep, and other conditions. She challenged their claims that her charges for expenses were excessive.

Another problem associated with paying for life by the pint was its linkage with illicit sex and sexually transmitted disease. Charles Nemo, a professional donor in New York City, explicitly linked blood selling and prostitution in a compelling 1934 magazine article. Readers of the *American Mercury* learned how Nemo, down on his luck, took up residence in a Brooklyn boarding house operated by a former professional blood donor and inhabited by other members of "the blood-selling fraternity."[87] Not only did the proprietor remind him of a "retired harlot" but the boarding house "resembled an old-time whore-house. Instead of selling our bodies, we sold blood."[88] When he was sent on a call to the County Hospital, Nemo described how the two young interns assigned to perform the transfusion procedure questioned him minutely about the number of transfusions he had given, his usual occupation, and the reasons that led him to sell blood, "evincing all the unhealthy curiosity of a young novice about to embark on his adventure with a prostitute." These two inexperienced doctors bungled his bloodletting; Nemo sat up to discover the sheets "a scarlet welter" and his arm a "mass of punctures from shoulder to wrist." Even worse, the hospital, in a cost-saving measure, had ceased to provide donors with several ounces of "prescription whiskey." As a "tacit apology for the orgy of carving" he endured, the interns shared their own whiskey bottle with him. After changes in donor management reduced compensation to blood sellers, Nemo quit the business, even as he saw "new blood" being recruited for the trade.

Few blood sellers would have welcomed Nemo's linkage of blood money with prostitution. The association of their services, mediated by physicians and intended to restore health and life, was degraded by this association with illicit sexuality, lust, and sin. Prostitution served a similarly degrading function when it was deployed to disparage those individuals who served as research subjects for money rather than for altruistic purposes. In his sensationally popular book *Microbe Hunters* (1926), author Paul de Kruif distinguished between the "mercenary" and "money-loving" Spanish immigrants, "hardly more intelligent than animals," who received money to participate in Walter Reed's yellow fever experiments in Havana, and the American soldier volunteers, who reportedly refused to accept payment for sleeping in bed linens stained by the body fluids of men dead from yellow fever or by exposing themselves to infected mosquitoes.[89] In 1934, when playwright Sidney Coe Howard's *Yellow Jack* debuted on Broadway, his play, written in conjunction with de Kruif, invoked prostitution to ennoble the heroic American volunteers. "Did you refuse compensation, like the two of us," demands the character Sergeant O'Hara, "or are you selling your bodies like a couple of whores?"[90] The two American soldiers who accept money are no heroes—one is a frightened, immature boy, the other is a Jewish Communist, who rejects the role of "bourgeois hero" and takes the money "for the wherewithal to further the radical movement."[91]

Invoking prostitution in the context of blood selling raised the specter of sexually transmitted disease, especially syphilis. Even before Nemo's exposé, concerns about professional donors "too often recruited from the less responsible elements of the community" prompted calls for greater control over the safety of the blood supply.[92] The "less responsible" members of the community presumably included men with low moral standards. But the system itself encouraged the over-frequent donation of blood. In some cases, doctors complained that the donor was in greater need of the transfusion than the purported recipient. One solution was the formation, in 1929, of the Blood Transfusion Betterment Association (BTBA).[93] Based in New York City and advised by a distinguished panel of medical experts (including Karl Landsteiner, who received the Nobel Prize in 1930 for his work on blood groups), the association guided the formulation of a new set of sanitary code regulations for professional blood donors in New York City.

In November 1930, the New York City Department of Health, working in cooperation with the BTBA, adopted new regulations to govern the activity of commercial blood agencies. Each individual who received a fee for blood was compelled to undergo a physical examination by certified physicians. His blood was typed, a Wassermann and Kahn test (for syphilis) performed, along with a determination of the hemoglobin content.[94] The Health Department "followed the modern passport book, even to the photograph of the legitimate holder."[95] This passbook, carried at all times, recorded examinations, donations, and other information. The Association also required donors to sign a form absolving the hospital from any liability as a result of injury from donating blood.

One consequence of these new sanitary regulations was a decline in income for professional donors. To support its activities and research, the Association reduced the usual compensation for blood donation from $50 to $35 (based on a rate of $7 per 100 cc). New restrictions on time between donations also reduced compensation. In an effort to protect the health of the blood supplier from over-frequent depletion, he was required to refrain from donating 1 week for every 100 cc of blood supplied. The sellers also had to maintain a minimum hemoglobin reading of 85% (to supply oxygen-carrying blood to recipients). Dissatisfaction with the new regime of oversight and reduced earnings led blood sellers to organize. In 1938, they obtained an official charter from the AFL. Charles Vonie, regional organizer of the AFL, explained that the 150 members of the blood donors union pledged to refrain from strikes and to be guided by "the best interests of society."[96]

Banking on Blood

Before the 1930s, blood for transfusion was stored in bodies not banks. Long before this, physicians and surgeons recognized that tissues and body fluids could be stored in cold temperatures to be used at a later time. In 1914, for example, Alexis Carrel reported putting arteries and other tissue into cold storage for later use.[97] During World War I, a young physician, Oswald Hope Robertson, used preserved blood in treating battlefield casualties. Robertson's efforts earned him the title of "world's first blood banker" from the American Association of Blood Banks in 1958.[98] He was an innovator in using preserved blood, but he did not introduce the idea and language of the "blood bank."

In March 1937, Bernard Fantus, a Chicago physician, organized the blood collection and distribution system at Cook County Hospital that he identified for the first time as a "bank." When he offered a preliminary report of his "blood bank," Fantus acknowledged the Russian lead in the preservation and use of cadaveric blood. Observing that cadaveric blood was "revolting to Anglo-Saxon susceptibilities," Fantus advanced what he called the "blood bank" proposition, based on simple rules and policies for obtaining blood and dispensing it within the hospital setting. "Just as one cannot draw money from a bank unless one has deposited some," he insisted, "so the blood preservation department cannot supply blood unless as much comes in as goes out. The term 'blood bank' is no mere metaphor."[99]

At the Cook County blood bank, staff physicians deposited blood for credit. Fantus initially assumed that most of this blood would come from "healthy volunteers," from those patients with high blood pressure or cardiac problems undergoing therapeutic bloodletting, and from women who had recently given birth. He also proposed that a healthy patient planning for an elective surgical procedure could place a pint of blood on deposit, which would then be available should the need arise during the surgery. "We deposit in a bank money we do not at the moment need, to be able to draw on it when we do need it." Just as a bank with surplus money might loan some to an individual, so too the blood bank might "lend" blood to those in need. Those who received a loan had a duty to repay their debt: "Any one who owes his life to blood transfusion clearly owes some blood to someone else," Fantus argued, "who is in great need of this restorative." Although he had assumed that families would deposit blood for patients, this proved unfeasible as the demand for blood increased. The Hospital then instituted a "paid donor system," in which an intern collected $10 from the patient and paid a donor sent by the Christian Men's Industrial League (which aided transients and the unemployed). As word spread, "many skid row habitués, derelicts, alcoholics came to receive payment for giving blood, and the Blood Bank flourished."[100]

One of the great advantages of the banking system, Fantus suggested, was that any healthy volunteer could supply the deposit. Even if the blood type did not match the recipient, the bank would have on hand blood of the requisite type. This would simplify the procedure at the hospital by dispensing with the response to the call for blood donors in which "a horde of excited, noisy, gesticulating foreigners" allowed their blood to be tested to see whether it would match.[101] At the blood bank, an intern taking the deposit recorded his name, the date, the donor's name and address, and the donor's "color" (race). The banker maintained an account book in which blood credits and debits could be easily seen. The account book also recorded blood that was discarded because of age (more than 10 days old) or because of a positive test for syphilis and malaria.

Fantus's blood bank proposition was speedily adopted by other hospitals. The term "bank," as two St. Louis pathologists explained, was "a particularly fortunate choice, since it is almost self-explanatory; the bank implies the keeping of accounts, the deposition and withdrawal of blood, and conveys at once the principle that an account cannot be overdrawn without penalty."[102] The blood bank capitalized on American familiarity with banking in a decade characterized by sensational bank failures. Although some 9000 American banks—big and small—failed in the 1930s, by 1937, when Fantus introduced the term, the recovery of the banking system was well underway, one outcome of Roosevelt's New Deal policies.

The association of blood with political economy had a much longer history. In the seventeenth century, English physician William Harvey's demonstration of the circulation of the blood—published in 1628—prompted parallels between the human body and blood and the body politic and money. In *Leviathan* (1651), English philosopher Thomas Hobbes described "mony" as "the Bloud [sic] of a Commonwealth," in which gold, silver, and money were "reserved for Nourishment in time to come . . . : For naturall Bloud [sic] is in like manner made of the fruits of Earth; and circulating, nourisheth by the every Member of the Body of Man."[103] The association of blood with economic forces persisted well into the nineteenth century. In 1837, the pro-slavery southern Senator John C. Calhoun similarly linked the human body and the body politic, observing "The currency of a country is to the community what the blood is to the human system. It constitutes a small part, but it circulates through every portion, and is indispensable to all the functions of life."[104]

In the late nineteenth century, California journalist Adeline Knapp offered lessons in practical economics through a "fable for grown-up boys and girls." In this fable, a sick man's corpuscles debate his continued existence. The corpuscles are determined to aid the man, but are dismayed when they are confronted by the semi-lunar valve, the aorta, and other parts of the system who demand their own share of the oxygen needed for the good of the man. "What do all these fellows," asks a newly transfused "foreign" corpuscle of a "native" corpuscle, "want of so much oxygen? If the other corpuscles pay it over at the same rate I have, some one must get a good deal more than he can possibly use." The native explains:

Why . . . it is the great medium of exchange in the organism, and of course we all want as much as we can get. They re-invest it, turn it over, double it and quadruple it.

But is there more in the organism on that account?

No, but they have more, don't you see?

The new corpuscle soon learns that the richest corpuscles in the liver have great influence with the organism and would not permit interference. These richer corpuscles do not permit some of the cells to work, but these now poor cells are "supported by charitably disposed corpuscles who have been blessed by Providence with plenty." In an unsubtle stroke, the sick man succumbs to fatty degeneration of the liver, the result of those high-living, greedy corpuscles.[105] Knapp's lesson in practical economics may have mystified more than enlightened late nineteenth-century Americans. But they would have recognized the associations between currency and blood, and their respective circulation through the body politic and through the body.

Even before the introduction of blood banking, some American physicians employed monetary metaphors when discussing the movement of blood between bodies. Attempting to explain why direct transfusions sometimes failed, New York physician A.L. Soresi noted the possibility that the morphologic agents in the blood of the donor and recipient did not mix well. To make this point, he compared the blood of the donor to currency: "if bills were presented in a land where people did not appreciate their value, a person could not buy a loaf of bread with even a thousand dollars. Unless the value of the blood of the donor is 'appreciated' by the new organism, it will not only not be of any help to it, but become an element of danger."

Such associations may have explained the cogency of banking in blood.[106]

Accounting for Blood

After 1937, hospitals around the United States began organizing their blood repositories along the banking lines suggested by Fantus. In 1938, the surgical staff of the Philadelphia General Hospital opened its own "central repository" for blood, which they, following Fantus, renamed a "blood bank." The Philadelphia surgeons had made a preliminary experiment using cadaveric blood, along the lines established by the Russians. But the preference for "live blood" returned them to the blood bank. Surgeons Charles Cameron and L. Kraeer Ferguson extended the metaphor of banking in their description of the blood service; they identified the "vault" of their bank as "an ordinary electrical refrigerator" in which flasks of blood were stored. They maintained a "reserve" of 40 flasks of blood of different types for the 40 or so transfusions performed weekly at the 2700-bed hospital. The bankers maintained a visual index file so that "bank assets" could be seen at a glance. Withdrawals of blood were recorded in red ink, the blood bank ledger balanced monthly, and "interns owing blood requested to make up their indebtedness."[107]

Like the Philadelphia physicians, surgeons at Johns Hopkins Hospital (blood bank opened in March 1939) and physicians at the John Gaston Hospital in Memphis (blood bank opened April 1938) adapted the language of finance to their blood systems. Physician Lemuel Diggs described how the "capital" of the Memphis blood bank was nearly lost when the refrigerator where blood was kept failed, and the blood discarded. At the Hopkins blood bank, surgeon Mark Ravitch maintained a "bank board," which had a card for each bottle of blood on hand in the various ABO blood groups. The donors were also identified in a ledger and supplied a page of the record of blood on hand from the "small book" issued to each of the hospital services (surgical, obstetric, gynecologic, orthopedic, and otolaryngologic).

The principle of banking biologic materials quickly circulated among members of the medical community. In 1938, Philadelphia physicians floated the idea of an "eye bank," in which corneas taken from the newly dead could be maintained "similar to the method used in preserving blood for transfusion."[108] In 1944, 19 hospitals created the "world's first eye bank."[109] In 1943, a "skin bank" at the Eastern State Penitentiary furnished skin from a 23-year-old convicted robber to a severely burned boy. In 1950, as the nation prepared for an atomic attack on an American city, the *Los Angeles Times* reported the Navy's plan to create "live skin banks" for large-scale grafting in case of nuclear war.[110]

Another biologic material banked for future use was sperm for artificial insemination. In some of the earliest publicized cases of "ghost fathers," physicians obtained semen from professional blood donors, who were paid the conventional fee. In 1938, Georgetown University physician Ivy Albert Pelzman announced the creation of male "gene register," containing the names of football players and medical students who would serve as "synthetic fathers" for childless couples.[111] The register, explained one Washington reporter, was similar to the registries of professional blood donors kept by hospitals, but "eventually it may be possible to develop the method to the point where 'gene banks' can be established at hospitals similar to the blood bank at Gallinger Hospital."[112] References to gene banks allowed the newspapers to avoid mention of human sperm or sperm banks, or what the Georgetown University priests privately labeled "semen clinics."[113]

Although human milk had been collected and sold since the early twentieth century, the pediatricians who organized these services initially used words like milk bureau or milk stations to describe their operations. In 1923, when New York pediatrician Henry Dwight Chapin praised "the possibilities of the human breast under proper control" for decreasing infant mortality, he used the word "dairy" rather than "bank" to describe the collection and supply of breast milk. The metaphorical linkage between human breasts "under proper control" and the udders of cows and goats was not unique to Chapin.[114] Other descriptions of "human dairies" included references to credit, collection, the cost per ounce, and the income women received, but they did not encompass the financial language of lending, penalty, and withdrawal that characterized banking blood. After the successful launch of the blood bank in 1937, human breast milk programs came to be described as "milk banks." [115]

Blood behind Bars

Compensating blood suppliers for their vital fluid became the rule rather than the exception. Not all compensation was financial. Thousands of pints of blood came from American prisons, both state and federal. In 1941, the Central Howard Association in Chicago, an organization formed to rehabilitate prisoners, proposed a Prisoners' Blood Bank for Defense, drawing on the 165,000 inmates of American penal and correctional institutions. By October 7, 1945, some 71,350 felons had donated more than 100,000 pints of blood.[116] The men and women who donated blood to the Prisoner's Blood Bank received an honor certificate for their patriotic service. Prisoners also played a crucial role in wartime blood research; they participated in trials of various blood substitutes, including Harvard biochemist Edwin Cohn's bovine blood trials in Massachusetts (where one prisoner died as a result of his participation). [117] Blood donation, just as serving as a research subject, gave prisoners the opportunity to "pay" for their debts and those of their fellow prisoners, like the inmates of the Connecticut State Prison in Wethersfield, who, in 1947, not only repaid the "debt of blood" owed by a fellow inmate, but also donated 2 additional pints to be used for cancer patients.[118]

Compensating prisoners for their blood was similar to the practice adopted in some cities and towns whereby officials gave individuals the option of paying their fines in money or blood. In 1940, a Chicago judge ordered Thomas Donohue to contribute blood to the blood bank at Cook County Hospital in lieu of the alimony he owed his wife. (His wife did not welcome his "alcoholic transfusions.")[119] In December 1941, in the wake of the Japanese attack on Pearl Harbor, the mayor of Honolulu ordered that traffic violators donate a pint of blood in lieu of the usual fine. During the Korean conflict, a Long Island, New York judge not only required blood donations for traffic violations, but also required that vagrants and others "brought before the court on drunkenness charges" donate blood.[120] In Worcester, Massachusetts, sightseeing motorists attempting to view the damage from a 1953 tornado learned that "a pint of blood is your admission fee down here." After donating the blood at the local Veterans Administration Hospital, the so-called "tourists" were escorted out of the stricken area.[121] In October 1973, a Lexington, Kentucky judge offered "speeders, reckless drivers and those who have run through a stop sign or a red light" the option of giving a pint of blood or paying a fine and court costs. In the first week, 15 of the 190 traffic violators in Fayette County chose to give blood.[122]

The blood of prisoners continued to play an important role in the American blood system. Without the wartime incentive, prisoners received a variety of inducements, including small sums of cash ($4–$5 per unit), an explicit reduction of their sentence, or an implicit advantage at parole hearings. In the 1950s, prisoners in the Virginia state penitentiary received days off their sentence for each pint of blood donated. Even in those prisons that insisted that blood donation would not affect release, parole boards did take blood donation into consideration when evaluating early release for felons. In 1965, the Massachusetts legislature passed a law whereby a prisoner sentenced to imprisonment for 30 days or more could have his sentence reduced by 5 days for each pint of blood donated.[123] Prisons in South Carolina, Mississippi, and Virginia offered a similar reduction of 5 days for each pint of blood donated.

In the 1960s, the safety of prison blood became an issue for some transfusionists. Stanford University professor of surgery Garrott Allen warned that prison populations had a higher incidence of narcotic drug users and higher rates of hepatitis. For some blood bankers, this raised the issue of liability if a recipient developed hepatitis. The editors of *Transfusion* cautioned about the use of blood from prisoners: "blood banks should consider whether hepatitis might not be more prevalent amongst a prisoner population, and whether adequate measures may be taken to eliminate persons who are potential carriers." Prisoners, the journal warned, were more likely to be drug users and more likely to conceal this information if they received remuneration for blood.[124]

One outcome of the reliance on paid donors was debate over the status of blood. Was it a commodity to be bought, sold, and taxed? Was it a gift of the body that transcended the commercial fetish of American consumer society? Would putting a price on blood reduce social investment in blood donation? Who should set the price for blood donation? The United States Congress offered some guidance to the question about price. In 1926, for example, Congress ratified a payment scale in legislation that set a price "not exceeding fifty dollars to persons in Government service submitting to transfusion."[125] But in 1933, the U.S. Comptroller General ruled that giving blood was a personal service rather than the sale of a commodity; therefore, the standard government price for blood was reduced 75 cents for 100 cc of blood (from \$5 to \$4.25).[126] During World War II, Congress considered legislation that authorized the Price Administrator to offer "meat- and fat-ration tokens, shoe-ration coupons, and sugar-ration coupons" to Americans who donated blood for use of the armed forces. Referred to the Senate committee on Banking and Currency, Senator Langer's bill (S-1262) did not pass.[127]

State and local governments sent different messages. In 1941, for example, the Colorado state treasurer's office declared that blood removed from the body, typed, and stored, would be subjected to taxation when it was purchased or sold. By order of the Colorado legislature, however, blood passed directly from donor to recipient was not taxed. Three decades later, the Louisiana State Revenue Department ruled that blood, as a living human tissue that, when taken from the body, could be seen, weighed, measured, felt, and touched, was "tangible personal property" and therefore subject to the Louisiana Sales Tax Law.[128]

One arena in which these issues were debated was whether giving blood should be regarded as a charitable gift for income tax purposes. In 1948, at the final Plenary Session of the American Red Cross Convention, the delegates entertained a resolution asking that Federal law be amended to allow a deduction for "income tax purposes the fair value of blood so donated to the American Red Cross."[129] One observer described the tenseness of the audience, the almost universal opposition to the resolution, and the handful of delegates who voted for it. The issue was an important one for the Red Cross because it touched on the crucial matter about donor motivation. Before the American entry into World War II, and during the war years, patriotic appeals to citizens brought large numbers of donations. But the war was over, and the National Blood Program required an ongoing supply of blood donors for the program's success. What incentives, if any, would ensure the blood supply?

Officials at the national headquarters of the American Red Cross continued to confront the issue of the income tax deduction in the 1950s and 1960s. "I am surprised at the number of people who have inquired of me," wrote the chairman of the Hartford, Connecticut Red Cross Chapter, "whether the donation of blood could be treated as a charitable deduction on the individual income taxes." Although he conceded that the Treasury Department would resist such a measure, the chair explained that many members believed that "every form of stimulation" to obtain the necessary blood would be welcome. In 1951, the medical staff at the Veteran Administration Hospital in St. Louis raised the question of a $25 deduction for each pint of blood donated to the Red Cross, taking the question to the St. Louis office of the Internal Revenue Service (IRS) for a response. (The local collector was not certain it was a valid deduction.) When similar inquiries came from South Carolina and Los Angeles, Red Cross attorney Howard J. Hughes approached the IRS for a ruling and was informed that, in May 1943, the Internal Revenue Bureau had ruled that "such a blood donation does not constitute an allowable deduction as a charitable gift under the Internal Revenue Code." In 1953, members of the American Legion in San Francisco sought the help of the American Red Cross when they tried to challenge the ruling with the help of a member of the Bar of the Tax Court of the United States. In this case, the Red Cross looked to the AMA's Committee on Blood for guidance. The AMA Committee Chair rejected the idea of a tax deduction: "permitting a deduction from income taxes for donations of blood would place a commercial, monetary value upon this donation." [130] In the 1950s, congressmen from Delaware and Missouri pressed the Red Cross about offering a bill to allow charitable deductions for blood donated. Representative Thomas B. Curtis endorsed the zeal with which one of his constituents made the case for allowing a tax deduction on blood.

> Why does the fact that an operation must be performed on the donor before his blood can be given render his blood gift any more a personal service than a manuscript gift, representing the literary efforts of the donor? If Ernest Hemingway had given the manuscript of his Pulitzer Prize winning "Old Man and the Sea," the product of his brain to charity, why would it be any the less a personal service than Mr. Powers' gift to the Red Cross of his blood, the product of his body?

Curtis continued to offer the Red Cross the opportunity to revisit the issue of a tax deduction for blood gifts. In the Senate, Lister Hill received requests from his constituents to sponsor a bill to allow a tax deduction of $25 per pint of blood, not to exceed $100 in any year, as a stimulus to blood drives. In 1961, Congressman Walter L. McVey (Kansas) introduced H.R. 6416, a Bill to amend the Internal Revenue Code of 1954 to provide that blood donations be considered as charitable contributions deductible from gross income. Unlike previous efforts, McVey sought to value the pint of blood at $50, with a maximum total deduction of $200 per year. In 1962, the House Ways and Means Committee entertained additional bills calling for the amendment of the tax code to permit charitable deductions for blood in order to stimulate greater donor interest in the national blood program.

The contest over blood's status as a commodity or gift received a mixed hearing in American courts. In 1954, for example, a New York court held that moving blood between bodies for transfusion represented a service, rather than the sale of blood. In Florida, the courts ruled that transfer of blood from a blood bank to a hospital was a sale (although not subject to the rule of strict liability for a faulty product). In 1967, a New Jersey court ruled that the transfer of blood between patient and doctor, blood bank and hospital, or hospital and physician represented a sale of blood. Three years later, a New York court argued that public need for blood made it necessary to exempt blood infected with hepatitis from the legal doctrine of breach of warranty of merchantability. Legislatures increasingly weighed in on this issue; by January 1970, 28 American states had passed laws that defined the movement of blood for transfusion as a medical service, not a sale. By 1975, another 15 states had adopted this approach.[131] At the federal level, the Internal Revenue Service similarly ruled that providing blood was a service, not the sale of a product, when it charged a New Orleans woman, Dorothy Garber, with tax evasion. Garber's blood contained an antigen so rare that a commercial company paid her $25,000, 1000 shares of stock, the use of an automobile, and an additional $200 per week for supplies of her blood. Although Garber claimed that she provided a product (which was taxed differently), the IRS rejected this argument, contending that the money she received for providing the blood was taxable income.

The Gift Relationship

In 1970, a British professor of social policy roiled the American blood establishment with his analysis of blood safety, altruism, and paid donation. In *The Gift Relationship*, Richard Titmuss compared the safety and sufficiency of the blood programs of Britain and the United States as part of a far-reaching critique of paid blood donation. In response to proposals for market-based blood collection from the Institute of Economic Affairs, "an ideological repository of Thatcherism," Titmuss spent seven years collecting materials on the collection, processing, distribution, pricing, and transfusion to advance his argument that the profit motive contaminated health care in general and the blood system in particular.[132] Because the United States relied almost exclusively on people paid either in cash or in some other form of credit (time off, vacation days, other incentives), Titmuss argued, that the American blood supply was inefficient, wasteful, unsafe, and expensive. Moreover, he insisted, the American model threatened more than Americans; the commercialization of the blood system fostered "the immeasureable effects of exporting as models to economically poorer countries the values and methods of commercialized blood markets; the cumulative effects of maximizing profits in hospitals in one country on the international distribution of doctors and nurses."[133]

Titmuss's critique ignored many factors, as science journalist Douglass Starr notes. Still, his book generated scores of exposés in which skid-row denizens, often sick and drunken, sold their blood. Newspaper columnist Ann Landers explained in a response to one reader that people who were paid for their blood were "sometimes boozers and junkies who are desperate for a fast dollar." Supporting the idea of voluntary, unpaid donation, Landers concluded her column noting "the more voluntary donors, the less need to buy blood from addicts who are the greatest hepatitis spreaders of all." In January 1972, the *National Observer* reported on several investigations of commercial blood banks and their lax practices. In his article "Blood That Kills," journalist August Gribben described how patients in American hospitals were unaware that they received "cheap, possibly contaminated blood from skid-row addicts and bums." This blood, along with the blood of prisoners and blood from "impoverished, medically backward Haiti," carried the threat of serum hepatitis.[134]

In the wake of these scandals and the lawsuits against commercial blood banks, President Richard Nixon declared blood "a unique national resource," the collection of which required extensive overhaul by the Department of Health, Education and Welfare (DHEW).[135] Elliot Richardson, HEW Secretary, ordered that supervision of the blood banks be moved from the Division of Biologics Standards to the Food and Drug Administration (FDA). One of the reforms adopted by the FDA in May 1978 was the requirement for new labels on all shipments of blood and blood components that indicated whether the supplier was a "paid donor" or a "volunteer donor."[136] The market for whole blood in the United States dried up. By 1976, less than 3% of all whole blood collected in the United States came from paid suppliers. At the same time, paid suppliers furnished 70% of the plasma collected in the United States.

Plasma (the liquid portion of the blood after the red blood cells have been removed) provided a range of therapeutic products, including albumin used in the treatment of shock, clotting factors (for hemophiliacs), and the gamma globulins used to prevent hepatitis, measles, mumps, rabies, tetanus, whooping cough, and Rh disease in newborns. The U.S. plasma industry not only furnished plasma products for American consumers and patients, but also supplied the majority of the plasma products used worldwide. By 1997, over 400 plasma collection centers operated in the United States in some 200 American cities. These centers offered compensation ranging from $9 to $20 to plasma donors, and collected some 35,000 units of plasma daily, accounting for $4 billion of the $7 billion worldwide sales in blood products. The for-profit plasma centers typically located in two areas: "downtown or ghetto neighborhoods" that attracted unemployed and underclass individuals or "college towns," which attracted students. Sociologists who have studied the paid plasma donors of the 1980s and 1990s have called attention to the remarkable diversity among Americans who sold their plasma. In his participant-observer study of paid donors, Martin Kretzmann described his encounters with "alcoholics, felons, ex-addicts, and those who lived on the street," as well as his encounters with young drifters, unemployed men and women, students, and "older Hispanic women who looked like grandmothers in their black dresses as they quietly sat and read their Bibles."[137] Money continues to play a critical role in the blood supply system.

Cashing in on Organs

If the market value of solid body tissues waned by the 1930s, the resurgence of solid organ transplantation, the successful kidney transplants performed at the

Massachusetts General Hospital in the 1950s and especially Christiaan Barnard's 1967 heart transplant, revived speculation and concern about the buying and selling of human organs from both the living and the dead. Some state legislatures took steps to restrict payment to individuals during their lifetime for their postmortem body parts. Between 1967 and 1969, five state legislatures (Nevada, Delaware, Hawaii, New York, and Oklahoma) adopted such laws. In 1969, Mississippi's legislature passed a bill to permit its citizens to receive money for body parts acquired by hospitals after death, and even a monetary penalty if the citizen's family failed to honor the contract. That same year, Massachusetts legislators banned the sale of body parts from the dead (both the premortem sale by the supplier and the postmortem sale by the next of kin).[138]

As in the early twentieth century, enterprising individuals sought to market their body parts. In May 1968, the following advertisement appeared in the *San Gabriel* (California) *Tribune*:

Need a Transplant?

Man will sell any portion of body for financial remuneration to person needing an operation. Write Box 1211–630, Covina.[139]

Physician-author Robin Cook cited this advertisement in his author's note to the novel *Coma*. But the idea of an elaborate medical conspiracy to provide wealthy recipients with the organs of healthy young people had already surfaced.

Just 1 month after Christiaan Barnard performed a heart transplant in December 1967, Moscow newspaper correspondent Geinrikh Borovik speculated that Barnard's success would become a social tragedy: "imagine a bandit corporation which deals with the murder of people only for the sake of selling their organs on the black market."[140]

The *Pravda* writer went on to warn that physicians would register deaths prematurely in order to make organs available to rich clients. Although some American newspapers dismissed his warnings as "the Communist view on heart transplants," Borovik pointed out that his comments about a murder ring to supply black market organs followed an editorial in the *New York Times*, which noted "One need not be a science-fiction writer to envision the possibility of future murder rings supplying black-market surgeons whose patients are unwilling to wait until natural sources have supplied the heart or liver or pancreas they need."[141]

The most vehement denunciation of paying for life by the part came in response to the proposal by H. Barry Jacobs to broker human kidneys. In 1983, Jacobs, a physician in Reston, Virginia who lost his license to practice medicine in Virginia following a conviction and prison sentence for Medicare fraud, launched the International Kidney Exchange. In letters to some 7500 hospitals, he explained his plan to purchase kidneys from individuals in need of money and provide them to Americans able to purchase the needed organ. Jacobs cited the serious shortfall in kidneys that resulted from a voluntary system. In 1982, some 10,000 Americans waited for an available kidney for transplant; more than 4000 people did not receive the needed organ. "Where is the wind blowing?" Jacobs told one reporter. "It is the money wind."[142] In his testimony before the Subcommittee on Health and the Environment of the Committee on Energy and Commerce in 1984, Jacobs was somewhat more formal: "What I am proposing is simply a monetary program. Where people fully informed, consenting adults, could give up a kidney if they wanted to, and more importantly, and the major thing is for the Government to offer the incentive to people to sign up while they are healthy."[143]

Leaders of the National Kidney Foundation blasted Jacob's plan: "It is immoral and unethical to place a living person at risk of surgical complication and even death for a cash payment."[144] Not everyone was critical. *Fortune* magazine challenged the National Kidney Foundation's stance by quoting the Foundation's own claims about the relative safety of live kidney donation. The magazine offered a ringing endorsement of selling kidneys: "that's what markets are for—to give people, desperate and otherwise, a chance to optimize their own situations. Most people don't need two kidneys but do need to pay the rent occasionally."[145] Everyone conceded that no existing American law prevented a plan like Jacobs' kidney exchange. Although nearly every American state had adopted some form of the Uniform Anatomical Gift Act by 1973, these statutes did not explicitly ban the sale of human tissue or organs.[146] The publicity generated by Jacobs' plan and other stories about traffic in organs in developing countries informed the public hearings in the U.S. House of Representatives' Committee on Science and Technology. Chaired by Representative Albert Gore, Jr. (Democrat, Tennessee), the Subcommittee on Investigations and Oversight heard testimony about the difficulty families faced in procuring organs and the lack of a coherent nationwide system. Gore, along with 89 fellow representatives, sponsored the National Organ Transplantation Act. Passed in 1984, this legislation funded the creation of a nonprofit organ procurement organization and criminalized the transfer of organs "for valuable consideration in use in human transplantation."[147] Gore expressly warned about the dangers posed to society by plans like Jacobs to supply human kidneys for transplantation. "We must not allow technology to dehumanize people so that we erode the distinction between things and people. People should not be regarded as things to be bought and sold like parts of an automobile. If this were allowed, it would seriously undermine the values of our society."[148]

This law did not prevent Americans and other wealthy Westerners from going abroad to purchase organs for transplantation. In 1990, reporter Raj Chengappa claimed that his country, India, dominated the market in the buying and selling of kidneys (an estimated 2000 such sales in 1990).[149] Although this trade was denounced as "vile, deplorable and morally reprehensible" by health professionals and transplant surgeons, the possibility that financial incentives might increase the number of kidneys—live and cadaveric—has not disappeared.

Even in the United States, the ongoing shortfall in available kidneys has prompted some reconsideration of the ban on organ sales. In 2002, the Council of Ethical and Judicial Affairs of the AMA called for more research studies into the potential harms from the use of financial incentives for organ donation that have been traditionally advanced against organ sales.[150] Several states have experimented with ways to provide some incentives for organ donation; in 1999, Pennsylvania sponsored a pilot project in which organ donors received a $300 payment toward funeral expenses and, in 2004, Wisconsin became the first state to offer living donors a tax deduction of up to $10,000 for medical costs, travel, and lost salary. In April 2004, President George W. Bush signed the Organ Donation and Recovery Improvement Act. The act continued the ban on buying or selling organs, but it also authorized the federal government to reimburse living donors for expenses and to offer project grants aimed at increasing donations and improving organ preservation and compatibility.[151] Such leading bioethicists as Robert M. Veatch, who opposed economic transactions in the procurement of organs in 1983, have argued for a reassessment of the ban on marketing organs. In light of the persistent American failure to provide for the basic needs of some of its citizens, Veatch has advanced lifting the ban, noting "If it is immoral to make an offer to buy organs from someone who is desperate because those making the offer refuse to make available the alternative solutions, it must be even more immoral to continue under these circumstances to withhold the right of the desperate to market the one valuable commodity they possess."[152] Perhaps in the near future, the prospect of auctioning one's bodily assets on e-Bay will be commonplace.

$$$

Money and its management played a significant role in the network of blood relations in twentieth-century America. Just as money itself was subjected to remarkable variety in the ways in which Americans identified, classified, organized, segregated, manufactured, designed, stored, and decorated it, blood too accreted value in its donation, collection, grouping, storage, and transfusion. Unlike money, however, which had been assumed to be interchangeable, impersonal, cold, distant, and calculating, blood was never "colorless."[153] Blood never remained free of value—it retained its racial, religious, social, cultural, and political meanings. These values have not remained static over the course of the twentieth century. Much of the symbolic power of blood as the vehicle for the transmission of heredity, for example, has been overtaken by the gene and more recently, by DNA.[154]

The movement of blood between bodies and the transplantation of tissues, organs, and other parts, especially between people of dissimilar backgrounds, challenged the stability of identities grounded in flesh and blood. What did it mean to one's identity to receive blood from someone of a different race, sex, religion, or even political affiliation? Although some recipients reportedly relished their new identifications (like the "Hebrew merchant" who received blood from a young man claiming to be descended from Irish kings), others apparently did not (the woman "so unpleasant that none of her family would donate" was angry to learn that she had received blood from a prizefighter, but it wasn't clear whether this resulted from his occupation or his sex). The boundaries of difference are explored in the next chapter.

Notes

1. Margaret Jane Radin, *Contested Commodities* (Cambridge: Harvard University Press, 1996).
2. See Nancy Scheper-Hughes, "Theft of Life: the Globalization of Organ Stealing Rumors," *Anthropology Today* 12 (1996): 3–11.
3. Véronique Campion-Vincent, "Organ Theft Narratives," *Western Folklore* 56 (1997): 1–33.
4. Cuba outlawed slavery in 1884; Brazil became the last nation to outlaw slavery in 1888; see Robert W. Fogel, *Without Consent or Contract* (New York: W.W. Norton, 1989).
5. Sharla M. Fett, *Working Cures* (Chapel Hill: University of North Carolina Press, 2002).
6. Susan E. Lederer, *Subjected to Science: Human Experimentation in America before the Second World War* (Baltimore: Johns Hopkins University Press, 1995).
7. "Shipped Bodies in Trunks," *New York Times*, 15 Nov. 1899, p. 1. "Dead Bodies are Drug on Market," *Chicago Daily Tribune*, 2 Feb 1902, p. 41.
8. Michael Sappol, *A Traffic of Dead Bodies: Anatomy and Embodied Social Identity in Nineteenth-Century America* (Princeton: Princeton University Press, 2001.)
9. Erasmus Darwin, *Zoonomia; or, the Laws of Organic Life* (1803).
10. James Blundell, *Researches physiological and pathological* (London: E. Cox, 1825), p. 116.
11. William Stanton, *The Leopard's Spots: Scientific Attitudes Toward Race in America, 1815–1859* (Chicago: University of Chicago Press, 1960), 6.
12. Lederer, *Subjected to Science*, p. 115.
13. Mark Blackwell, "'Extraneous Bodies": The Contagion of Live-Tooth Transplantation in Late-Eighteenth-Century England," *Eighteenth-Century Life* 28 (2004): 21–68.
14. "Selling Human Hair a Traffic of Tragedies," *New York Times*, 27 Mar. 1904, p.12; Peter S. Jowe, "China's Human Hair Market," *Millard's Review* 10 (1919): 253–255. For allusions to *Les Miserables*, wherein Cosette sells her hair and bargains to sell her teeth in order to feed her baby, see "Can One Sell Part of His Body?" *Washington Post*, 29 Nov. 1903, p. C8.
15. Janet Golden, *A Social History of Wet Nursing in America: From Breast to Bottle* (Cambridge: Cambridge University Press, 1996).
16. Charles Mixer, "The Transposition of Stomachs," *The Black Cat* (April 1900): 39–42.
17. In November and December 1903, the *New York Times* printed six articles about the ear graft; the *New York Tribune* published 10 articles about the episode. "Offers $5000 for an Ear," *New York Times*, 8 Nov. 1903, p.1. According to the Inflation Calculator, $5000 in 1903 would be $101,000 in 2003.
18. "Offers $5000 for an Ear," *New York Times*, 8 Nov. 1903, p. 1.
19. "Ear Seller a German," *New York Tribune*, 13 Nov. 1903, p. 6.
20. "Lend Me Your Ears, Price of One $5000," *Philadelphia Inquirer*, 19 Nov. 1903.
21. See "Ear Grafting Accomplished," *The State* (Columbia, SC), 5 Dec. 1903, p. 3; and also "Here with New Ear," *New York Tribune*, 3 Dec. 1903; and "Ear Grafting Operation Is a Success," *San Jose Mercury News*, 3 Dec. 1903, p. 8.
22. "Ear Grafting," *New York Times*, 6 Dec. 1903, p.6
23. "The Replacement of a Lost Ear," *New York Medical Journal* 78 (1903): 948–949.
24. See "A Strange Problem of Ear Surgery," *British Medical Journal* 1 (1902): 161.
25. Maurice Renard, *New Bodies for Old* (New York: Macauley, 1923), 203–204. This quotation comes from the "chaste" English translation of Renard's, *Le Docteur Lerne Sous-Dieu* (Paris: Société du Mercure de France, 1908). The only difference between the French

and English version of the ear grafting reference is that "le roi des conserves" is called Lipton in the 1908 text rather than X; see *Le Docteur Lerne*, p. 209.

26. "Pianist Buys Finger: Replaces Stiff One," *Washington Post*, 27 Mar. 1927, p. 12.

27. Arthur Train, *Mortmain* (New York: Charles Scribner's Sons, 1918).

28. Robert Abbe, "The Surgery of the Hand," *New York Medical Journal* 59 (1894): 33–40.

29. Arthur C. Train, *My Day in Court* (New York: Charles Scribner's Sons, 1939), 221–222.

30. "Mortmain," *Variety*, 3 Sep. 1915, p. 40; and "Mortmain" in American Film Institute Catalog, online. I have not been able to locate a copy of this film.

31. A.C. Train, *My Day in Court*, p. 222.

32. *The Blind Bargain*, movie, Goldwyn, 1922; "Monkey Gland Transferred to Make New Chaney Film," *Washington Post*, 31 Dec. 1922, p. 38.

33. "Boys Furnish Cuticle at Five Cents a Patch," *Los Angeles Times*, 3 Dec. 1889, p. 2.; "Successful Skin Grafting," *Wheeling (W.Va.) Register*, 15 Jul. 1891, p. 7.

34. "Skin Grafting," *Washington Post*, 25 Mar. 1903, p. 6.

35. "Would Sell Part of Body," *Washington Post*, 23 Dec. 1906. p.5. "Offers to Sell Skin," *New York Times*, 5 Oct. 1907, p. 6; "The Active Woman," *New York Times*, 6 Oct. 1907, p. 10.

36. "Skin-grafting in a Workhouse," *The Lancet*, 3 Jun. 1899: 1505–1506.

37. F. Gregory Connell, "Removal of Skin from the Abomen during Laparotomy as a Source of Material for Grafting," *International Journal of Surgery* 22 (1909), p. 359.

38. "Sell Skin for Revenue," *Los Angeles Times*, 17 Aug. 1910, p. II9.

39. "Kaplow, Altruist, A Puzzle to Nutley," *New York Times*, 15 May 1913, p. 20.

40. Mrs. William Chalmar to A. Carrel, 31 Mar. 1913, Alexis Carrel Papers, box 45, sec. 15–1, f. 18. Georgetown University Library.

41. See Max Thorek, *The Human Testis and Its Disease* (Philadelphia: J. B. Lippincott Co., 1924), 426–444.

42. P. Kammerer, *Rejuvenation and the Prolongation of Human Efficiency* (New York: Boni and Liveright, 1923), 62. For reports of gland theft, see "Youth Robbed of Glands: Attack in Chicago Believed Perpetrated by Rich Aged Man's Hirelings and Surgeon," *Los Angeles Times*, 22 Nov. 1923, p. I2.

43. "Plan Law to Forbid Human Gland Sales," Atlanta Constitution, 23 Jun. 1922, p. 14; "Women Seek Glands Now," *Los Angeles Times*, 23 Jun. 1922, p. 11; "Offers Glands for Best Bid," *Los Angeles Times*, 22 Dec. 1922, p. I11; Editorial cartoon, "the Unknown Soldier," *Chicago Tribune*, 22 Jun. 1922, p.1

44. "Material for Experiment," *Boston Globe*, 19 Jun. 1922, p. 12.

45. "Sale of Living Human Tissue to be Object of New Bureau," *Washington Post*, 20 Aug. 1937, p. 5.

46. "The Value of Human Blood," *New York Times*, 13 Jul. 1883, p. 8.

47. "City and Suburban News—Suit to Recover Pay for Transmission," *New York Times*, 21 Jul. 1883, p. 8.

48. "Medical Fees and Millionaires," *Pacific Medical Journal* 42 (1899): 108–111.

49. George W. Crile, *Hemorrhage and Transfusion: An Experimental and Clinical Research* (New York: D. Appleton, 1909), 301.

50. F. D. Gray, "Direct Transfusion," *Medical Record* 79 (1911): 198–201.

51. See R. Ottenberg, "Transfusion and Arterial Anastomosis," *Annals of Surgery* 47 (1908): 486–505.

52. "Hero Sells His Blood," *Washington Post*, 18 May 1914, p. 10.

53. Bertram M. Bernheim, *Adventure in Blood Transfusion* (New York: Smith & Durrell, 1942), 74.

54. "Homeless Men Sell Blood," *New York Times* 15 Jan. 1917, p. 9.

55. "Many in District Sell Their Blood for Transfusion," *Washington Post*, 28 Sep. 1930, p. M13.

56. For compensation to research subjects, see Susan E. Lederer, *Subjected to Science*.

57. "Retails His Blood at $600," *New York Times*, 14 May 1920, p. 21.

58. "Sells His Blood to Wed," *New York Times*, 20 Sep. 1923, p. 4.

59. Lewis Thomas, *The Youngest Science* (New York: Viking Press, 1983), 37. For an English protest against the use of medical students, see "Blood-Donors," *The Lancet* 2 (1921): 1123.

60. "Columbia Blood in Demand," *New York Times*, 17 Jan. 1915, p. C1. Advertisements continued to appear in the college newspapers seeking students willing to sell blood. See "150 Men at Columbia Sell Blood for Living," *New York Times*, 2 Nov. 1928, p. 18.

61. "Yale Lists Blood Selling," *New York Times*, 17 Oct. 1925, p. 3.

62. "College Youth Not As Painted," *Los Angeles Times*, 10 Jan. 1927, pp. A1–A2.

63. Helen Murray, "What Profit?" *Christian Century* (1 Jun. 1932): 703.

64. "Feats of a Champion Blood-Donor," *The Literary Digest* 97 (5 May 1928): 65.

65. B.M. Bernheim, *Adventure in Blood Transfusion*, p. 87

66. Henry M. Feinblatt, *Transfusion of Blood* (New York: Macmillan, 1926), 44.

67. Herbert Z. Giffin and Samuel F. Haines, "A Review of Professional Donors," *Journal of the American Medical Association* 81 (1923): 532–535.

68. "Rewards Doctor with Car," *New York Times*, 29 Apr. 1924, p. 21.

69. "Caruso Paid $1,500 for Quart of Blood," *New York Times*, 18 Jan. 1923, p. 16.

70. "Court Releases Drinker Who Gave Blood for 206," *Washington Post*, 29 Jan. 1923, p. 3.

71. "Blood Donor Freed in Row," *New York Times*, 12 Jul. 1929, p.46.

72. "$1,000 For Her Blood," *New York Times*, 27 Sep. 1911, p. 22.

73. "Claims $5,800 for Blood Given Man on his Deathbed," *Chicago Daily Tribune*, 2 Feb 1918, p. 2; and "Pint of Blood to Save Life Cause of Suit," *Los Angeles Times*, 22 Nov. 1923, p.13.

74. "College Youth Not As Painted," *Los Angeles Times*, 10 Jan. 1927, pp. A1–A2.

75. Herbert Harlan, "This Business of Selling Blood," *Hygeia* 7 (1929): 471.

76. For Flower Hospital, see "Stop Profiteering in Transfusion," *New York Times*, 15 Jan. 1920, p. 17; and "The Strike That Failed," *Washington Post*, 18 Jan. 1920, p. 24.

77. "Funds Requested for Blood Transfusions," *Journal of the American Medical Association* 90 (1928): 1296.

78. Jean Begg, "Blood by Donor: The Growth of Organized Transfusion Here and Abroad," *Medical Economics* 13 (1935–6): 33–34.

79. "Everyday Heroism," *Washington Post*, 26 Oct. 1908, p. 6.

80. "Wills Money to Blind Newsboy," *Los Angeles Times*, 20 May 1919, p. 110.

81. "Grateful for Gift of Blood," *New York Times*, 27 Jan. 1915, p. 9.

82. "World's Champion Blood Donor," *Life* (28 Feb. 1938).

83. H. Russell Fisher, "The Record of a Blood Donor," *Journal of the American Medical Association* 116 (1941): 2101.

84. "Gen. Mitchell's Son Gets 'Golden Blood,'" *Philadelphia Evening Bulletin*, 26 Oct. 1942. "Lieut. Mitchell, General's Son, Dies at Camp," *Washington Post*, 28 Oct. 1942, p. B15.

85. "Champion Donor," *Time*, 36 (29 Jul. 1940): 38.

86. David Camelon, "Blood Donor Fights High Fee Charges," *Chicago Herald American*, 5 Mar. 1941, clipping from Historical Health Fraud and Alternative Medicine Collection, Box 495, Folder 1: McMullin, Mrs. Rose, 1940–1955, American Medical Association, Chicago, Illinois.

87. Charles V. Nemo, "I Sell Blood," *American Mercury*, 31 (1934): 194–203. This magazine began publication in 1924 as a quality monthly for educated readers. By 1934, its original

editor, American man of letters H.L. Mencken, had resigned, signaling the decline of the magazine. See Frank Luther Mott, *A History of American Magazines* vol. 5 (Cambridge: Harvard University Press, 1968), 3–26.

88. C.V. Nemo, "I Sell Blood," p. 196.

89. Paul de Kruif, *Microbe Hunters* (New York: Blue Ribbon Books, 1926), 322–324.

90. Sidney Coe Howard, *Yellow Jack: A History* (New York: Harcourt, Brace, 1934), 135.

91. Ibid.

92. E. H. L. Corwin, "Community Control of Professional Blood Donors," *New York State Journal of Medicine* 35 (1935): 317.

93. H. Harlan, "This Business of Selling Blood," p. 470.

94. Jean Begg, "Blood by Donor: The Growth of Organized Transfusion Here and Abroad," *Medical Economics* 13 (1935–6): 33–34.

95. "'Passport' Planned For Blood Donors," *New York Times*, 15 Sep. 1929, p. 19.

96. "Blood-Givers Form a Union in A.F.L.," *New York Times*, 15 Sep. 1938; see editorial 25 Sep. 1938.

97. Alexis Carrel, "The Preservation of Tissues and Its Applications in Surgery," *Journal of the American Medical Association* 59 (1912): 523–527.

98. C.L. Hoag, "The World's First Blood Banker—Oswald Hope Robertson," *Bulletin of the American Association of Blood Banks* 11 (1958): 95–97.

99. Bernard Fantus, "Cook County's Blood Bank," *Modern Hospital* 50 (1938): 57–58.

100. M. Telischi, "Evolution of Cook County Hospital Blood Bank," *Transfusion* 14 (1974): 623–628.

101. Bernard Fantus, "Cook County's Blood Bank," *Modern Hospital*, 50 (1938): 57–58.

102. R.O. Muether and K.R. Andrews, "Studies on 'Stored Blood,'" *American Journal of Clinical Pathology* 11 (1941): 307–338.

103. C. George Caffentzis, "Medical Metaphors and Monetary Strategies in the Political Economy of Locke and Berkeley," *History of Political Economy* 35 (2003): 204–233.

104. Michael O'Malley, "Specie and Species: Race and the Money Question in Nineteenth-Century America," *American Historical Review* 99 (1993): 369–395.

105. Adeline Knapp, *One Thousand Dollars a Day: Studies in Practical Economics*, (Boston: Arena, 1894). Knapp is better known today as the intimate companion of feminist Charlotte Perkins Gilman; see Ann J. Lane, *To Herland and Beyond: The Life and Work of Charlotte Perkins Gilman* (New York: Pantheon Books, 1990).

106. A.L. Soresi, "Why Is Direct Transfusion of Blood often a Failure?" *New York Medical Journal* 96 (1912): 936–941. For earlier references to nonbiologic materials in banks, see "Now the Radium Bank: Wherein Is Kept the Almost Priceless Metal," *New York Times*, 23 Jan. 1910, p. SM10; and "Women as Radium Porters," *New York Times*, 12 Feb. 1911, p. C2.

107. Charles S. Cameron and L. Kraeer Ferguson, "The Organization and Technique of the Blood Bank at the Philadelphia General Hospital," *Surgery* 5 (1939): 237–248.

108. "Physician Suggests 'Eye Bank,'" *New York Times*, 22 Jun. 1938, p. 25; "'Eye Bank' is Set Up to Preserve Cornea Tissues to Save Sight," *New York Times*, 9 May 1944, p. 21.

109. Lois Mattox Miller, "Banks of Human Spare Parts," *Readers Digest* 45 (Nov. 1944): 25–26.

110. "Convict First Skin Bank Donor," *New York Times*, 3 Nov. 1943, p. 17. "Live Skin Banks Seen in Atom War," *Los Angeles Times*, 17 Mar. 1950, p. 13.

111. Ed Neff, "Fathers Corps is Formed to Aid Childless," *Washington Herald*, 13 Sep. 1938. See also "Proxy Fathers," *Time* (26 Sep. 1938): 28.

112. Thomas R. Henry, "Gene Register Planned Here," *Washington Star*, 13 Sep. 1938; clipping from Georgetown Medical School, Box 1938–1949, folder 1938.

113. Memorandum on Statements Attributed Doctor Ivy Albert Pelzman, Clinical Instructor in Urology, Georgetown University School of Medicine, 12 Nov., 1938. David V. McCauley, the Dean of the Medical School, expressed displeasure that the first paper to take up the story was a Catholic newspaper *The Tidings*, from Los Angeles. Archives, Georgetown Medical School, Box 1938–1949, folder 1938.

114. Henry Dwight Chapin, "The Operation of a Breast Milk Dairy," *Journal of the American Medical Association* 81 (1923): 200–202.

115. Mary D. Blankenhorn, "A Breast Milk Dairy," *Hygeia* 11 (1933): 411–412. For milk banks, see "Mother's Milk Bank in Milwaukee," *Chicago Daily Tribune*, 8 Dec. 1942, p. 5; and "Quadruplets Well and 'Mother Is Fine,'" *New York Times*, 3 Nov. 1944, p. 23.

116. Eugene S. Zemans, *Prisoners' Blood Goes to War* (Chicago: Central Howard Association, 1945).

117. For Cohn's work, see Angela N. H. Creager, "Biotechnology and Blood: Edwin Cohn's Plasma Fractionation Project, 1940–1953," in *Private Science: Biotechnology and the Rise of Molecular Science*, ed. Arnold Thackray (Philadelphia: University of Pennsylvania Press, 1998), 39–64; and "From Blood Fractions to Antibody Structure: Gamma Globulin Research Growing Out of World War II," in *Singular Selves: Historical Issues and Contemporary Debates in Immunology*, ed. Anne-Marie Moulin and Albert Cambrosio (Paris: Elsevier, 2001), 140–154.

118. "Prisoners Repay Blood," *New York Times*, 9 Nov. 1947, p. 3.

119. "Husband Ordered to Donate Blood in Lieu of Alimony," *Los Angeles Times*, 21 Nov. 1940, p. 23.

120. American Red Cross, Thomas H. Evans to Dr. James W. Davis, 28 Mar. 1956, ARC 505.1.

121. See "Yankee Ingenuity Aids the Blood Drive," *Saturday Evening Post* 226 (12 Sep. 1953): 10–12 for description of another New England town which offered "New York city slickers" who went a trifle above the speed limit the opportunity to donate a pint of blood or pay a fine of $50.

122. "Blood Money," *Time* 102 (1 Oct. 1973): 113.

123. Richard M. Titmuss, *The Gift Relationship: From Human Blood to Social Policy* (New York: Vintage Books, 1971), 138.

124. "Medicolegal Questions Answered," *Transfusion* 6 (1966): 613–614.

125. "No Payment for Donors," *Journal of the American Medical Association*, 87 (1926): 2008. See "The Price to be Paid for Blood Transfusions," *Boston Medical and Surgical Journal* 196 (1927): 251.

126. "Awards to Blood Donors," Excerpt from Congressional Record, volume 91, Washington D.C. Thursday, July 12, 1945, No. 139, p. 7552. ARC RG 200, Group 3, f: 505.05 legislation.

127. Ibid.

128. "Blood for Transfusions Subject to Sales Tax," *Science Newsletter*, 39 (1941): 184; and L.A. Hines and H.B. Alsobrook, "Should Blood Sales Require Sales Tax?" *Journal of the Louisiana State Medical Society* 122 (1970): 321–322.

129. H.F. Thompson to Dr. Ross McIntire, 2 Jul. 1948, ARC 505.1, Box 1201, Blood Donors Income Tax Deduction for Blood Donations, Proposed.

130. American Medical Association, 6 Apr. 1953, ARC 505.1, Blood Donors: Income Tax Deductions for Blood Donations Proposed.

131. "Sale of Blood," *The New Physician* 19 (1970): 267–268.

132. R.M. Titmuss, *The Gift Relationship*, pp. 245–246.

133. Ann Oakley and John Ashton, eds. *The Gift Relationship* (London: London School of Economics, 1997), p. 7.

134. Ann Landers "Disease Risk Greater in Paid Blood Donor," *Oakland Tribune;* letter from George M. Elsey to Ann Landers, 10 Nov. 1971; and August Gribben, "Blood That Kills," *The National Observer*, 29 Jan. 1972; ARC Record Group 200, Group 5, 020.101 folder Blood Program Hepatitis Material.

135. Douglas Starr, *Blood: An Epic Story of Medicine and Commerce* (New York: Knopf, 1998), 229.

136. See *The Gift Relationship*, ed. Ann Oakley and John Ashton (London School of Economics, 1997).

137. Martin J. Kretzmann, "Bad Blood: The Moral Stigmatization of Paid Plasma Donors," *Journal of Contemporary Ethnography* 20 (1992): 416–441; and Leon Anderson, Kit Newell, and Joseph Kilcoyne, "Selling Blood: Characteristics and Motivations of Student Plasma Donors," *Sociological Spectrum* 19 (1999): 137–162.

138. Russell Scott, *The Body as Property* (New York: The Viking Press, 1981), 190.

139. See Author's Note in Robin Cook, *Coma (Boston: Little, Brown,* 1977), p. 278.

140. "Russian Sees Threat of Heart Sale Racket," *Washington Post*, 8 Jan. 1968, p. A12.

141. "Black Market for Transplants," *New York Times*, 18 Jan. 1968, p. 38.

142. Walter Sullivan, "Buying of Kidneys of Poor Attacked," *New York Times*, 24 Sep. 1983, I: 9.

143. National Organ Transplant Act: Hearings before the Subcommittee on Health and the Environment of the Committee on Energy and Commerce, House of Representatives, Ninety-eighth Congress, first session, on H.R. 4080. July 29, October 17 and 31, 1983. (Washington: U.S. Government Printing Office, 1984).

144. "The Crisis in Human Spare Parts," *New York Times*, 4 Oct. 1983, p. 26.

145. "A Little Organ Music," *Fortune* 108 (31 Oct. 1983): 31–32.

146. Renée C. Fox and Judith P. Swazey, *Spare Parts: Organ Replacement in American Society* (New York: Oxford University Press, 1992), 65.

147. "Regulating the Sale of Human Organs," *Virginia Law Review* 71 (1985): 1015–1038.

148. "Network Is Proposed for Organs Transplants," *New York Times*, 6 Oct. 1983, p. I19.

149. Raj Chengappa, "The Great Organ Bazaar," *India Today* (31 Jul. 1990): 60–67.

150. Sara Taub, Andrew H. Maixner, Karine Morin, Robert M. Sade, "Cadaveric Organ Donation: Encouraging the Study of Motivation," *Transplantation* 76 (2003): 748–751.

151. "What Is a Kidney Worth?" *Christian Science Monitor* (9 June 2004); Madhay Goyal, et al. "Economic and Health Consequences of Selling a Kidney in India," *Journal of the American Medical Association* 288 (2002): 1589–1593; David J. Rothman, "Ethical and Social Consequences of Selling a Kidney," *Journal of the American Medical Association* 288 (2002): 1640–1641.

152. Robert M. Veatch, "Why Liberals Should Accept Financial Incentives for Organ Procurement," *Kennedy Institute of Ethics Journal* 13 (2003): 19–36.

153. Viviana Zelizer, *The Social Meaning of Money* (New York: Basic Books, 1994).

154. Dorothy Nelkin and M. Susan Lindee, *The DNA Mystique: The Gene As a Cultural Icon* (New York: W.H. Freeman, 1995), 15.

4

Lost Boundaries

Race, Blood, and Bodies

In the 1949 "social message" film *Lost Boundaries*, Scott Carter, a Negro physician, his wife, and children pass for white in a New Hampshire town. When the physician seeks to enlist during World War II, his request for a commission is rejected when his old college records reveal his Negro blood. Before this revelation, in a dramatic scene in the film, a nurse holds a bottle of blood. When someone mentions "Negro blood," she drops the bottle, it crashes to the floor and the blood splashes over the white hospital tiles.[1] *Lost Boundaries* was based on a "true story." First published in *Readers Digest* and later as a slim book, the story of Doctor Albert Johnston (an African American radiologist) described the light-skinned physician's inability to find a hospital position (he was rejected by both Southern "black" hospitals and by Northern "white hospitals").[2] He eventually located in a small New England town where he and his wife passed as white and raised their children as white. *Lost Boundaries* focused on the politics of skin color, and it also recognized that blood too was colored—not red, but black and white. During World War II, blood was collected, labeled, and segregated by race. The American Red Cross maintained racial tags on blood until 1950. In the wake of the 1954 Supreme Court ruling on *Brown v. Board of Education*, blood labeling by race became another symbolic battlefield in the fight over civil rights, desegregation, and integration that convulsed American society during the 1950s and 1960s. This chapter considers the role of race and assumptions about racial identity in the movement of blood between bodies and in the collection, storage, banking, and provision of blood.

One Blood

In the late nineteenth century, the transfusion of blood remained a rarely undertaken operation. In these cases, the desperate circumstances of the patient seemed to trump concern about differences between the giver and the recipient of blood. In 1883, when a Western Union Telegraph clerk fell sick in a New York City hotel, his doctors insisted that he needed blood. The only person willing to provide the blood was a "colored porter." Edward Banks agreed to supply the blood at 10 cents a drop. This was a problematic case, not because the transfusion crossed the color line, but because the clerk refused to pay for the blood after his recovery. Indeed Joseph Howe, a New York physician, told a reporter that he had performed several transfusions using blood from "a young Negro man" for white gentlemen. Noting that, in most cases, family members provided blood, the doctor explained that blood was easily obtained from laborers and others, many of whom could recall the times when they had paid physicians to take their blood. When the reporter asked whether it made a difference if the blood was taken from a black man or a white man, the doctor answered no. He explained, "the Negro is a human being and all human blood is alike in its constitution." Howe did concede one curious aspect of "Negro blood"—it was much darker in color than white blood.[3]

The idea that human blood was alike in its biologic constitution would be directly challenged in 1900 with Karl Landsteiner's discovery of the ABO human blood groups (see Chapter 5). Landsteiner's discovery prompted the search for greater blood-borne differences, including the putative test to distinguish bloods from individuals of different races. In 1907, German physician Carl Bruck maintained that he could reliably distinguish the blood serum of a Caucasian, a Negro, a Malayan, a Chinese, and an Arab.[4] Five years later, A. L. Bennett, a physician and Japanese Consul of Denver, claimed that through exhaustive experimentation, he was able to discern whether a drop of dried blood came from "the body of an Oriental, a Negro, or a white man."[5] In 1926, *Hygeia*, the American Medical Association (AMA)'s magazine for laymen, printed the letter of one reader seeking to know whether the blood of the "colored races, such as the Negro, the Japanese, and the Chinese" differed from the blood of whites, and whether the blood of the "colored man" more closely resembled the blood of an animal rather than a white man. The editor explained that all human beings contain the same kinds of blood. Still, *Hygeia's* readers continued to learn of new tests whereby biologists could demonstrate "striking difference" between Gentile and Jewish blood.[6]

Most investigators rejected such claims. John G. Fitzgerald, at Harvard Medical School's laboratory of serum diagnosis, reported that his efforts to demonstrate racial differences in blood were unsuccessful.[7] In the 1920s, Landsteiner challenged the claims about racial differences in human blood, even as he reserved the possibility that such differences had yet to be detected. In studies of the differences between the blood of humans and the nonhuman primates, Landsteiner and C. Philip Miller noted:

> if serological differences do exist between the bloods of white men and American Negroes—no longer a pure race—they are much smaller than those between man and the anthropoid apes. So far we have been unable to demonstrate any characteristic difference. It's not impossible, however, that slight difference might be found if individuals of several races preferably of pure blood were carefully studied by this method in all of its modifications.[8]

In the 1940s, serologist Alexander Wiener, like Landsteiner, reached a similar conclusion about the repeated failures to produce a serum test that distinguished the blood of individuals of different races. "By means of serological tests, the proteins and cells of animals of any species can be differentiated, as a rule, from those of animals belonging to other species," Weiner observed in 1943, "attempts to produce sera which would serve to differentiate bloods of different races particularly in the human species have been unsuccessful."[9] Despite the lack of confidence on the part of leading serologists in any race-specific blood test, some researchers continued to hunt for the elusive means to separate the bloods of different races. At Yale University School of Medicine, immunologist George Smith used white and black blood sera from New Haven Hospital, black sera from Howard University School of Medicine, and Native American sera from Albuquerque, New Mexico. He argued that chemical tests with the sera from the "white, black, and red races" suggested the existence of cellular components distinctive of the three races. (He did express skepticism that the test would be readily adaptable for mass purposes.)[10]

In the United States, the search for the test for racial specificity of blood was largely overtaken by research on the differing frequencies of the ABO groups in populations. In 1919, physicians Ludwig and Hannah Hirszfeld, compelled by wartime circumstances to locate in Salonica, typed the blood drawn from Allied forces, including Serbian, French, and British soldiers, as well as soldiers from colonial Africa. Tests on some 8000 soldiers demonstrated that, although all human groups possessed the same four ABO groups, the frequencies of these groups differed. Europeans showed a higher frequency of blood type A, whereas people from Eastern Europe and Asia had a higher percentage of type B blood.[11] This discovery prompted extensive testing of bloods from groups—near and far—in search of a racial blood index. In the United States, allergist Arthur Coca, for example, tested the blood of children at Indian schools in Oklahoma, Kansas, and New Mexico, and discovered that nearly 80% of the children had blood type O.[12] Some researchers seized the opportunity to apply the blood group ratios to distinguish "racial types," including the New York transfusionist Reuben Ottenberg, who identified six "racial types" based on ABO blood frequencies. When biologist Julian Lewis surveyed the "widespread intermixture of Negroes and Caucasians" in America, he expressed the hope that racial distribution of the blood groups would be useful. He typed blood from 270 African Americans and found that the distribution of Group II and III (B and O) in this population was very different from that of American whites. Although the race index for "American Negroes" approximated the distribution in "African Negroes," it remained different. Lewis concluded that the change in the race index of "American Negroes" resulted from racial mixing in the United States.[13]

Science, Sexuality, and Sensibility

The idea that more than red cells and serum were transmitted through transfusion was centuries old. In the 1660s, diarist Samuel Pepys, a witness to demonstrations of early transfusions at the Royal Society, had mused about the implications of transfusing blood from a Quaker into the Archbishop of Canterbury. In 1789, a writer in the *Massachusetts Magazine* reflected on the ways in which the skillful mixture of various bloods would benefit individuals: "The fire of youth might be tempered with some of the calmness of age, and the languour of age be stimulated with some of the impetuosity of youth . . . The plodding blood of the lawyer might be enlivened by a few drops of the volatile blood of the poet; and the inspired poet be saved from that madness in which his poetick [sic] raptures are likely to end, by some portion of the half stagnant blood of the lawyer."[14]

Novelists in the nineteenth century eroticized the movement of blood between the male and female body. In one of the most famous novels of the nineteenth century, Bram Stoker's *Dracula* (1897), the transfusion of blood from three young men into the body of a sickly young woman (Lucy) signals a premarital sexual union. One of Lucy's donors notes, "this so sweet maid is a polyandrist." This marriage prefigures the literal penetration of Lucy's pale, deathless body with a wooden stake. The vampiric appropriation of the transfused blood (as Dracula completes Lucy's metamorphosis into the "undead") suggests that fluids and their movement collapse boundaries and cross the streams of unrelated individuals.[15] A far less sinister depiction of the implications of moving blood between the male and female body appeared in the 1912 American silent film, *The Hospital Baby*. In the film, an emaciated infant girl receives life-saving blood from a student doctor. After she grows to adulthood, she goes to work for Dr. Brown, who does not yet realize their blood relationship. After the girl saves the doctor from his own near-death experience, the two recognize their blood union and marry.[16]

Late nineteenth-century novelists explored the implications of moving blood between men and women of different nationalities and temperaments. In 1899, novelist Frank Kinsella depicted the grave consequences that result from the transfusion of Dolly Castlemaine, the daughter of an English professor. After a fall during a bicycle lesson, Dolly—injured and close to death—receives the "disturbing, vile-germed life fluid" of her Spanish admirer, Senor Manuel de Castro. Following the transfusion, Dolly's character and disposition change dramatically; she abandons her puzzled English husband and runs off with the "swarthy Spaniard." Acknowledging his own responsibility for the life changes in Dolly, her physician explains how "like Frankenstein" he had "literally created a monster" when he took blood from:

> the native of a country where the national sport is bull fighting,—a sport
> so characteristic of the degraded instincts of the race,—and where
> superstition, viciousness and lasciviousness are prevalent to an appalling
> degree. It is a race, cunning, deceitful, and treacherous as has been proved time
> and time again. Imagine such tainted blood in the veins of a young girl! [17]

Although Dolly enjoys a temporary respite when she receives a transfusion of blood from her own husband, she becomes delirious and dies, a woman broken by the "unlucky transfusion." Although one Chicago reader blasted Kinsella's "bizarre straining after effect" in his portrayal of transformation via transfusion, a Philadelphia reader praised the novel as a "mental champagne cocktail," not unlike the strangeness of the fictional Dr. Jekyll and Mr. Hyde.[18]

How the early recipients of blood from racially dissimilar individuals regarded their transfusions in fact rather than fiction is impossible to know. Despite the newer scientific knowledge about blood, it seems clear that older associations of blood with ethnicity persisted. As Stanford University President David Starr Jordan explained in 1902, "We know that the actual blood in the actual veins plays no part in heredity, that the transfusion of blood means no more than the transposition of food, and that the physical basis of the phenomena of inheritance is found in the structure of the germ cell and its contained germ-plasm." Still, Jordan insisted:

> The blood which is "thicker than water" is the symbol of race unity. In this
> sense the blood of the people concerned is at once the cause and the result
> of the deeds recorded in their history. For example, wherever an Englishman
> goes, he carries with him the elements of English history. It is a British
> deed which he does, British history that he makes. Thus, too, a Jew is a
> Jew in all ages and climes, and his deeds everywhere bear the stamp of
> Jewish individuality. A Greek is a Greek; a Chinaman remains a Chinaman.
> In like fashion, the race traits color all history made by Tartars, or Negroes,
> or Malays.[19]

Stories in the popular press suggested that some people felt themselves trans-formed by the transfusion of new blood. When tenor Enrico Caruso received two blood transfusions in 1921 (from Harry Fenstad and Everett Wilkinson), he report-edly worried about the effects of receiving blood from people who were not Italian. His widow recalled his distress: "I have no more my pure Italian blood," mourned Caruso. "What now am I?"[20]

More often, stories in the popular press about transformations wrought by transfusion conveyed wonder over blood mingling. In 1927, a white boy in a Long Island hospital for an operation became "fast friends" with an 11-year-old African American boy also hospitalized for a surgical procedure. When Jim Blunt's opera-tion went badly, Jimmy Murphy volunteered immediately to provide the necessary blood. After the successful transfusion, Jim told a reporter: "I've got Irish blood in me. Just wait till I get back to Harlem and give them a look at a colored boy with Irish blood in him!"[21]

In some cases, these stories about the effects of mingling strange blood func-tioned to convey the unscientific assumptions of lay people. "Laymen have great difficulty believing that sex and skin color have nothing to do with blood," wrote journalist J. C. Furnas in 1938. In addition to describing women of the "limb-not-leg" school who refused blood from male donors, Furnas described how one orthodox Jewish woman adamantly refused blood from a non-Jewish donor. When the doctor phoned the commercial blood agency for a "kosher substitute," the only donor available with her blood type was a Swede, who was instructed to introduce himself as Isaac Goldberg. "He was blond and ruddy and talked like Minnesota broadcasting but the name was right, the blood was given and the lady was happy."[22] The journal-istic portrayal of this incident as humorous reflected a scientific consensus that human blood was human blood, regardless of the ethnic or sexual container it flowed in.

Moving blood across racial and ethnic lines remained newsworthy in the decades before World War II. When a white man supplied blood to a "Negress" in 1909, a "case without precedent," the story of this successful transfusion in New York's Bellevue Hospital appeared not only in the New York press, but in small-town newspapers like the *Reading* (Pennsylvania) *Daily Times.*[23] In 1926, when a white ambulance driver provided blood to a Negro woman whose relatives and family declined to give blood, the paper described how he "volunteered without inquiring what the patient's station in life or color."[24] If such reports highlighted the incongruity of the blood exchange, there were few, if any, reports that suggested this movement threatened the social order and the stability of racial classifications.

At the same time, some physicians seemingly used the bloods from whites and blacks without comment about differences. In 1912, Johns Hopkins Hospital physicians interested in developing a skin reaction for cancer studied the use of blood injections in both whites and "colored patients." They stopped further observations on patients with "Negro blood" not because of any difference in the blood, but because the desired skin reaction "could not be recognized in them, because of the pigmented skin."[25] When Parke Davis researchers William Culpepper and Marjorie Ableson reported the typing of 5000 different bloods, they noted that they used both white and Negro bloods without comment.[26]

Brothers in Blood

In 1942, science journalists Noah Fabricant and Leo M. Zimmerman described the American public's investment in blood donation and blood banking. In the months following the Japanese attack on Pearl Harbor, the American Red Cross and other organizations begged for blood donations to provide blood and plasma for American and Allied troops. "There is something about the exchange of blood which accentuates belief in democratic processes," gushed the two journalists.

> Most people are willing donors to members of their own family. But how do they react to the proposal that the blood they give may go to a stranger? Who will get the blood? White man, black, or yellow? Christian or Jew? Fortunately, the blood bank has great appeal to the popular imagination, and the vast majority of donors are undisturbed by the thought that another's child or another's uncle may receive their blood. There is an unusual spirit of cooperation and amiability in accepting the notion that we are all brothers-in-blood.[27]

Fabricant and Zimmerman exaggerated the extent to which Americans participated in a blood brotherhood independent of race, religion, or family. Even before American preparations for the war in Europe and Asia, signs of segregation in the American blood supply were evident. When the first American blood bank opened at Cook County Hospital in Chicago in 1937, doctors registered the patient's race, in addition to his name, address, and the name of the intern who took the blood. Although the published reports from the Cook County blood bank did not indicate whether blood was transfused between individuals of different racial groups, other blood banks explicitly observed the color line. In 1938, when white physician Lemuel Diggs opened the blood bank at the John Gaston Hospital in Memphis, Tennessee, he recorded the racial origins of the blood donors and maintained separate stocks of blood collected from whites and blacks. In routine cases, he explained that he matched donors and recipients by race, although Diggs explicitly noted in print that, in cases of emergencies, "the color line does not hold, for when a patient of either race needs blood, any available compatible blood is used."[28]

At the Johns Hopkins Hospital blood bank, opened in 1939, surgeon Mark Ravitch described how "the considerable proportion of Negro patients at the Johns Hopkins Hospital constituted one of the primary problems for establishing the bank."

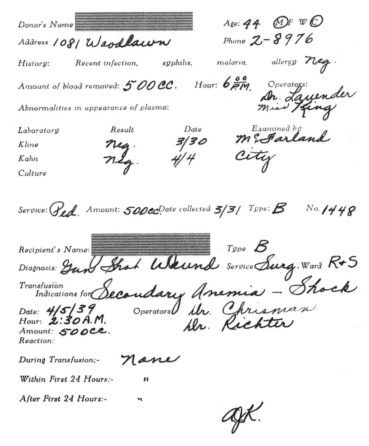

Figure 4.1 This donor card from a 44-year-old "colored man" shows his blood was administered to a man who received a gunshot wound in 1939 (Reproduced with permission of the L.W. Diggs Collection, Health Sciences Historical Collections of the University of Tennessee Health Science Center).

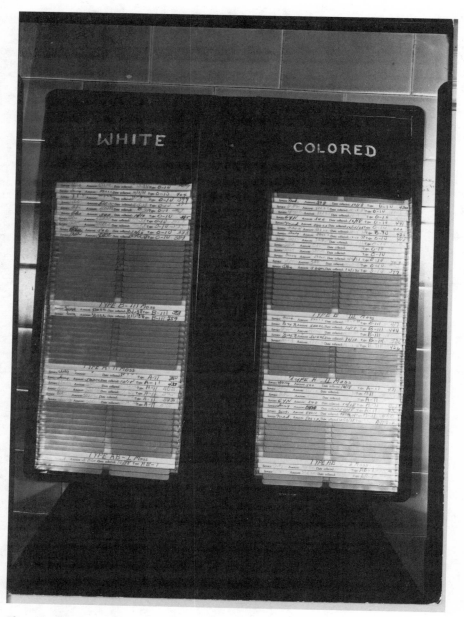

Figure 4.2 The names of white and black donors were maintained in two separate files (Reproduced with permission of the L.W. Diggs Collection, Health Sciences Historical Collections of the University of Tennessee Health Science Center).

Even though there was "no valid objection on biologic or physiologic grounds for transfusing patients of one race with blood from another," the surgeon conceded that "it was deemed best to avoid the issue."[29] Ravitch strove to maintain the segregation of the banked blood to ensure that blood from black donors would not be used for white patients. Although blood collected from white and black donors was stored in the same refrigerator, for example, the flasks were maintained on separate shelves. The record-keeping and administration similarly reflected the efforts to maintain the separate (and initially equal) stocks of black and white blood. Ravitch's initial "quota system" entailed stocking five flasks of O blood, four flasks of A blood, three flasks of B blood, and no AB blood for each race. (The quota system was later changed for "the Negro race" to six O, four A, and two B flasks). The "bank board" conveyed this information visually. Cards for blood from white and Negro donors were filed on a board (white background for white blood; black background for Negro donors).

Separating the bloods of whites and blacks represented more than a cultural preference. It reflected assumptions about blood purity and disease, especially the concern about syphilis. The administrative forms developed by blood bankers exemplified the nexus that physicians saw between African Americans and syphilis. At the Memphis blood bank, Diggs explained that the high rate of syphilitic infection and the inadequate treatment available to black donors made it efficient to perform Kline tests on all "Negroes" before they were selected to supply blood. When they processed white donors, Diggs and his staff questioned them about any disease lesions, tests, and treatments, but the initial tests for syphilis were not made until their blood was taken. At the Hopkins blood bank, Ravitch developed a record to account for blood deposits. In the form he published, entries identified two lots of blood as "out of date" or "spoiled." The first, from a donor identified as w (for white) was labeled "out of date." The second, from a donor identified c (for colored), was recorded as "spoiled," with the entry "S.T.S. positive" (the serologic test for syphilis was positive for the disease). In the widely used 1942 textbook on the blood bank, serologist Robert Kilduffe and surgeon Michael DeBakey reproduced the Hopkins's form, together with form sent biweekly to Hopkins resident physicians reporting the blood in the bank: "The blood bank has on hand the following bloods, Colored: O___ A___ B ___ AB ___. White: O___ A ___ B___ AB___, which will be out of date on _____. We should be glad to have this blood used."[30]

Kilduffe and DeBakey followed Ravitch's lead and created an additional form to account for every flask or container of stored blood. This "master record" was maintained in the laboratory to show blood charged out and its disposition. In their textbook example, three entries appeared on the record, displaying one colored donor and two white donors. Of the blood from these donors, two were discarded. Blood from the colored donor carried the notation "positive serology," the indications of a Wassermann +4 and Kline +2 demonstrating syphilitic infection, and was discarded. The blood from one white donor was discarded not because of syphilis but because the cells had broken up in the flask.[31]

In the 1930s, syphilis became the explicit focus of the United States Public Health Service. Surgeon General Thomas Parran led the crusade against syphilis, calling attention to the starkly higher rates of the disease in African Americans. "The Negro is not to blame because his syphilis rate is six times that of the white. He was free of it when our ancestors brought him from Africa," Parran wrote in his popular book, *Shadow on the Land*. "It is not his fault that the disease is biologically different in him than in the white; so that his blood vessels are particularly susceptible so that late syphilis brings with it crippling circulatory diseases," Parran explained.[32] Such assumptions about syphilis and racial differences continued to inform policies about blood. Although historians such as Spencie Love and Sarah Chinn have discussed the segregation of the blood supply during World War II, they have overlooked the extent to which concern about syphilis informed the decisions made by the Surgeons General of the Armed Forces and the American Red Cross in the 1940s.[33]

Blood and War

By 1940, American physicians viewed the transfusion of blood as crucial to the practice of modern medicine and surgery. In the face of the European war, the National Research Council (NRC) Committee on Transfusion and the Surgeons-General of the Army and the Navy began making plans to supply military hospitals with blood. Given the choice between providing whole liquid blood or plasma (the serum without the red blood cells), the authorities opted for plasma, which entailed blood collection and processing through freeze-drying to provide a powder that was easy to ship and safe to use—even after several years—once it was reconstituted with sterile water. Such a project depended on the generosity and compliance of large numbers of American blood donors.[34]

To some extent, the Red Cross and other agencies already knew how to mobilize Americans to supply blood. In 1940, the Blood Transfusion Betterment Association and the NRC launched the Blood for Britain project, selecting a young African American physician, Charles R. Drew, as its medical supervisor. A graduate of McGill University Medical School, Drew had enrolled at Columbia University's College of Physicians and Surgeons, where, together with surgeon John Scudder, he set up a blood bank at the Presbyterian Hospital. This experience became the basis of Drew's dissertation "Banked Blood." Drew proved enormously successful in achieving the goals of the Blood for Britain project. During the period between August 1940 and January 1941, 17,000 New Yorkers and nine hospitals supplied blood plasma for the British.[35] In the wake of the project's success, Drew served as the director of a pilot blood collection unit for the United States Navy at New York's Presbyterian Hospital. In April 1941, he returned to Howard University School of Medicine to head the department of surgery.[36]

In the summer of 1941, the American Red Cross began its large-scale effort to collect blood to process into plasma for Allied and American troops. In so doing, they chose to ignore the policy Drew had administered in the Blood for Britain project, namely accepting all donors regardless of their race. Drew's program collected blood from "Negro donors" and used it "with the proviso that the plasma therefrom should be specially labelled as to its origins."[37] In 1941, officials from the

Red Cross lacked a national policy about African American donors. Some centers refused African American donors; others accepted the donations, but transferred the blood to other programs. In New York City and Philadelphia, the blood collection centers accepted blood from a few "colored volunteers," but sent the blood to local hospitals and not to the plasma processing plant. In late July, when five "colored volunteers" appeared at the Baltimore chapter of the Red Cross to donate blood for plasma, they were informed that their blood would be used for the regular blood transfusion service. These volunteers left without giving blood, and the local black newspaper, *The Afro-American*, published several articles attacking the Red Cross for its "Jim Crow" blood policy.[38]

African American organizations and individuals challenged the exclusion of Negro donors from the Red Cross program and the ongoing association of Negro blood with sexually transmitted disease. The blood donation issue represented only a small part of the segregation, discrimination, and mistreatment that black servicemen experienced during World War II. But the powerful appeal of blood sacrifice and blood imagery and its implications for the body politic intensified the bitterness over policy. As one angry African American college student observed, "the Army Jim-Crows us. The Navy lets us serve only as messmen, the Red Cross refuses our blood, employers and labor unions shut us out. What more could Hitler do than that?"[39] Working within the War Department, William Henry Hastie, a graduate of Harvard Law School and the first black jurist on the federal bench, sought to persuade Army and Navy officials to reverse the decision to segregate blood by donor race. Despite his efforts, Army Surgeon-General Norman T. Kirk maintained as late as April 1944 that there was no reason to reverse the blood segregation policy.[40]

Amid the protests, letters, and debate, the Red Cross announced on January 21, 1942 a new policy: blood collection centers would accept Negro donors but the blood, carrying the label "N" (or "AA" for Afro-American), would be processed separately into plasma. Facilitating the separate processing of plasma required some additional organization. Physician G. Canby Robinson, the national director of the Blood Donor Service, explained that Negro blood would have to be processed in groups of 8–25 donors. He asked the blood collection centers to enroll Negro donors in groups, provide designated sessions at the centers, or arrange for a mobile blood unit to make a special trip to collect Negro blood. Aware that this was a sensitive issue, Robinson warned that it would be undesirable to designate blood collection sessions for Negro donors only, and "unsatisfactory to attempt to question prospective donors regarding color over the telephone."[41]

Red Cross officials publicly acknowledged that the reasons for segregating blood from Negro donors were social rather than scientific. "It must be recognized that there are many people in this country who object to having Negro blood used for transfusion of white persons. This is a matter of tradition and sentiment rather than of science, as there is no known difference in the physical properties of white and Negro blood," Red Cross chairman Norman H. Davis explained to First Lady Eleanor Roosevelt. "Neither the American Red Cross nor the Medical Departments of the Armed Forces have considered that this feeling can be disregarded."[42] In private letters, however, Davis, who regarded the issue of "Negro blood" as a problem "loaded with dynamite," expressed some reservations about using black donors because of syphilis. In response to an offer from the editor of *Colliers*, a popular weekly magazine, to run an editorial clarifying the Red Cross position, Davis signaled that the issue of syphilis remained part of the decision. "I am informed by medical advisers that there is no chemical difference, insofar as they can see, between blood plasma processed from white blood and that from Negro blood but some of them are not sure some effect will not be registered in later years (the high syphilitic rate among Negroes, for instance.)" In a telephone conversation with the chairman of the Princeton Red Cross chapter, Davis similarly explained that, while doctors agreed that there was no chemical difference between white and Negro blood, physicians "did recognize that, on account of the Wassermann test, it would be most expensive and difficult to take Negro blood, and that there was no certainty that in subsequent years something might not show up that would not appear by any tests made now."[43]

Amid the criticism of the racial segregation of blood, Red Cross officials sought to blame the armed services for the policy. They were surprised when Rear Admiral Ross T. McIntyre, Surgeon General of the Navy, vehemently insisted that the Navy had never asked the Red Cross to refuse blood from Negro donors. Recognizing a classic political move, the Red Cross acknowledged that the Navy had not explicitly asked that Negro donors be refused. However, the Navy stated that "Negro blood" would not be necessary (presumably, because the Navy did not allow Negroes to serve as sailors, gunners, or officers.)[44] Although some Red Cross officials were not pleased with segregating the blood supply, they considered it preferable to the alternatives: either refusing Negro blood altogether or accepting the blood and discarding it. In a private letter to the Secretary of the World Council of Churches, G. Canby Robinson explained, "The deep-rooted sentiments and emotions regarding the Negro in this country are survivals of slave days, especially strong in the South as of course you know. They cannot be swept away suddenly because we are now fighting Hitlerism, as they are not rational or suddenly controllable by the individual."[45] Robinson was well aware that Nazi practices often framed American support for and opposition to the segregation of blood. Stories about "Nazi blood" peppered the newspapers. The Nazis reportedly created regiments of soldiers with the same blood type (presumably to allow anyone to serve as a source of blood); they developed a biologic test to distinguish Aryans from non-Aryans, and Nazi experts challenged the claim that transfusions of "alien blood" could not alter the racial origins of the individual.[46]

Medical and scientific organizations protested the Red Cross decision. "The transfusion of Negro blood into white persons and that of white persons into Negroes has been repeatedly performed in civil practice without any evidence of harm or aversion on the part of the recipients," protested the AMA.[47] Other organizations, including the National Medical Association, the American Public Health Association, and the American Association of Physical Anthropologists similarly opposed the ban. "One objection to the indiscriminate use of Negro blood in the blood bank is the somewhat higher incidence of syphilis among them and the erroneous notion that the disease can be transmitted by means of dried blood of a luetic [syphilitic] donor to a nonluetic recipient," noted the Committee on Race Relations of the

Physical Anthropologists. The editors of *Scientific American* echoed the argument about exclusion based on sexually transmitted diseases: because all syphilitic blood was excluded by testing, "the rate of syphilis in Negroes is of no concern in this connection."[48] Several groups pointed to the increased use of products made from the blood of horses, rabbits, and other animals, as well as those obtained from the urine of stallions and pregnant mares.[49] They also pointed to the longtime intimacies of Southern life. "It is interesting in this connection," observed the Committee on Race Relations, "to recall that the practice of using colored women as wet nurses was at least formerly quite widespread among the better circumstanced families in the Southern part of the country. It is quite certain that, along with the nutritious elements in the milk of those colored women, the white infants ingested many of the same substances which were circulating in the blood stream of the women who suckled them. It is most unlikely that it did them any harm."[50] On scientific grounds and on the basis of social practices, these organizations argued for the end to the ban on Negro donors.

Organizations such as the National Association for the Advancement of Colored People (NAACP) and its secretary Walter White continued to pursue the blood segregation issue. White took issue with the Red Cross's position that respect for the preference on the part of some recipients dictated the segregation of blood. In a series of letters to the Red Cross, he continued to point out how honoring racial preferences made little sense. He quoted from a letter written by the editor of a New York publishing house: "I saw no Negroes [at the blood collection center] today, although I was followed by Wellington Koo, Jr. Whether he stipulated that his blood be given to Chinese I do not know. I intend, upon my next visit to stipulate that my blood be given only to the American males of Scotch-Irish extraction, with Moustaches, and coming preferably from Bradford County in Pennsylvania."[51]

Implementing the segregation policy continued to cause problems for some Red Cross collection centers. How should the blood of other nonwhite donors be handled? Members of the Women's Auxiliary of the National Maritime Union of America registered a complaint in March 1942, after the Red Cross opened a blood collection unit in the Los Angeles County Jail. 29 men—10 Negroes, 3 Japanese, and 16 whites—donated blood on the first day. Red Cross workers pooled the blood of the white and Japanese donors, and processed separately the blood from the Negro donors. "Are we to assume," asked Vivian Warner and Mall Vaida, "that the Red Cross considers the Japanese as members of the white race?" On behalf of their organization, the two women withdrew the offer to donate blood to the Red Cross, "since we cannot ask our Negro members—wives of seamen who are daily risking their lives in the merchant marine—to submit to such a gratuitous insult." At the Boston Red Cross collection center, officials expressed confusion about processing blood from Filipino and Chinese donors. When they wrote to the national headquarters seeking clarification, they were informed that these groups were "whites."[52] In other cities, labeling the blood by race also posed problems. In Pittsburgh, for example, the staff of the mobile blood units informed blacks that the blood was not labeled, but told whites that it was so tagged. In a number of cases, the blood collectors failed to label the blood altogether "making a farce of the order scientifically, and leaving only the unnecessary humiliation" of African American donors.[53]

Not everyone of course opposed the segregation of blood. Sam Hobbs, a Congressman representing Alabama, praised the Red Cross's stand. Even as he acknowledged that there existed no biologic basis for separating the blood, Hobbs defended the right of individuals to take plasma and blood from members of their own race. "This may not be scientific," Hobbs conceded, "but it is very positive and strong." The Congressman described how one mother with a son in the United States Army "was driven into hysterics by the thought that her son might be given an injection of plasma derived in part from the blood of another race."[54] In June 1942, Mississippi Congressman John E. Rankin blamed "radical communistic elements" for spreading the "the false propaganda" that the Red Cross was sending racially unlabeled blood to the troops. He blasted the radical New York paper *PM* for its claim that the Red Cross was mixing the blood of whites and Japanese: "In the name of all the gods at once," Rankin asked his colleagues, "when did it become a discrimination against a colored person to refuse to pump white blood or Japanese blood into him or to refuse to pump Negro blood or Japanese blood into white people without their knowledge or consent, to probably have it crop out in their children?"[55]

As the war drew to a close in Europe, Americans remained mixed over transfusing across the color line. There were apparently dramatic differences by region. In Honolulu, for example, the optimistically named Honolulu Peacetime Blood Plasma Bank issued donor registration cards in 1944 stating "Blood from all races is equally good." In July 1945, 1 month before the bombing of Hiroshima and Nagasaki, a popular women's magazine, *Glamour*, published a "tolerance quiz." Among the questions they posed for their readers was: "How does it happen that a number of Americans of pure Caucasian parentage have Chinese blood in them?" The answer, according to the magazine, was "blood plasma from Chinese donors is often used for wounded American soldiers in the China-Burma-India theater."[56]

American educators like Eugene Lavine, from the Northern State Teachers College in South Dakota, offered curriculum materials to teach tolerance and racial harmony. *All Blood Is Red*, Lavine's play, made the point that "a bullet or bomb fragment don't draw no color line and it hurts just as much to die if your skin is black."[57] Elsie Austin's play, *Blood Doesn't Tell*, offered a similar educational message for the members of the Young Women's Christian Association. The play "about blood donors and blood plasma" featured "four colored and nine white teenagers," including such "various types" as a Jewish boy, Irish girl, Spanish girl, and Italian boy. The teenagers visit a blood bank center where they learn about the ABO blood types, including the response—certainly—to the question: "Could an Eskimo or a Zulu, for instance, have the same type of blood as an Englishman or an Indian?" The teenagers, impressed by their visit and the need for blood, begin a community campaign in which all races can participate: "this battle against ignorance is just as important as any battle on the war front. It can mean victory over hatred, division, prejudice, and distortion."[58]

The American government and American labor unions also participated in efforts to promote "the brotherhood of man" and blood unity. Drawing on the 1943 pamphlet authored by anthropologists Ruth Benedict and Gene Weltfish entitled "Races of Mankind," the United Auto Workers sponsored the production of an animated cartoon that included discussion of blood types and racial difference. "Brotherhood of Man" had a distinguished pedigree; screenwriters for the cartoon included Ring Lardner, Junior (a recent Academy Award winner for *Woman of the Year*); Maurice Rapf, whose writing credits included *Song of the South;* and Phil Eastman, a writer for animated training films released by the Army Signal Corps during World War II. In the cartoon, a patient who needs a transfusion receives blood from his own brother and dies. "Brother or no brother," the narrator intones, "what he needs is type A. And the right blood donor for him could belong to any race, since the four blood types appear in all races." When the patient receives the right blood type, he recovers. "We're not really so different at all," Henry, one of the cartoon character concludes.[59] Blood is red—not white, yellow or black.

Red, White, and Black

The issues raised by the racial segregation of blood during the war continued to fester in the postwar years. In 1948, the absence of racial labels on blood created controversy at Gallinger General Hospital. Health care in the nation's capital was marked by highly racialized boundaries. Although Gallinger Hospital admitted "Negro patients" (70% of the patients were African American), the District of Columbia Medical Society, which controlled the hospital, opposed the admission of Negro physicians. Just 2 years earlier, a young Negro woman in labor attempted to reach the maternity ward at Gallinger Hospital. Realizing the birth of her child was imminent, she sought admission to a church-supported hospital in the District, but was refused. The woman delivered her baby on the sidewalk in front of the hospital, where they waited for an ambulance to take them to Gallinger.[60] In 1948, Gallinger made headlines when the hospital's chief of staff rejected offers of free blood from the District Red Cross Blood Center because the center refused to designate the racial origins of the blood and plasma it supplied. According to the chief of the hospital's blood bank, transfusions of white blood to Negro patients or Negro blood to white patients was expressly forbidden by order of the hospital's executive committee. Several days later, the hospital lifted the ban on Red Cross blood despite the telephone call to a District Health Officer from an unidentified man who "threatened to take him across the river and fill him full of lead if he dared to allow 'mixed blood' transfusions."[61]

Several months after the controversy over Gallinger blood, the issue of race, loyalty, and the blood bank arose in a different context. In the face of concern over communist threats to the American government, members of a regional loyalty review board asked a federal employee for her opinion of the separation of white and black blood in the Red Cross blood bank. Harry W. Blair, a member of the Loyalty Review Board, explained that he had asked Dorothy Bailey, an African American woman: "Did you ever write a letter to the Red Cross about the segregation of blood?"[62] Once Bailey's suit against the board was settled, Blair explained that "one of the principal projects of the Communist Party has been to inveigle

Negroes into joining the Party. All 'front and Communist dominated organizations play up and emphasize all the wrongs with regard to discrimination, segregation, etc., of which the Negro race so rightly complains." He described how "alert officers of the Metropolitan Police Force" had recognized the objection to blood segregation as "'party line' technic [sic]." The police made a record of the letter signed by Bailey because of her association with United Public Workers, a group suspected of Communist domination.[63]

The ongoing controversy over racializing the blood supply continued to create problems for the American Red Cross. In 1947, the organization announced a new policy in which blood would no longer carry labels identifying the racial origins of the donor. Although this step was hailed by many African American and white groups, the controversy did not disappear. One of the issues that faced the Red Cross was how or whether to designate race on the proposed Blood Donor Master Card. Initially, the Red Cross planned to offer a choice between five group designations: Caucasian, Negro, Indian, Mexican, and Japanese and others. Jesse Thomas, assistant to the Red Cross vice-president for public relations and liaison to the African American community, warned about the fallout from such a plan: "I believe Jews, Greeks, Irish, Germans, and Italians and other ethnic groups are to be included in the Caucasian column." Thomas predicted "We may, therefore, not only expect violent reaction from Negroes and interracially minded white persons in organizations, but from the Indians, Mexicans, Japanese, and others and their friends and supporters."[64] The issue of racial labels on blood continued to arise.

In 1948, officials from the Red Cross decided that no designation of racial origins would appear on the labels of blood bottles. They made an exception when the local medical advisory committees requested such a designation. The medical advisory committees of all Southern blood centers voted to require some means to identify the racial origins of the blood donor. In 1949, the District of Columbia Red Cross made news when it rejected blood from the Interchurch Fellowship of Washington, a group including native Americans, Catholics, African Americans, Nisei, Chinese-Americans, Asiatic Indians, Jews, Mennonites, and Seventh-Day Adventists. The fellowship had requested that their blood be accepted as "human blood" without identifying the racial origins of the donor. The District Red Cross refused reportedly because they sought to maximize the choices of both doctors and patients. For this reason, they recorded "the color of the blood donor and their race, as American Indian, Japanese, Caucasian, or 'all other.'"[65] In addition to the labeling issue, Southern blood centers faced the problem of complying with the segregation laws of several states. In compliance with state law, for example, the Red Cross built separate toilets for whites and blacks, although these groups could donate blood in the same donor rooms. In cities with strict laws about the separation of the races, white and Negro blood donors were processed on different days. At the Birmingham, Alabama blood center, for example, Thursdays were reserved "only for Negroes." The blood center in Memphis, Tennessee also restricted Negro donors to specific days to ensure racial segregation.

The issue of race recurred in 1950, when staff at the United Nations (UN) offered to provide blood for UN forces stationed in Korea. The blood donor committee informed Trygve Lie, the first United Nations Secretary-General, that they would not cooperate with any Red Cross agency that required racial designations on its donor cards. Suggestions that the category "nationality" be substituted for race; that race be noted with a symbol "such as 'X,' 'Y' or 'Z' be used to designate blood from a Caucasian, Negro or Mongolian"; and even the substitution of numbers for racial group were floated between the Red Cross and the medical staff at the UN. When the blood bank opened, the UN maintained a separate set of donor cards without racial classifications.[66] In December 1951, the daughter of Japanese premier Hideki Tojo appeared at the UN blood bank in Tokyo to donate blood for UN troops in Korea. Kimie Tojo made two trips to the blood bank; the first time the crowd of photographers and reporters caused a rise in her blood pressure. Her second trip was more successful. Transfusions with American plasma was credited with saving her father's life after his failed suicide attempt in September 1945. Tojo was convicted of war crimes and executed in 1948.[67]

Human Blood Is Human Blood

In 1950, following a decade of strife over racial classifications, the Red Cross's Board of Governors voted to eliminate all racial designations for blood donors. Welcoming the decision, a *New York Times* editorialist explained "human blood is human blood regardless of the degree of pigmentation in the skin."[68] But the ongoing social pressures to remove race as a category in the blood supply encountered new resistance amid claims for a scientific justification for same-race transfusions. In 1941, scientific assumptions about the blood supply (the failure to detect differences in the bloods of whites and blacks) lost out to social preferences for same-race transfusions. In 1959, scientific assumptions about blood again took a back seat to social pressures; this time, to ignore the putative biologic differences in the blood of whites and blacks.

In November 1959, Dr. John Scudder, director of a prominent New York blood bank, offered a "new philosophy" of blood transfusion at the annual meeting of the American Association of Blood Banks (AABB). Together with three colleagues at New York City's Presbyterian Hospital, Scudder recommended that blood donors be selected with a view to minimizing sensitization to the growing list of blood factors. The ideal blood donor for the patient was the patient or, if not possible, from his or her identical twin. The next best donors would be compatible blood relatives and compatible blood from donors of the same ethnic group. Using blood from members of the patient's own race would increase the safety of transfusion. "It was wrong," he explained to a *New York Times* reporter, "to give the blood of a white donor to a Negro patient. In some particular groups, such transfusions would be six to eight times more dangerous than would be the transfusion of a Negro's blood to a white patient."[69]

Scudder directed the blood bank at Presbyterian Hospital. A one-time supervisor and later collaborator with Charles Drew, Scudder realized the political consequences of his call for a new philosophy. As he explained to the reporter, "the nub of the problem" was the fact that no two persons possessed blood that was "exactly alike," except for identical twins. "This may sound wrong sociologically," Scudder insisted, "but it is scientifically correct." Blood banks, he explained, could not possibly catalogue all the known variations in human blood, which included 12 main blood groups systems and more than 20 rarer blood groups. Scudder explained that Negroes would be the beneficiaries of the new philosophy, inasmuch as giving white blood to Negroes was more dangerous than transfusing Negro blood into whites.

The blood banker was reportedly surprised when, 3 days after this initial report, the *New York Times* published a story about how 7 members of the Columbia University Seminar on Genetics and the Evolution of Man publicly challenged the race-to-race transfusion policy of their medical colleagues. Prominent members of the Seminar, some 30 Columbia faculty members, including geneticists L.C. Dunn and Theodosius Dobzhansky, denounced the race-to-race policy: "The so-called new philosophy serves no useful purpose except to reinforce the old philosophy of race prejudice, which has been shown repeatedly to rest on ignorance rather than biological or medical knowledge." On November 12, 1959 administrators at Presbyterian Hospital issued a press release affirming the medical center's policy of accepting donors of all races and explaining that medical compatibility between donors and recipients was the sole criterion used in making blood transfusions.[70] In Washington, D.C., researchers at the National Institutes of Health, Georgetown University Medical School, and the Red Cross Regional Blood Center agreed that blood differed between individuals, but argued that racial differences were no more likely to create problems than other factors.[71]

What scientific evidence prompted Scudder's call for same-race transfusions? In the 1950s, researchers had discovered several new blood groups, many of which were distributed along racial lines. These blood groups included the Kell blood group (found in the serum of Mrs. Kell in 1946) and the Duffy system (found in 1950 in the serum of Mr. Duffy, who apparently gave his permission for his name to be used). In 1951, the Kidd blood group was named for a factor found in the blood of a newly delivered woman, Mrs. Kidd, whose infant son developed hemolytic disease of the newborn.[72] In 1953, blood specialist Alexander Wiener and his colleagues reported that a "Negroid woman, aged 35" suffered a fatal transfusion reaction when she received blood from a second donor. The researchers pointed to a new, previously unknown blood factor, which they designated with the letter "U" (they noted that no "satisfactory symbol" could be devised from the patient's name). After the woman's death, they obtained blood postmortem and used it to test over 1000 individuals. "Since the patient herself was Negroid, it was anticipated that such persons would be more apt to occur among Negroids than among Caucasoids, so that both Negroids and Caucasoids were included in the study." Of the nearly 1100 persons tested, the blood factor U was present in every white persons and in 421 of the 425 black persons tested.[73] This report of a new antigen U was quickly followed by a report of another "new" antigen "common in Negroes, rare in white people." Mr. V, a patient at St. Luke's Hospital in New York City, suffered from an "obscure anemia," which physicians treated with multiple transfusions. When blood from his 27th donor was cross-matched, the bloods were not compatible. His prospective donor was Negro, as were six of his previous donors. When their blood was checked, the antigen was discovered; rare in whites, it was found frequently in New York Negroes, and even more frequently in West Africans. (The researchers explained that in selecting New York Negroes to be tested, they used "darkness of skin" as a criterion.)[74] Other reports of variations in the Rh factor among both American Negroes and Africans also peppered the literature.

As the number of blood transfusions increased, the possibility of sensitizing someone to one of these and other blood groups increased. As a blood banker, Scudder was concerned about the implications for trying to find compatible blood for those individuals who had been sensitized by previous transfusions. To make this point, Scudder and his co-author William Wigle, medical director of the Canadian Red Cross Blood Services in Hamilton, Ontario, published case reports from their respective practices to illustrate the need for greater selectivity in selecting donors.

Scudder described a recent case from Presbyterian Hospital in which a "white war veteran" became sensitized by a previous transfusion given him during exploratory open-heart surgery. The man, whose blood was established as group B, Rh positive, received blood from a seemingly compatible B-positive "Negro donor" whose blood was also Kidd positive. This initial transfusion produced no adverse reactions; but the surgical patient subsequently developed a protective antibody belonging to the Kidd system (a rare agglutinin occurring only once in every 30,000 cross-matches). When the surgical team prepared to undertake open-heart surgery on the war veteran to correct the defect found in the initial surgery, the surgeon asked the blood bank for 14 pints of compatible blood (the surgery was very blood intensive). Meeting this request required extensive networking within the eight metropolitan blood banks. To ensure that the donated blood would be compatible with the newly sensitized surgical patient, blood bank personnel had to obtain antiserum in sufficient quantities to screen potential blood. The need for antiserum required repeated bleedings of the patient, who then required retransfusion in light of his loss of red blood cells. Some 700 donors had to be screened and processed to obtain the necessary 14 pints for the operation to proceed. "In summary," Scudder noted, "the mischief done by a single blood transfusion necessitated this herculean endeavor to secure compatible blood for the open-heart operation."[75]

Canadian physician William Wigle offered a case report from his blood banking experience intended to illustrate the virtues of same-race transfusions. The patient was a 38-year-old black woman with sickle cell anemia. As treatment for her condition, she had received an estimated 72 units of blood between 1940 and 1958. As a resident of Hamilton, Ontario, she had received transfusions of blood donated by whites. Wigle assumed that none of the blood she had received came from "Negro donors" since only 1 in every 2500 donors in Hamilton was a "Negro." By 1956, she had developed an antibody detectable only by a special test (the Coombs test). When she received a transfusion of 1000 cc of blood in 1957, she experienced severe complications. In 1959, she survived another severe transfusion reaction when she entered Hamilton (Ontario) General Hospital for treatment of pain, and doctors detected the presence of another antibody in her blood. "It was difficult to find any blood compatible with hers (84 bottles of A positive blood were cross-matched to find two compatible ones.) Future transfusions will be limited by the fact and also by the dangers of developing other antibodies." In other words, the lesser-known blood groups represented an important potential source of difficulty for blood bankers and for patients, especially those in need of multiple transfusions.

Employing the "new philosophy" of selecting donors from the same family and the same race, Scudder and Wigle argued, would benefit such patients as the woman with sickle cell and the war veteran undergoing heart surgery. In the selection of blood donors, the physicians concluded, "'Unto each his own,' with the family relative assuming a far more important role, is the future pattern of blood transfusions."[76] Perhaps one of the strangest things about this paper was its publication in the journal of the National Medical Association (the NMA was established in 1895 as a professional forum for black physicians, who continued to be excluded by the AMA through 1968). The Howard University anatomist Montague Cobb, the journal's long-time editor, explained that his decision to publish the controversial paper reflected Scudder's personal association with one of the century's preeminent black physicians. "Because, as is well known to readers of this journal, the late Dr. Charles R. Drew of Howard University, who directed the Blood for Britain project and set up the first American Red Cross Blood Bank during World War II, did his doctoral thesis on 'Banked Blood' under the supervision of Dr. Scudder, it could not be readily inferred that racial bias played a part in the authors' conclusions. Such bias, indeed, Dr. Scudder straightaway denied."[77] The two physicians had collaborated on 12 scientific papers published between June 1939 and June 1941, and Drew also contributed to Scudder's 1940 book on *Shock—Blood Studies as a Guide to Therapy*.[78]

Scudder continued to argue that science, rather than stereotypes, prompted the new philosophy of blood transfusion. "There is no racial bias in this," he informed a reporter from *Jet*. "It is purely a medical fact."[79] But Scudder must have been aware that the concept of race was itself in flux. One of his colleagues at Columbia University was the geneticist Leslie Dunn, a contributor to the UNESCO's 1950 Statement on Race. However, Scudder chose a second, perhaps even stranger, publication in which to pursue the potential for racial incompatibilities in blood transfusion. His paper appeared in the first volume of a new professional journal—*Mankind Quarterly*—dedicated to discussions of race and ethnology.[80] Promoted by the newly formed International Association for the Advancement of Ethnology and Eugenics, the quarterly was ostensibly founded to "permit a free and open discussion of racial and related problems." The founders of the association and the journal were closely aligned with the Liberty Lobby, a neo-Nazi organization, and other proponents of the Radical Right. Instead of an open and scientific discussion about race, the journal offered a "respectable academic platform for ideas about scientific racism more akin to the publications of the Ku Klux Klan and the Nazi party."[81]

A number of critics assailed Scudder's new philosophy and its social and political implications. Edward Mazique, president of the NMA, dismissed press reports of same-race transfusions as "fantastic."[82] In a widely reported statement, Mazique compared the efforts of the New York blood banker to the antebellum Southern physician Samuel Cartwright and his creation of the notorious disease category "drapetomania" (the disease causing slaves to run away from their masters). The physician challenged the scientific basis for the claims that the bloods of whites and blacks could be so readily distinguished in light of the considerable "cross-breeding between colored and whites since 1619."[83] Mazique blasted Scudder's effort as a political ploy to foster the development of segregation among northern whites. "There is nothing new in the application of the scientific approach for segregation purposes, and such findings can have no effect but to continue our people in an inferior role," Mazique noted. "Chattel slavery was conceived of and supported in its time by religious leaders on moral grounds, by scientists for physical reasons; statistically documented by the social scientists and politically activated by the politicians."[84]

Leaders of the American blood banking community similarly rejected the Scudder plan for same-race transfusion. E. R. Jennings, president of the AABB, emphasized that the Association and the majority of its members did not share the Presbyterian banker's views. Acknowledging that some races do have higher frequencies of certain blood factors, which made matching bloods easier, the organization's leadership categorically denied any justification for Scudder's conclusion that intermixing the blood of racially dissimilar individuals represented a danger. "The segregation of blood on a racial basis," Jennings remarked in a press release, "is unnecessary and would do more harm than good."[85]

Scudder's own institution, Presbyterian Hospital, moved swiftly to separate its policies in blood transfusion from the philosophy Scudder outlined. Less than a week after Scudder's address, Presbyterian Hospital, in response to repeated inquiries about the doctor's remarks, released a statement confirming that their blood bank not only welcomed donors of all races but also did not use racial origins when determining the medical compatibility of blood in transfusions.[86] At Columbia University, geneticists Theodosius Dobzhanksy and Leslie C. Dunn, as well as Dr. Philip Levine, one of the discoverers with Karl Landsteiner of the Rh factor, conceded Scudder's point that there existed a number of blood factors not tested in routine blood bank preparation, which could sensitize a blood recipient and cause difficulty in subsequent transfusions: "These other blood types, like the better-known blood types, do tend to occur in different frequencies in different human populations." But they challenged Scudder's contention that estimates about the probability of incompatibility between the races were greater than intragroup incompatibility estimates. "Since even the patient's own mother or brother often differs from him in many blood factors, and a person of a different race may well possess compatible blood, the only satisfactory criterion in blood transfusion is the testing of the blood for the standard factors and as many others as practical, plus actual testing by cross-matching of the proposed donor blood and a sample of the patient's own blood. With these tests passed, the blood of any persons of any race will be satisfactory for transfusion."[87]

Montague Cobb offered members of the Columbia Seminar on Genetics the opportunity to comment on Scudder and Wigle's article. Geneticist Leslie Dunn rejected the statistical basis for the new philosophy of blood transfusion and the rule about using members of the same race. Analyzing a chart supplied by Scudder and Wigle, Dunn pointed out that a person of whatever race, negative for any one of the 19 listed antigens (except c, P, and Jk[a]) could more safely receive blood from a Negro donor than from a white donor. This was true because Negroes were more likely to be negative for these antigens. White blood was better only in the case of individuals negative for the types c, P, and Jk^a. Thus, if a negative patient were white, preferring a Negro donor would lead to less risk than following the rule of transfusing only within the white races.[88] At the same time, Dunn praised Scudder and Wigle for urging that doctors use blood transfusion only when necessary in light of the fact that a single blood transfusion had the potential to sensitize some individuals and thus create potential problems for future transfusions. Doctors from both Howard University Medical School and Meharry Medical College (two historically black medical schools) also endorsed this position, including Howard's William Bullock, who agreed that autotransfusion (the use of the patient's own blood), blood from a twin, and blood from a compatible family member were preferable to using blood from random donors. Like Dunn, he challenged the claim that blood donors selected from the same race or same ethnic group would necessarily be safer than blood from a person of a different race.

Dunn thanked Scudder for bringing the issue of interracial blood transfusion once again to the headlines. Dr. Edward Mazique was far less thankful.[89] Mazique organized a meeting with the Manhattan Central Medical Society, a constituent society of the National Medical Association, where Scudder publicly retreated from his earlier statements about the need for a new philosophy in blood transfusion. He reportedly conceded that his references to race were unfortunate and that the popular press had grossly exaggerated his discussion of the potential dangers of transfusing across the color line.[90] In some ways, it is difficult to believe that Scudder had not anticipated the adverse reaction that his call for same-race transfusions would foster. In the paper he co-authored with William Wigle, they had cited I. Dunsford's analysis of the racial aspects of blood transfusion in South Africa, where the Medical and Dental Council discussed, in late 1956, a recommendation that labeling be introduced to distinguish the donated blood of Europeans and non-Europeans. Even within South Africa, the recommendation for same-race transfusions and its scientific basis had been hotly disputed. Whereas the head of the Blood Research Group Unit of the South African Institute of Medical Research insisted that it would be sounder medical practice to transfuse African patients with the blood of Africans and Europeans with the blood of Europeans, the Director of the Johannesburg Blood Transfusion Service argued that "Any discrimination in the form of the label for European blood cannot be justified on scientific grounds, and such distinction should not be enforced by regulation."[91]

Scudder may not have anticipated how readily segregationists would take up his call for same-race transfusion. In December 1959, Charles Smith, editor of the *Truth Seeker*, a self-proclaimed journal for "reasoners and racists," described Scudder's presentation to the AABB and emphasized his warning that the call for same-race transfusions was wrong sociologically but nonetheless scientifically correct. "The war on physics," Smith noted, "is perpetual. Led by certain Jews, the Brotherhood Boys, the repeaters of slogans, such as, We are all one, Togetherness, and No discrimination, suppress the truth when it does not fit in with their socialized biology and genetics."[92] Smith concluded by identifying the names of the majority of the participants in the Seminar on Genetics who had condemned Scudder as Jewish. In January 1960, another publication, *The American Nationalist*, praised Scudder for his courage in defying the conventional wisdom in the centers of higher learning by identifying the hazards of cross-race transfusions. "The time is near," the paper warned

> when Americans will discover that for years the health of their families and loved ones has been deliberately placed in danger by blood banks who for "sociological reasons" (or under pressure of propaganda) have failed to protect them from tainted Negro blood transfusions. No one can say how many thousands of critically ill patients have been made sicker, or even killed, by this evil practice, but one thing is certain: what has been perpetuated in the sweet name of racial "equality" and "democracy" is one of the most vicious scandals in all American history.[93]

Scudder's call for a new philosophy on racial lines offered a scientific justification for laws requiring that bottles of blood be labeled with the donor's race. But the members of White Citizen's Councils hardly needed such a justification for what they saw as "unnatural" and "unhealthy"—the movement of blood between white and black bodies.

There Ought to Be A Law!

In 1954, the United States Supreme Court rocked American society with its landmark decision in *Brown v. Board of Education*, finding that segregation in education was inherently unequal. Although the Court did not require the immediate desegregation of all schools, allowing a "deliberate speed" approach to integrating the American educational system, the so-called "Black Monday" (the day the Court announced its school decision) became a rallying cry for southern segregationists. In the wake of the Brown decision, segregationists organized White Citizens' Councils throughout the South to oppose integration, revived the Ku Klux Klan, and encouraged southern legislators to preserve the traditional institutions of southern life.[94]

Amid the turbulence over desegregation, legislators in southern states turned their attention to the blood supply and the need to ensure the physical separation of the races. As in World War II, blood carried enormous symbolic weight for those on both sides of the segregation issue. "The blood of one people is no darker or more virile than that of another, but the racially prejudiced, their fears intensified by hate, have magnified the image of the Negro from a conscience-burdened shadow into a seven-tailed monster about to destroy the sacred world of white. To them, one drop of the potent stuff [Negro blood] is more powerful than the Jupiter 'C' rocket, more threatening than atomic fallout, more dreaded than a universe dominated by communists."[95] Some southern legislators regarded the transfusion of such blood as a fate worse than death, including South Carolina Representative George S. Harrell, who informed his colleagues in the House of Representatives that he would refuse the blood from a black donor even it if meant his own certain death.[96]

The legislation regarding racial designations on blood represented only a footnote to the larger battles being fought over the desegregation of American schools, health care, and the Civil Rights movement.[97] But symbolic battles can be satisfying to those who wage them, and the victories and losses all the sweeter for their simplicity. Blood donation and transfusion offered an arena for some southerners to demonstrate the inherent weakness of "Negro blood" and the need to preserve blood purity in the face of threats from physicians and organizations like the American Red Cross.

In 1957, Red Cross officials from the southeastern United States called attention to publications like *The White Sentinel*, which called on the Red Cross to reverse its policy of pooling white and black blood. The reasons for segregating the blood were twofold: the hereditary disease sickle cell anemia found "only in Negroes" and the fact that no studies had been done to ensure the safety of interracial transfusion. "Until it is definitely established that no harm can come to a White person or his descendants from the infusion of negroid blood into his veins, the Red Cross should stop mixing the blood collected in its blood program." Because there was no cure for sickle cell anemia and because there was no evidence that the transfusion of blood from those sick with sickle cell anemia was safe for recipients, the *Sentinel* warned "If the Red Cross continues to racially mix the blood it collects, then it will be up to states to pass legislation forbidding it."[98] In 1958, Red Cross officials monitored the distribution of pamphlets such as "Sickle Cell Anemia: Found in Negro Blood," that were distributed in churches in Lexington, Kentucky. The anonymous author of the pamphlet blamed "Communists, religious leaders and others" who claimed that all blood was the same, but failed to explain why the "dread sickle cell anemia" is found principally among Negroes. The pamphleteer insisted that "White America" was vulnerable because, when they needed blood, they were too sick to know or care that they were getting the "right type" of white blood.[99]

Southern state legislatures quickly turned their attention to such legislation. In January 1958, Georgia became the first state to consider blood labeling laws. When Senator Quill Sammon sponsored the bill requiring all blood to bear a label indicating the racial origins of the donor, he explicitly identified the legislation as a "segregation move."[100] The bill stipulated that any person about to receive a blood transfusion or their next of kin be informed about the racial origins of the donated blood. The legislation further required that all collected human blood be labeled either "Caucasian, Negroid, or Mongoloid," and specified that violators would be guilty of a misdemeanor and sentenced up to 18 months in jail or a $1000 fine for violating the law. In February 1958, the Georgia State Senate voted unanimously (35–0) to require that all blood be labeled with the race of the donor. "This is not a prejudice bill," Sammon informed reporters. "It is a precaution to preserve the dignity and identity of each race and prevent the mixing of the races."[101] When the House took up the bill, representatives voted to table the bill, killing its chances for passage. "If I were dying," House Representative W.C. Parker explained, "I wouldn't care what kind of blood I got if it saved my life."[102] (The legislature was also preoccupied with legislation that would do away with using different colored paper to distinguish the tax returns of white and Negro citizens. The segregationists successfully maintained the right to keep whites and blacks from filing returns on the same colored paper.)[103]

In March 1958, the Mississippi House of Representatives passed without a dissenting vote a bill requiring that blood for transfusions be labeled to show the race of the donor. The Mississippi law required that recipients of blood transfusion be informed of the race of the donor. However, in the event of an emergency, the attending physician was free to waive this notification, but was nonetheless required to prepare a certificate stating the race of the donor that would become part of the patient's case record. Blood was not the only bodily substance that concerned the Mississippi White Citizens' Council. In 1958, when a scientist suggested the stockpiling of human sperm to counteract radiation damage caused by nuclear warfare, the organization demanded racial labels on sperm to permit repopulation along racial lines.[104]

Representative Elmo Anderson, sponsor of the Mississippi race blood label, insisted that blood must be labeled because of the potential threat of disease transmission. The disease here was not syphilis, but a disease newly visible to the medical establishment. Anderson put it more bluntly: "Negroes were susceptible to a disease, sickle cell anemia, which was not known to any other race."[105] The Mississippi legislator's concern with the "Negro" malady of sickle cell anemia reflected intensifying interest in the disease during the 1950s. The first disease known in terms of its molecular biology, sickle cell anemia, as historian Keith Wailoo has argued, transformed the disease from an invisible plague into an "archetypal disease—with different lessons for different observers."[106] For white segregationists like Elmo Anderson, developments in molecular biology offered an illustration grounded in modern biology for the need to maintain the separation of the blood of the three races. But there were apparently other physiologic reasons as well. Segregationists cited the research of Dr. William Levin at the University of Texas, whose work on behalf of the U.S. Air Force School of Aviation Medicine reportedly revealed that Negroes with sickle cell trait suffered damage to the spleen and other complications at high altitudes.[107] These arguments appeared in segregationist literature exhorting voters to push for federal law to prevent intermarriage and reduce the burden of sickle cell anemia.

Red Cross officials continued to insist that sickle cell anemia was a hereditary disease and not communicated via the blood. Still, the medical director of the American National Red Cross asked the Committee on Blood and Related Problems of the National Academy of Sciences to issue an expert statement on transfusion and sickle cell trait blood. (Sickle cell anemia occurs when both parents provide the gene for the sickle-shaped hemoglobin; sickle cell trait could be distinguished from the anemia by the quantity of hemoglobin S in the blood.) The Committee on Blood endorsed the Red Cross position that persons with sickle cell anemia would not qualify to donate blood; moreover, even if by chance they did so, sickle cell anemia was a hereditary disease—it was not acquired. The blood from an individual with sickle cell trait could pose problems if the recipient also possessed the sickle cell trait or had chronic lung disease. But even in such cases, the Committee on Blood insisted that transfusions with sickle-cell trait blood would be "normally effective for acute blood replacement and cause no untoward clinical reactions."[108]

Unlike the Mississippi and Georgia legislators, lawmakers in Louisiana, spurred by the White Citizens Council, enacted a law in June 1958 requiring human blood donated for transfusion be labeled as "Caucasian, Negroid, or Mongoloid, or some equivalent designation." The law further specified that a recipient must be informed whenever blood from a "racially different" donor was to be used, except in cases of emergency, when interracial transfusions without patient consent was permitted. Violation of the blood label and notification law carried a penalty of $100, 30 days in jail, or both.[109]

In 1959, legislatures in four southern states again took up the issue of laws to require racial labels on blood. In May 1959, the Florida Senate voted 76–0 to require labels on bottled human blood to indicate the race of the donor, but the bill failed to pass in the House of Representatives.[110] In the Georgia legislature, which had considered such legislation in the preceding year, the measure was also defeated. In South Carolina, State Representative George S. Harrell sponsored House bill H-1024 to require blood banks to label all blood showing the race and sex of the donor. "The Supreme Court and Eisenhower are going to beat you on integrating the schools," Harrell informed his fellow legislators, "but that is no reason why we should mix the blood in South Carolina."[111] Later that year, Alabama's House Bill #227 requiring labeling of blood by race "quietly passed away" when the legislature adjourned in October 1959.[112]

Lawmakers in Arkansas were the only legislators to follow Louisiana's lead in enacting legislation requiring hospitals and physicians to inform transfusion recipients about the racial origins of the blood donated for transfusion. In April 1959, Arkansas Governor Orval E. Faubus signed into law a bill to require that blood for transfusions be labeled by the race of the donor. Two years earlier, in 1957, Faubus had garnered national attention when he called in the Arkansas National Guard to forestall the integration of Central High School in Little Rock. When rioting erupted in the city, President Dwight D. Eisenhower sent U.S. troops to Little Rock and placed the National Guard under federal command in order to ensure the integration of the high school. Known for his political expediency, the Governor offered various explanations for his support of the blood-labeling act. Citing a "a great demand by the public" for the adoption of the racial blood label law, Faubus dismissed the opposition of the medical profession and others, which "boiled down mainly to objections to the administrative detail of labeling."[113] In an "exclusive" interview with *Jet*, Faubus claimed that he had little interest in the measure, which had been introduced independently of his administration. But like the Mississippi legislator, Faubus cited sickle cell anemia as one of the reasons for the need of the law. The legislation, he argued, would do much to "relieve the fears of white patients about getting diseases like 'sickel [sic] cell anemia' from Negro blood."[114] In the 1960 legislative sessions, bills for blood labeling by race were considered in Virginia and once again in the Georgia legislature.[115] Although the Georgia House voted 107–2 in favor of a "racial blood ban," the bill failed for the third year in a row to pass the Senate.[116] But even though the Georgia bill failed three times, blood continued to be labeled and segregated along racial lines. According to a 1967 *Wall Street Journal* article, the director of the blood bank at a large Atlanta hospital reported that they used Red Cross blood (which remained unlabeled by racial origin of the donor) only when absolutely necessary. "We keep our blood that we get from donors coming here segregated. When we have Negro patients we use Negro or Red Cross blood, and when we have white patients we definitely use white blood."[117]

The African American press followed the legislative efforts to achieve and enforce blood-labeling laws. In September 1958, the Baltimore *Afro-American*, for example, reported that the "Jim-crow blood policy" in Louisiana would contribute to the death of a 3-year-old boy in a New Orleans hospital. Already the veteran of two major heart operations, the boy required extensive blood transfusions. But his parents were not able to pay the necessary fees for blood ($45 a pint), and the Red Cross, which had adopted a policy of race-blind blood collection in 1951, refused to participate in the blood labeling required by Louisiana law and would not donate blood to the child.[118] Nine months after Governor Faubus signed the Arkansas blood bill into law in 1959, the same newspaper reported few signs of white anxiety about the possibility of developing sickle cell anemia through receiving a transfusion from a Negro donor. The *Afro-American* did note that permitting recipients to reject blood from racially dissimilar donors produced an unexpected result. "Given the bill's sponsors and backers, the biggest slap in the face was the fact that in 9 months, there have been more rejections of white blood by colored persons than the other way around."[119]

In the 1960s, changes in civil rights compelled some reexamination of blood segregation policies. After 1964 and the passage of the Civil Rights Act, the Public Health Service ordered hospitals to desegregate blood supplies or risk the loss of Medicare, Medicaid, and Hill-Burton funds. In 1969, Arkansas repealed its blood labeling law.[120] In Louisiana, where the law remained on the books, the Office for Civil Rights at the Department of Health, Education, and Welfare (HEW) investigated the separation and identification of blood by race. When Leon Panetta, the special assistant to HEW Secretary Robert Finch, informed Louisiana Senator Russell Long's office of this practice, one of his aides snorted, "Wouldn't you know it—we're number 50 again."[121] Panetta and his health division director Lou Rives also informed Governor John McKeithen that the Louisiana blood statute was unconstitutional and violated Title VI of the Civil Rights Act. McKeithan was "clearly from the old school in terms of politics in Louisiana," Panetta recalled in 2002. "He knew that ultimately things would have to change."[122]

An investigation into hospital practices in Louisiana in 1969 indicated considerable variability in the implementation of the blood label statute. Some hospitals, fearing a lawsuit from a segregationist patient, followed the law to the letter. At another hospital, every transfusion was regarded as an "emergency," and emergency transfusions did not require patient consent or patient notification. At another hospital, which remained unintegrated, the hospital refused to accept as a blood credit the donation of blood from a Negro friend of one of the patients. When the patient refused to pay for the blood, the hospital apparently obtained a debtor's judgment against the patient and was able to collect the fee.

Complying with the requirement for racial designation on donated blood created difficulties when blood was shipped into the state. For example, some Louisiana hospitals only accepted blood from out-of-state hospitals if the blood carried a racial label. The American Red Cross, which officially maintained a policy of nondiscrimination in blood banking, did permit its blood collection agencies in Mobile and Birmingham, Alabama to send racially labeled blood in response to requests from Louisiana hospitals. The Public Health Service (PHS) hospital in New Orleans reported frustration with the blood segregation policy. Although the PHS hospital generally sought out-of-state and unlabeled blood, officials reported that blood from the New Orleans Blood Bank and other local hospitals was sometimes used. The PHS removed the information about the racial origins of the donor from the blood. More frustrating to PHS officials was the fact that the hospital was not able to trade expiring stock with local hospitals since the racial origins of the PHS blood were not recorded. For that reason, the PHS was often forced to throw out blood and, lacking blood for trade, was forced to purchase blood.[123]

In 1970, Representative Ernest Morial, "Louisiana's only Negro legislator," urged his fellow lawmakers to repeal the blood labeling statute.[124] Despite Morial's warning about the loss of up to $50 million in federal funds, the legislature rejected the bill. "I don't want no nigger blood in my veins, and I refuse to have it," insisted Representative Archie Davis, a white legislator. "I would see my family die and go to eternity before I would see them have a drop of nigger blood in them." In light of the vote, an African American soldier in Vietnam described how his friends from Louisiana were altering their dog tags to reflect their new blood type, from

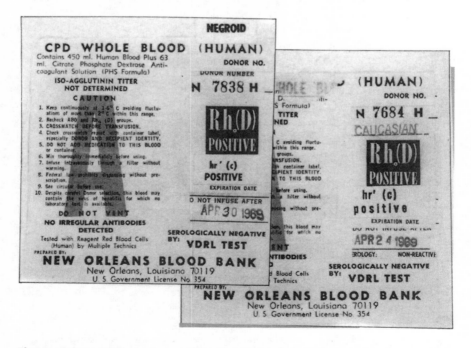

Figure 4.3 In 1969, the journal *Hospital Practice* noted the ongoing controversy over racial labels on blood in Louisiana blood banks (*Hospital Practice* [July 1969]: 21.)

"O Positive" to "O Pos-N" for O Positive Negro. "Any joker who want to lay there dying while I have life-sustaining blood or life-saving blood running warm in my body," the solider observed. "May God have Mercy on his soul and grant his wish. I can stand there and watch him die."[125] Morial tried a second time to gather the votes necessary to repeal the racial blood labeling law. Despite the support of some white legislators, including New Orleans Representative Edward Booker, who acknowledged that there were "more Negroes on the front lines in Vietnam right now in proportion to their part of the population than whites," and despite the fact that the blood of African Americans was "just as red, just as American, just as precious," Morial's bill was defeated.[126]

In light of the federal government's investigation into the blood segregation practices and the threatened loss of Medicare revenues, the Governor, who was reportedly surprised to learn of the existence of the law, promised to repeal the measure when the legislature met the following year. In June 1972, Louisiana legislators repealed the blood label laws, as well as laws restricting race mixing in dancing, marriage, seating on trains, restrooms, and water fountains.[127]

Seeking Minority Donors

John Scudder's call for a new philosophy of same-race transfusions was soundly rejected. Yet, the issue of sensitizing transfusion recipients, especially those who received large numbers of transfusions from different donors, did not go away. As William Wigle had pointed out in 1959, one of the populations most likely to become sensitized were patients with sickle cell anemia. One significant therapy for sickle cell anemia was transfusion; patients received large numbers of transfusions. In 1959, *Ebony* magazine profiled a young sufferer with the disease. As a 21-year-old college student in Huntington, West Virginia, Marclan Walker had already received more than 250 pints of blood from parents, friends, doctors, nurses, and hundreds of blood donors. The only treatment for her disease was transfusion, but she ran the risk of becoming sensitized to blood antigens and suffering a transfusion reaction.[128]

Some physicians opted to use only blood donated by African Americans for their patients with sickle cell anemia. (In other words, it was safer to use same-race transfusions, just as Scudder had proposed.) In 1968, the American Red Cross established a Rare Donor Registry to help local blood banks identify individuals with unusual blood proteins. In 1986, when the American Red Cross sought to broaden the base of a program to recruit donors of rare blood types, they recruited a black pediatrician, who headed a local Sickle Cell Foundation. This pediatrician explained that patients with specific antibodies created serious logistical problems when doctors sought to provide compatible blood for chronically ill sickle cell patients who underwent repeated blood transfusion. He called for African Americans to donate blood to make it easier for such patients to receive blood for the treatment of their disease. In 1990, physicians at Children's Hospital in Oakland, California described their program for treating patients with sickle cell anemia with "racially matched blood." Elliott Vichinsky explained that they did not want to return to the 1950s and 1960s, when blood was labeled by race; instead they sought to recruit minority-group blood donors to identify their blood antigens and thus provide safer blood for the long-term transfusion of sickle cell patients. As Johns Hopkins hematologist Samuel Charache noted, "Most of us react with instant hostility to any suggestion that our skin color, our religion, or the shape of our nose might determine whether we have access to public facilities or new neighborhoods—or blood. And yet, giving black patients blood from black donors would probably save time and money and avoid medical problems."[129] In 1990, for the first time, the New York Blood Center began asking its donors to volunteer information about their racial and ethnic background, to speed the identification of specific rare blood types, especially from groups under-represented in the blood donor population.[130] The history of blood and its segregation by race continued to feature in the treatment of patients and the understanding of ways to promote medical safety and to prevent societal injustice.

Cultures of Blood

In the 1970s, a popular television situation comedy—*All in the Family*—featured a bigoted, white, working-class man and his racial and ethnic prejudices. Producer Norman Lear used the symbolic power of blood to make a point about its universality; in the first season, Archie Bunker donates blood but expresses concern that it will be mixed with the blood of other races.[131] Lear revisited blood symbolism in a 1976 episode of the popular television program when Bunker enters the hospital for an operation and experiences the bigot's triple threat: a Puerto Rican nurse, a Jewish doctor, and a blood transfusion from a black Caribbean woman. *All in the Family* portrayed for laughs the bigot's discomfiture at receiving blood from someone of another race. (Another popular sit-com, *M*A*S*H*, featured an episode in 1973 in which a soldier who insists that he receive the "right color blood" learns a lesson from the surgeons; they paint his face with iodine, serve him watermelon, and lecture him about Charles Drew and the blood bank.)[132] But for some Americans, the character of the blood they received was no laughing matter. For some whites, black blood reeked with disease. In the 1930s and 1940s, the disease was syphilis, the sexually transmitted "shadow on the land." In the 1950s and 1960s, the disease was sickle cell anemia, which despite its hereditary status, offered a biologic basis for not transfusing across the color line.

By the 1980s, a new blood-borne and sexually transmitted disease appeared in the United States and around the world. When the first cases of acquired immune deficiency syndrome (AIDS) were initially identified, researchers implicated four major groups in the spread of the disease: homosexuals, heroin users, hemophiliacs, and Haitians. Despite the fact that the transmission of AIDS and human immunodeficiency virus (HIV), its causative agent, remained little understood, between 1983 and 1985, the Centers for Disease Control defined Haitians as one of the four high-risk groups for AIDS. To ensure the safety of the blood supply, the Food and Drug Administration (FDA) acted to prevent Haitians from serving as blood donors. Initially, the FDA banned blood from those Haitians who arrived in the United States after 1977. In 1990, the FDA extended the ban to prohibit all Haitians from donating blood. Haitians, both those living in the island nation and those living in the United States, were understandably outraged by the lurid media associations of bad blood, black skin, and bizarre (voodoo) sexual practices. Following large demonstrations and marches in Miami, New York City, and Washington, D.C., the FDA formally removed Haitians from the list of barred blood donors in December 1990. But considerable damage had already been done.[133]

When he ran for president in 1996, Senator Bob Dole appeared before the National Association of Black Journalists, where he recalled his World War II experiences. "When Senator Dan Inouye was badly wounded [in World War II], he looked over at the transfusion he was being given, which was marked with the words 'Black Blood.' He recalled how, at the time, he thought to himself: 'I don't care who that blood came from.' And likewise, I have no idea who gave the blood that may have helped save my life." (Dole was also wounded in World War II.)[134]

Blood retained its power to provoke and to provide opportunities for redrawing and reinscribing the limits of community, the dimensions of safety, the desires for purity, and the drama of peril. Over the course of the twentieth century, blood, once a universal red fluid, became an increasingly specific fluid. As physicians and researchers accumulated greater knowledge about the variety of proteins on the surface of the red blood cell and their clinical implications, there developed new ways of understanding blood relations.

Notes

1. Thomas Cripps, *Making Movies Black: The Hollywood Message Movie from World War II to the Civil Rights Era* (New York: Oxford University Press, 1993), 226–232.

2. See "Albert Johnston, 87, Focus of Film on Race," *New York Times,* 28 Jun. 1988, p. D25. Johnston was refused a commission in the U.S. Navy in 1940, when he revealed his mixed-race heritage. See W.L. White, "Lost Boundaries," *Readers Digest* (Dec. 1947): 135–154. See W.L. White, *Lost Boundaries* (New York: Harcourt, Brace, 1948).

3. "Transfusions of Blood," *Washington Post,* 14 Oct. 1883, p. 6. Another apparent curiosity of "Negro blood transfusion" in the nineteenth century was the superstitious beliefs of the participants. When "an aged Negro, at the point of death" received 8 ounces of blood from his wife, his wife experienced a "curious decline." She whispered to the doctor that her ailment was the result of the blood she had given her husband, and she demanded that it be returned. Against the physician's judgment, he complied with her request, replacing 1 ounce of the lost 8 ounces. When the old woman recovered, she credited her recovery to the return of her blood.

4. Carl Bruck, "Die biologische Differenzierung von Affenarten und menschlichen Rassen durch spezifische Blutreaktion," *Berliner Klinische Wochenschrift* 44 (1907): 793–797.

5. "Separates Blood of Races," *New York Times,* 5 Dec. 1912, p. 6.

6. "Letter to the Editor: Blood Differences of White and Colored Races," *Hygeia* 4 (Oct. 1926): 607. And see "Jewish Blood and Gentile Blood," *Literary Digest* 107 (1930): 27.

7. John G. FitzGerald, "An Attempt to Show Specific Racial Differences in Human Blood by Means of the Reaction of Fixation," *Journal of Medical Research* 21 (1909): 41–45.

8. Karl Landsteiner and C. Philip Miller, Jr. "Serological Studies on Blood of Primates," *Journal of Experimental Medicine* 42 (1925): 841–852.

9. Alexander S. Wiener, *Blood Groups and Transfusion* (Springfield, Illinois: Charles C. Thomas, 1943; 3rd ed.), 295.

10. George H. Smith, "Antigenic Patterns in Human Sera: Race-Specific Antigens," *Yale Journal of Biology and Medicine* 11 (1938–9): 629–643.

11. William Schneider, "Blood Group Research in Great Britain, France, and the United States Between the World Wars," *Yearbook of Physical Anthropology* (1995): 87–114; and also by the same author "The History of Research on Blood Group Genetics: Initial Discovery and Diffusion," *History and Philosophy of Life Sciences* 18 (1996): 277–303.

12. Arthur F. Coca and O. Diebert, "A Study of the Occurrence of the Blood Groups among American Indians," *Journal of Immunology* 8 (1923): 487–491.

13. Julian H. Lewis and Deborah L. Henderson, "The Racial Distribution of Iso-hemagglutinin Groups," *Journal of the American Medical Association* 79 (1922): 1422–1424.

14. "On the Transfusion of Blood," *The Massachusetts Magazine: Or, Monthly Museum of Knowledge and Rational Entertainment* (Dec. 1789): 762–64.

15. Bram Stoker, *Dracula* (New York: Signet, 1992), 82; and Troy Boone, " 'He is English and Therefore Adventurous': Politics, Decadence, and *Dracula*," *Studies in the Novel* 25 (1993): 76–90.

16. *"The Hospital Baby,"* *Chicago Daily Tribune*, 4 Feb. 1912, p. G7. For similar depictions of surgery replicating the romantic penetration of the body, see Susan E. Lederer, "Repellent Subjects: Hollywood Censorship and Surgical Images in the 1930s," *Literature and Medicine* 17 (1998): 91–113.

17. Frank Kinsella, *The Degeneration of Dorothy* (New York: D. W. Dillingham, 1899), 201–204.

18. "The Degeneration of Dorothy," *New York Times*, 9 Dec. 1899, p. BR863.

19. David Starr Jordan, *The Blood of the Nation* (Boston: American Unitarian Association, 1906), 8–9.

20. "Caruso Paid $1500 for Quart of Blood," *New York Times*, 18 Jan. 1923, p. 16 (for Fenstad); see also Robert W. Prichard, "The Death of Enrico Caruso," *Surgery, Gynecology & Obstetrics* 109 (1959): 117–120 (for Wilkinson). For Caruso's own descriptions of the torments he experienced, see Francis Robinson, *Caruso: His Life in Pictures* (New York: Studio Publications, 1957), 137–140.

21. "Crippled White Boy Gives Blood to Negro," *New York Times*, 11 Jul. 1927, p.7.

22. J.C. Furnas, "Blood from a Stranger," *Saturday Evening Post* 211 (1938): 8–12.

23. "Negro Woman's Life Is Saved by White Man," *Reading* (Pennsylvania) *Daily Tribune* 27 Feb. 1909.

24. "Negro Saved by White's Blood," *Los Angeles Times,* 12 Apr. 1926, p. 10.

25. L.W. Gorham and Hans Lisser, "Hemolysis in Vivo and in Vitro as Diagnostic of Cancer," *American Journal of the Medical Sciences* 144 (1912): 103–116.

26. William L Culpepper and Marjorie Ableson, "Laboratory Methods: Report on Five Thousand Bloods Typed Using Moss's Grouping," *Journal of Laboratory and Clinical Medicine* 6 (1921): 276–283.

27. Noah Fabricant and Leo M. Zimmerman, "The Cry for Blood," *Hygeia* 17 (1939): 881–884, 936–937.

28. L.W. Diggs and Alice Jean Keith, "Problems in Blood Banking," *American Journal of Clinical Pathology* 9 (1939): 591–603. Diggs did not capitalize "negroes"; see p. 594.

29. Mark M. Ravitch, "The Blood Bank of the Johns Hopkins Hospital," *Journal of the American Medical Association* 115 (1940): 171–178.

30. Robert A. Kilduffe and Michael DeBakey, *The Blood Bank and the Techniques and Therapeutics of Transfusions* (St. Louis, C.V. Mosby, 1942), 257–258.

31. R.A. Kilduffe & M. DeBakey, *The Blood Bank and the Techniques*, p. 263.

32. Thomas Parran, *Shadow on the Land* (New York: Reynal & Hitchcock, 1937), 175.

33. See Douglas Starr, *Blood: An Epic History of Medicine and Commerce* (New York: Alfred A Knopf, 1998); Sarah E. Chinn, *Technology and the Logic of American Racism: A Cultural History of the Body as Evidence* (London: Continuum, 2000); and Spencie Love, *One Blood: The Death and Resurrection of Charles R. Drew* (Chapel Hill: University of North Carolina Press, 1996).

34. Douglas B. Kendrick, *Blood Program in World War II* (Washington, D.C.: U.S. Government Printing Office, 1964).

35. American Red Cross. Earl S. Taylor, "Blood Procurement for the Army and Navy: Preliminary Report," 23 Mar. 1939, F. 505.08, Box 908, Group 3, Record Group 200.

36. S. Love, *One Blood*, p. 7.

37. DeWitt Stetten, "Blood Plasma for Great Britain Project," *Bulletin of the New York Academy of Medicine* 17 (1941): 27-38, on p. 34.

38. Albert McGown, "Visit to Baltimore, Md.," 12 Aug. 1941, F. Negro Blood 1941–43, Box 909, Group 3, Record Group 200.

39. Dwight Macdonald, *The War's Greatest Scandal: The Story of Jim Crow in Uniform:* (1941), 2–15.

40. Phillip McGuire, "Judge Hastie, World War II, and the Army's Fear of Black Blood," *Review of Afro American Issues and Culture* 1 (1979): 134–151.

41. G. Canby Robinson to Laboratories Processing Dried Human Plasma for the United States Army and Navy, 24 Jan. 1942, F. Negro Blood 1941–43, Box 909, Group 3, Record Group 200.

42. Eleanor Roosevelt to Norman H. Davis, 20 Dec. 1941, F. Negro Blood 1941–43, Box 909, Group 3, Record Group 200; Norman H. Davis to Eleanor Roosevelt, 30 Dec. 1941, F. Negro Blood 1941–43, Box 909, Group 3, Record Group 200.

43. Norman H. Davis to William L. Chenery, 12 Mar. 1942; "Telephone Conversation with Dr. Arthur Lee Kinsolving," 20 Apr. 1942; Arthur Lee Kinsolving to Norman Davis, 14 Apr. 1942, Arthur Lee Kinsolving to Mrs. Leon, 4 Apr. 1942, all in F. Negro Blood 1941–43, Box 909, Group 3, Record Group 200.

44. "No Bar to Negroes as Blood Donors," *New York Times,* 18 Jan. 1942, p. 16.

45. G. Canby Robinson to Henry Smith Leiper, 19 Jan. 1942, F. Negro Blood 1941–43, Box 909, Group 3, Record Group 200.

46. "Nazis Test Blood for 'Non-Aryanism.'" *New York Times,* 23 Sep. 1942, p. 11.

47. "Use of Negro Blood for Blood Banks," *Journal of the American Medical Association,* 119 (1942): 308.

48. "Not Scientific: Aversion to Non-Caucasian Blood is Emotional, not Factual," *Scientific American* 167 (1942): 173-174.

49. "The Segregation of Bloods," *Science* 96 (1942): 8.

50. William K Gregory, Harry L Shapiro, Franz Weidenreich, W.W. Greulich, "Opposition to Segregation of Bloods from White and Negro Donors in Blood Banks," *Journal of the American Medical Association* 119 (1942): 801.

51. Walter White to Norman Davis, 15 May 1943, F. Negro Blood 1941–43, Box 909, Group 3, Record Group 200.

52. Vivian Warner and Mall Waida to Norman H. Davis, 6 Mar. 1942; Walter Davidson to B. D. Thomas, 12 Mar. 1942, F. Negro Blood 1941–43, Box 909, Group 3, Record Group 200.

53. R. Maurice Moss to Jesse O. Thomas, 12 Jul. 1943, F. Races and Racial Matters, Box 1, Group 3, Record Group 200.

54. Sam Hobbs to Canby Robinson, 20 Jun. 1942, Folder: Negro Blood 1941–43, Box 909 Group 3, RG 200.

55. John E. Rankin, "Slandering the Red Cross," 5 Jun. 1942, F. Blood Donor Service 1935–42, Box 3, Group 3, Record Group 200.

56. "Miscellaneous Information," 21 Jan. 1942, F. 020.101, Box 4, Group 3, Record Group 200.

57. Eugene Lavine, "All Blood Is Red," *Education* 66 (Jan. 1946): 292–296.

58. Elsie Austin, *Blood Doesn't Tell* (New York: The Womans Press, n.d.).

59. Ring Lardner, Jr., Maurice Rapf, John Hubley, and Phil Eastman, "Brotherhood of Man: A Script," *Hollywood Quarterly* 1 (1946): 353–359.

60. Joseph D. Lohman and Edwin R. Embree, "The Nation's Capital," *Survey Graphic* 36 (Jan. 1947): 33–37.

61. "Gallinger Rejects Blood of Red Cross," *Washington Post*, 22 July 1948, p. B1; "Gallinger Ban on Red Cross Blood Lifted," *Washington Post*, 24 July 1948, p. B1.

62. Loyalty boards asked a variety of questions, including some about the Soviet Union, NATO, the Marshall Plan, and even about possession of Paul Robeson records, the opera "The Cradle Will Rock," and the Ballet Russe in Russia. See Eleanor Bontecou, *The Federal Loyalty-Security Program* (Ithaca: Cornell University Press, 1953), 141–142.

63. E. Bonteco, *The Federal Loyalty-Security Program*, p. 139.

64. Jesse O. Thomas to Mr. Howard Bonham, 19 Dec. 1947, 505.09 Negro Blood

65. "Red Cross Rejects Blood Gift of Multiracial Fellowship," *Washington Post*, 23 Feb. 1949, p. B1. See Thomas P. Moore's response, "Segregated Blood," *Washington Post*, 28 Feb. 1949, p. 8.

66. "Rift on Blood Bank for U.N. Is Healed," *New York Times*, 9 Sep. 1950, p. 4.

67. "Tokyo Gesture," *Washington Post*, 9 Dec. 1951, p. B4.

68. "Race and the Blood Bank," *New York Times*, 12 Sep. 1950, p. 25.

69. Austin Wehrwein, "Blood Expert Says Transfusion between Races May Be Perilous," *New York Times*, 7 Nov. 1959, p. 1.

70. "Race No Barrier, Blood Center Says," *New York Times*, 12 Nov. 1959, p. 23.

71. "Experts Here Discount Blood Mixing Warning," *The Sunday Star* (Washington, D.C.), 8 Nov. 1959.

72. R. R. Race and Ruth Sanger, *Blood Groups and Man*, 4th ed. (Oxford: Blackwell Scientific Publications, 1962), 275. The reference to patient permission appears only for Duffy, not for Mrs. Kell or Kidd (see p. 261).

73. A.S. Wiener, L.J. Unger, E.B. Gordon, "Fatal Hemolytic Transfusion Reaction Caused by Sensitization to a New Blood Factor U," *Journal of the American Medical Association* 153 (1953): 1444–1446.

74. Albert DeNatale, Amos Cahan, James A. Jack, Robert R. Race, "V, a 'New' Rh Antigen, Common in Negroes, Rare in White People," *Journal of the American Medical Association* 159 (1955): 247–250. See Eloise R. Giblett, Jeanne Chase, Arno G. Motulsky, "Studies on Anti-V: A Recently Discovered Rh Antibody," *Journal of Laboratory and Clinical Medicine* 49 (1957): 433–439.

75. John Scudder and William D. Wigle, "Safer Transfusions through Appreciation of Variants in Blood Group Antigens in Negro and White Blood Donors," *Journal of the National Medical Association* 52 (1960): 76–80.

76. J. Scudder & W.D. Wigle, "Safer Transfusions," p. 79.

77. "Scudder Blood Transfusion Controversy," *Journal of the National Medical Association* 52 (1960): 57.

78. Drew's publications are listed in Charles E. Wynes, *Charles Richard Drew: The Man and The Myth* (Urbana, University of Illinois Press, 1988), 125–126. Most of the papers on which Scudder and Drew collaborated involved blood preservation studies, including the preservation of placental and cadaveric blood.

79. "Says Negro Blood Bad for Whites, Expert Brews Storm," *Jet* 17 (26 Nov. 1959): 7.

80. J. Scudder, S. B. Bhonslay, A. Himmelstein, and J.G. Gorman, "Sensitising Antigens as Factors in Blood Transfusions," *Mankind Quarterly* 1 (1960): 99–100.

81. William H. Tucker, *The Science and Politics of Racial Research* (Urbana: University of Illinois Press, 1994), 170–174.

82. "Negro Scores Data on Blood-Giving," *New York Times*, 15 Nov. 1959, p. 67; "Mazique Rips Into Scudder's Blood Theory," *Pittsburgh Courier*, 28 Nov. 1959, p. A2, and "Reviving the 'Racial Blood' Fiction," *Pittsburgh Courier*, 21 Nov. 1959, p. A4.

83. For drapetomania, see Samuel A. Cartwright, "Report on Diseases and Physical Peculiarities of the Negro Race," *New Orleans Medical and Surgical Journal* 7 (1851): 691–715.

84. "Statement of Edward C. Mazique, President, National Medical Association," *Journal of the National Medical Association* 52 (1960): 57–58.

85. "Statement of E.R. Jennings," 14 Nov. 1959, in "Briefs," *Journal of the National Medical Association* 52 (1960): 295.

86. "Race No Barrier, Blood Center Says," *New York Times*, 12 Nov. 1959, p. 23.

87. "Seven at Columbia Doubt Peril in Bi-Racial Blood Transfusion," *New York Times* 10 Nov. 1959, p. 49.

88. For the statistics, see Louis S. Marks, "Blood Types and 'Race:' An Unfortunate Controversy," *Inter-racial Review* (Jan. 1960): 21.

89. Florence Ridlon, *A Black Physician's Struggle for Civil Rights: Edward C. Mazique, M.D.* (New Mexico: University of New Mexico Press, 2005).

90. "Blood Separation Advocate Backing away from Theory," *Afro-American* (Baltimore; 7 May 1960): 5.

91. I. Dunsford, "Racial Aspects of Blood Transfusion," *New Biology* 29 (1959): 63–74.

92. "Jewized Science vs. Physical Science," *The Truth Seeker* 86 (1959): 180.

93. "Blood Bank Scandal Exposed," *American Nationalist* (Jan. 1960).

94. James Graham Cook, in *The Segregationists* (New York, Appleton-Century-Crofts, 1962), credited Mississippi Representative John Bell Williams and the book—*Black Monday*—by Judge Tom Brady with resurrecting "almost forgotten doctrines of Negro inferiority and rekindled old white sexual fears of the Negro" (p. 14).

95. "Power in the Blood," *Ebony* (Sept. 1958): 70–71; the accompanying photograph depicts an Army medic performing blood transfusion for a wounded soldier on the battlefield.

96. "S.C. Legislator Fights for Negro Blood Label," *Washington Post*, 13 Feb. 1959, p. A13.

97. See W. Michael Byrd and Linda A. Clayton, *An American Health Care Dilemma: A Medical History of African Americans* (New York, Routledge, 2000), 135–140. This work recaps some of the health-care civil rights movement.

98. *White Sentinel*, p. 8.

99. American Red Cross pamphlet, folder. Negro Blood Sickle Cell Anemia, Box 1199, Group 4, Record Group 200.

100. "Bill Segregates Blood," *New York Times*, 22 Jan. 1958.

101. "Racial Step Voted," *New York Times*, 13 Feb. 1958, p. 16.

102. "Racial Bill Killed," *New York Times*, 21 Feb. 1958, p. 14.

103. "Voter Curb and Mental Bills Pass," *Atlanta Constitution*, 22 Feb. 1958. See "Tax Forms Stay Segregated in Georgia," *Pittsburgh Courier*, 27 Feb. 1960, p. 3.

104. "Power in the Blood," *Ebony* (Sept. 1958): 70–71.

105. "Blood Label Voted," *New York Times*, 25 Mar. 1958, p. 25.

106. Keith Wailoo, *Dying in the City of the Blues: Sickle Cell Anemia and the Politics of Race and Health* (Chapel Hill: University of North Carolina Press, 2001), 116.

107. See "Negroes Have Diseased Blood," *The Thunderbolt*, August 1963. I am grateful to Professor James Jackson for this shared material and the *American Nationalist*.

108. American Red Cross, Statement on Transfusion of Sickle-Cell-Trait Blood, 13 Feb. 1959; Folder: Negro Blood, Sickle Cell Trait Blood, Box 1199, Group 4, Record Group 200.

109. "Segregated Blood: A Backlash Backfires," *Hospital Practice* 4 (1969): 21.

110. "Florida Acts to Label Blood," *New York Times*, 30 May 1959, p. 10.

111. "S.C. Legislator Fights for Negro Blood Label," *Washington Post*, 13 Feb. 1959, p. A13.

112. See American Red Cross; Carlton W. Winsor to Paul W. Yost, 17 Nov. 1959; RG 200, Gr. 4, Box 1199, F: Negro Blood Segregation, Racial Designation, etc. 1950–1963.

113. "Arkansas Blood Law," *New York Times*, 7 Apr. 1959, p. 24.

114. "Little Rock Whites and Negro under Faubus 'Blood' Law," *Jet* 15 (23 April 1959): 24–27.

115. See "Race Tags for Blood Provided in Senate Bill," *Journal and Guide* (Norfolk, Virginia), 27 Feb. 1960.

116. "Racial Blood Ban Wins," *New York Times*, 17 Feb. 1960, p. 22.

117. "Some Hospitals Still Keep Negro, White Blood Apart," *Wall Street Journal*, 1 Mar. 1967, p. 1.

118. "Jim-Crow Blood Policy may Kill Youth in New Orleans," *Afro-American* (Baltimore; 13 Sept. 1958).

119. "Arkansas Blood Label Law 'Ridiculous,'" *Afro-American* (Baltimore; 23 Jan. 1960): 19.

120. "No Blood Labels," *Washington Post*, 17 Jan. 1969, p. A9.

121. Leon E. Panetta and Peter Gall, *Bring Us Together: The Nixon Team and the Civil Rights Retreat* (Philadelphia and New York: J.B. Lippincott Company, 1971).

122. Telephone interview with Leon Panetta, 29 May 2002.

123. "La. Hospitals Segregate Blood While Receiving Federal Funds," *Washington Post*, 6 Jul. 1969, p. 2.

124. Morial went on to become the first black mayor of New Orleans in 1977; he died in 1989 at age 60. "Blood Labeling Law Debated in La.," *Washington Post*, 21 Jun. 1970, p. 19.

125. "Letter to the Editor," *Negro History Bulletin* 33 (Nov. 1970): 164.

126. "Legislator Gives Up on Racial Blood Labeling," *Los Angeles Times*, 28 Jun. 1970, p. 8.

127. "Segregated Blood: A Backlash Backfires," *Hospital Practice* 4 (1969): 21–25, 82–83. In 1970, the Louisiana legislature established a mathematical formula to determine whether a person was black. According to the legislators, anyone having one thirty-second or less of "Negro blood" should not be designated as black, and should be provided a means to legally alter one's racial designation. See "Louisianians Vote to Repeal Race Laws," *Washington Post*, 8 Jun. 1972, p. A23.

128. Marclan A. Walker, "I'm Living on Borrowed Time," *Ebony* Jan. 1959, pp. 40–46.

129. See Letters to the Editor, *New England Journal of Medicine* 323 (1990): 1420–1422; and D. Mallory, D. Malamut, and S.G. Sandler, "A Decade of Rare Donor Services in the United States. Report of the American Red Cross Rare Donor Registry (1981–1990)," *Vox Sanguinis* 63 (1992): 186–191.

130. Richard Severo, "Donors' Races to be Sought to Identify Rare Blood types," *New York Times*, 13 Jan. 1990, p. 29.

131. Norman Lear to the Editor," "Laughing While We Face Our Prejudices," *New York Times*, 11 Apr. 1971, p. D22.

132. James H. Wittebols, *Watching M*A*S*H, Watching America: A Social History of the 1972–1983 Television Series* (Jefferson, NC: McFarland, 1998), 171.

133. Eric A. Feldman and Ronald Bayer, ed. *Blood Feuds: AIDS, Blood, and the Politics of Medical Disaster* (New York: Oxford University Press, 1999).

134. Maureen Dowd, "Semi-Soul Brothers," *New York Times*, 25 Aug. 1996, p. F13.

5

Are You My Type?

Blood Groups, Individuality, and Difference

One of the great achievements in understanding blood and advancing transfusion in the twentieth century was the discovery of difference. As historian Pauline Mazumdar has noted in her elegant reconstruction of the early twentieth-century science of serology, "species and specificity are the concepts that lie at the heart of the modern science of immunology."[1] Earlier experiences with transfusion had already suggested that blood from one animal might be harmful when introduced into the body of an animal of another species. In the early nineteenth century, James Blundell offered this as rationale for his resolution to use only human blood when attempting a transfusion. The compelling demonstration of the differences in human blood came from Vienna in 1900, when a young pathologist, Karl Landsteiner, investigated how red blood cells from one person either reacted or failed to react with the serum (the liquid portion of the blood) from another individual. In 1901, he reported experiments with the blood of 22 different people, noting several patterns of agglutination (or clumping). Based on his results, Landsteiner divided human blood into three groups, which he designated A, B, and C (later changed to O). In 1902, one of Landsteiner's students, Adriani Sturli, and his colleague, Alfred von Decastello, identified the fourth and rarest group, type AB. Landsteiner's work on blood and his subsequent contributions to the understanding of blood differences earned him the Nobel Prize in 1930.[2] Recognition of the ABO blood types and the discovery by Landsteiner and others of additional blood systems would revolutionize transfusion by making the transfer of blood less dangerous. In the 1950s and 1960s, the discovery of the human leukocyte antigen (HLA) system would increase the success of transplantation.

The differences in human blood (the presence or absence of proteins on the surface of the blood cell) detected by immunologists and hematologists coexisted and melded with popular assumptions about the differences in blood between dissimilar individuals. As the previous chapter illustrated, assumptions about racial difference profoundly affected the social organization of the blood system, the blood bank, and the designations on bottled blood. This chapter considers how the introduction of new knowledge about the biologic differences in human blood—between individuals and groups and between members of the same family—influenced social and scientific policies about blood transfusion. The chapter also examines how the accumulation of technical knowledge about the blood and its components influenced public understanding of the differences between human beings and presented the opportunities to develop policies that incorporated this new knowledge, ranging from proposals to limit the marriage of Rh-incompatible couples to creating dog tags and tattoos documenting blood type affiliation as part of the civilian preparations for massive nuclear destruction of an American city. Blood groups, like blood itself, accumulated multiple meanings in American culture.

A and B and C

Landsteiner's laboratory work established that human blood was not the same, but could be effectively divided into two groups on the basis of the presence or absence of certain proteins on the surface of red blood cells and in the plasma or liquid portion of the blood. He identified two antigens, A and B, on the red blood cell and two agglutinins (anti-A and anti-B) in the plasma or serum. Landsteiner used the letter C to designate those red blood cells that failed to react with anti-A or anti-B. In 1910, Landsteiner published a paper demonstrating the ABC blood groups. A year later, in 1911, two investigators, E. von Dungern and L. Hirszfeld, introduced the term "O" for those blood cells that did not react to either anti-A or anti-B, and the letters AB to describe those cells that reacted to both. (It remains a matter of speculation whether the O was actually a zero or the first letter of "ohne," the German word "without.")[3] Working independently, in 1907, a Czech physician Jan Jansky similarly segregated human blood into four discrete groups; instead of ABO, he introduced Roman numerals (I designated the most common blood type, IV the least common). Published in an obscure Bohemian journal, Jansky's article received scant attention. Three years later, in Baltimore, Johns Hopkins physician Henry L. Moss similarly identified four blood groups and also adopted Roman numerals to identify the different groups. Moss used the Roman numeral I to designate the rarest blood group and IV to denote the most common—in other words, he reversed the Roman numerals adopted by Jansky.[4]

Consensus held that human blood could be reliably differentiated into four major groups, but little agreement was reached on how to designate blood belonging to the different groups. More familiar with the American medical literature, the English, for example, relied mainly on the Moss system to distinguish bloods of different types, but in the United States, there was much less standardization. Some American hospitals designated blood using the Moss numeration, but others preferred the Jansky system and, to avoid potential confusion, some hospitals employed both.

In an effort to resolve some of the confusion and to bring consistency to blood handling, special committees of the Society of American Bacteriologists and the Association of Pathologists and Bacteriologists recommended jointly in 1921 that, on the basis of priority, the Jansky classification be universally adopted.[5] But this pronouncement seemingly exerted little effect on hospitals and physicians. In 1922, after Landsteiner emigrated to the United States, he continued to pursue his blood researches at the Rockefeller Institute. As a member of the American National Research Council Committee on Blood, Landsteiner recommended that the competing systems of Roman numerals in the Jansky and Moss systems be abandoned in place of the designations, A, B, AB, and O (formerly C). Although this "international classification" was swiftly adopted in principle, in practice many American hospitals and physicians continued to use all three systems well into the 1950s.[6]

Landsteiner's work established that human blood could be differentiated biochemically, but he did not pursue the clinical significance of this finding. Working at the laboratory bench, he did not perform transfusions. Those surgeons who did transfuse blood initially played little heed to the potential adverse consequences of mixing human blood containing different proteins on the red blood cell. In 1907, Chicago pathologist Ludwig Hektoen suggested that careful selection of a blood donor could avert dangerous complications in transfusion.[7] That same year, two Philadelphia physicians, William Pepper and Verner Nisbet, reported the death of a patient who had undergone surgical transfusion. After receiving blood from his wife and his brother-in-law, Pepper's patient soon began to experience distress. He developed jaundice, his urine became bloody, and hemorrhages appeared under his skin, suggesting that his blood had reacted badly with the blood he had received. After the patient's death, his physicians warned that the confidence most surgeons held in moving blood from normal individuals into others was misplaced, and they advised caution until "knowledge of the hemolytic action of different sera is more exact."[8]

George Crile similarly recognized that red blood cells could rupture when donor blood reacted with the recipient's cells. In his 1909 textbook, he recommended preliminary hemolysis tests in all but the most dire emergencies. Crile insisted that the agglutination of the recipient blood cells by the donor serum was not an absolute bar to transfusion; instead, this knowledge allowed the surgeon to regulate the dosage of donor blood in order "to handle a given transfusion more intelligently and protect the recipient more fully." Crile did recognize that "serious hemolysis" could occur. He described one patient suffering with a suppurating cancer in the groin, who received blood from five different donors and died 10 days after his initial transfusion. Determining the cause of death for such a patient was not uncomplicated. "It is impossible to say," Crile explained, "whether death occurred from hemolysis (toxemia from the transfused serum) alone or from a combination of causes."[9] The patient's condition was extremely serious; his cancerous wound had become infected, and he had experienced severe blood loss before the transfusions. Crile's uncertainty about the cause of death was shared by other physicians; the moribund condition of many patients who received transfusions and died made it difficult to conclude whether the patients would have succumbed in any case or whether they died as a result of a transfusion reaction. Crile apparently did not embrace routine blood grouping (as opposed to cross-matching the bloods of donors and recipients) for some time. In 1917, Crile continued to advocate agglutination tests prior to transfusion if time permitted, and endorsed the method developed by Johns Hopkins physician Walter Brem.[10] During the Great War, Crile performed some 216 transfusions in European field hospitals. Many of these emergency surgeries did not permit the preliminary cross-matching tests he had endorsed, nor did they involve performing blood grouping. Crile acknowledged that some transfusion recipients experienced reactions from the unmatched blood. But not all Crile's mismatched transfusions ended badly. In 1962, 56 years after he underwent one of Crile's first person-to-person transfusions, Clevelander Joseph Miller learned that his blood had not been compatible with that of his donors, his brothers Samuel and Morris. "He was amazed to learn," noted reporter Don Dunham, that one of his brothers "has a different blood type than the other two." According to modern knowledge, Dunham concluded, the transfusion "shouldn't have worked at all." Nonetheless, Joseph survived the transfusion and lived at least 56 years in apparent good health.[11]

Crile did not readily adopt the use of blood grouping in transfusions, but other physicians did. At Mount Sinai Hospital in New York City, physician Reuben Ottenberg was perhaps the first transfuser to take blood type consistently into account when making a transfusion.[12] By 1920, both blood typing and cross-matching became more established in clinical practice. Yet, agreement about the stability and meaning of the four blood groups remained in flux.[13] As Brooklyn clinician Henry Feinblatt observed, muddles about blood groups and blood compatibility abounded. One contested issue was the blood types of a mother and her infant. "It has often been alleged," Feinblatt noted in 1926, "that, in the case of an infant, the mother may safely be used as the donor without preliminary compatibility tests. Reliance on the assumption that the mother and child are necessarily compatible may lead to disaster under certain circumstances," he warned.[14] Certainly, many physicians assumed that infants did not possess a blood type, and claimed on the basis of their clinical practices that "all mothers can be used as donors in transfusions of their newborn infants."[15] As late as 1942, for example, surgical transfusion pioneer Bertram Bernheim continued to insist that blood compatibility tests were unnecessary when transfusing babies because, not having a blood type, they could receive any blood.[16]

There was perhaps good reason for confusion about blood types in infancy. As some physicians noted, the agglutinins that determined blood group were not generally present in an infant's blood at birth or during the first month of life. Although they agreed that the percentage of children with a fixed blood group increased with age, physicians disputed the age at which the blood group was established in all children. Whereas Feinblatt, among others, claimed that by age 2 years, all children had a fixed blood group, others insisted the question was only settled when the child turned 10 years of age.[17]

The issue of blood compatibility was further complicated by the claims for what physicians called a "universal donor." Individuals with blood type O (Jansky I, Moss IV) had blood lacking the agglutinogens A and B; therefore, when cells from these individuals were mixed with sera from those of the other three blood groups, no clumping occurred. When a donor belonging to the same group as someone with A, B, or AB blood could not be located, blood group O could theoretically be used. Here again, however, the path was neither straight nor smooth. The blood of some "universal donors" possessed dangerous amounts of other agglutinating agents. If a transfusion proceeded without cross-matching, the use of blood from this so-called "dangerous donor" could lead to a massive hemolytic (cell-rupturing) crisis and even death. Some physicians also identified the so-called "universal recipient," the individual with type AB (Jansky IV, Moss I) blood. In an emergency, this person could theoretically receive blood from individuals with the three other blood groups. But, like the universal donor, the recipient could also be in a danger if his blood contained even trace amounts of other agglutinating agents.[18]

Other questions persisted about the blood groups. Did diet influence the blood grouping? Some said yes, insisting that Group III (B) blood in particular was influenced by a diet "insufficient in greens." This diet apparently reduced the ability of Group III (B) blood cells to clump when mixed with Group II (A) serum, leading to the possibility of misgrouping.[19] Did the use of anesthesia affect the stability of the blood type? Some contended that prolonged exposure to ether altered the clumping phenomena of red blood cells. Other investigators made similar claims about changes in blood group resulting from exposure to x-rays and the administration of such drugs as quinine, arsenic, and calcium lactate. These claims received little confirmation.[20] Still, the search for correlations between blood, body, and behavior persisted. Physicians reported that Group III (B) blood appeared more often than other blood groups in prison populations and in patients with nervous disease and, in 1922, New York physician William S. Bainbridge informed his fellow obstetricians and gynecologists that the blood groups would enable physicians to prevent unhappy marriages by ensuring the blood compatibility of a couple through premarital testing.[21]

Given the diverse and conflicting claims among physicians about blood groups, perhaps it was hardly surprising that lay people might be confused by their status and utility. As British surgeon Geoffrey Keynes noted in 1922, "Knowledge of the existence of the blood groups has become somehow mixed up with vague popular beliefs concerning 'affinities' and blood relations."[22] It was not straightforward that a mother would not be a compatible donor for her own child. Nor was it easy to accept that some brothers and sisters could be compatible blood donors and not others.

The initial efforts to popularize the blood types did little to dispel the complexities of blood groups. In 1922, in one of the earliest references to blood types in the popular press, reporter Ivan Calvin Waterbury attempted to translate "the ponderous cryptic terms that spell scientific precision to the medical men who discuss this subject of blood grouping" into layman's language. He explained Landsteiner's discovery that red blood cells could become clumped when mixed with serum from another person and how this clumping created problems for the blood recipient. He introduced the Jansky classification of Roman numerals to designate the four major human blood groups and explained how these blood types could be used in cases of disputed parentage.[23] The American Medical Association's lay magazine *Hygeia* spent several years trying to educate Americans about the blood groups and their vital importance in transfusion. Intended to convey in lay terms how some donors could not safely donate blood to some recipients, these articles offered complex diagrams of the competing Moss and Jansky systems for distinguishing the four blood groups.[24] *Hygeia*'s editors acknowledged the abundant confusion over transfusion persisted. In one 1934 illustration for an article on blood, a man and a woman stand near a seated, white-coated physician; after the thin woman learns that her blood would be acceptable for donation, the strong husky man alongside her asks: "Doctor, does that mean my blood is—is bad?"[25] In the article, reporter Clennie Bailey explained why tests were required before donation to match the bloods of donors and recipients, warning readers "not to become frightened and begin to wonder where you got that 'bad blood.'" What made people compatible donors was medical not political: "do not think that the refusal to use your blood was due to the fact that you did not work for the mayor in the last election!" The reason, Bailey explained, was simple: "the doctors are trying to save a life and they do not want the capillaries of their patient clogged with clumped red corpuscles, no matter how healthy those corpuscles might be." Not surprisingly however confusion persisted amid the multiple classification systems and the changing nomenclatures and methods. *Hygeia* may have even increased the confusion over transfusion with the reference to "bad blood," one of the synonyms for syphilis, the focus of intense popular fear and interest in the 1930s.

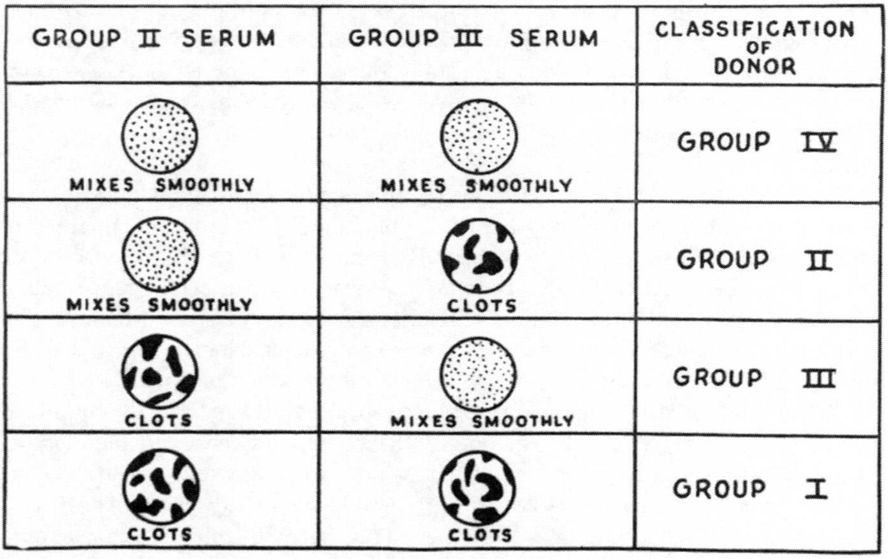

GROUP II SERUM	GROUP III SERUM	CLASSIFICATION OF DONOR
MIXES SMOOTHLY	MIXES SMOOTHLY	GROUP IV
MIXES SMOOTHLY	CLOTS	GROUP II
CLOTS	MIXES SMOOTHLY	GROUP III
CLOTS	CLOTS	GROUP I

Figure 5.1 In 1929, the American Medical Association's lay journal, *Hygeia*, illustrated the four blood groups using only the Moss system of Roman numerals, despite the efforts to standardize the blood groups with the ABO nomenclature (Source: H. Harlan, "This Business of Selling Blood," *Hygeia*, 7 [1929]: 470-471)

One index to the diffusion of knowledge about the different blood types was the reference to an individual possessing a particular type of blood. In 1926, for example, newspapers reported how one Pennsylvania war veteran succumbed to pernicious anemia after receiving some 107 transfusions. In his first forty transfusions, four of his brothers—"who possessed the same blood type"—supplied the blood. When more was needed, advertisements and radio announcements brought other donors with the necessary blood type to the hospital.[26] In 1928 when an article in *Popular Science Monthly* described the "extraordinary career" of professional blood donor Thomas Kane, the author explained that transfusion required "quality blood" from a donor whose blood had to match that of the recipient. Kane was Type 2, the article noted, and his blood was "typed up" at hospital laboratories and kept on file.[27] In the 1930s, American readers learned that physician Tsunemasa Niigaki urged the Japanese foreign office to select diplomats according to their blood type. "Only 'superior' men like Prince Fumimaro Konoye, the Premier, who possesses 'O' type blood, were fitted to fight Japan's diplomatic battles. These men combine level-headedness with quick, unerring decision, perseverance, and a gentle mien cloaking an iron will," the Japanese physician explained.[28] In 1938, when Hudson Grauert of Jersey City, New Jersey fell ill with bacterial endocarditis (an infection of the heart), doctors turned to the newspapers seeking donors with Grauert's blood type, "Jansky one."[29]

Popular authors began incorporating references to blood types in short stories and novels. In 1936 English novelist Dorothy Sayers made the uncertain nature of blood grouping central to her short story "Blood Sacrifice," in which a playwright remains silent when his despised patron is mistakenly given the wrong blood and dies.[30] In 1940 American novelist Carlton Williams invoked blood types in *Emergency Nurse*. When Mrs. Piper desperately needs a transfusion at Ellwood Memorial Hospital, there is no blood bank and the patient is Type AB, "the rare one." With no time to locate an outside donor, the surgeon prepares to administer a saline infusion, when Nurse Orpha Billman interrupts him to say that she has type AB blood. "Fortunate thing you knew your type," the surgeon opines. The nurse blithely replies, "Guess we all know our type these days." (And in one of those coincidences beloved by sentimental novelists, when the patient learns that she has received Nurse Billman's blood, she experiences a moral epiphany and confesses that her daughter, and not Orpha, stole money from the hospital and precipitated the nurse's expulsion.) That AB blood was the rare one was reinforced by newspaper accounts of such individuals as Mrs. Leo Vick, a Chattanooga housewife, and Janis Paige, a screen actress, who required transfusions of the rare blood "that occurs in only eight of one hundred persons."[31] Milton Propper, the author of numerous popular mystery novels, similarly demonstrated the diffusion of blood types in popular literature. In *The Blood Transfusion Murders* (1943), when a young man is injured in an automobile accident, his cousin Eugene agrees to act as a donor. He learns that he and his cousin both have Type B blood. And in another fillip of plausibility, Propper describes how Eugene must sign various papers before the transfusion, "releasing the hospital from liability for the projected operation [blood transfusion]" and allowing Eugene to forego the Wassermann test in light of his cousin's dire need of blood.[32]

In popular films, American moviegoers heard references to blood types in such diverse Hollywood productions as *The Return of Doctor X* and *The Sea Wolf*. In the 1939 Warner Brothers film, Humphrey Bogart (in his only role as a mad scientist!) played Doctor X, who required a particular blood type—Type I—to keep him alive. In an effort to insure an adequate blood supply, he roams the city identifying potential donors with blood type I, and secretly stealing their blood. In the 1942 adaptation of Jack London's *The Sea Wolf*, the screenwriter introduced a dramatic scene in which fugitive Ruth Brewster requires a blood transfusion. When the ship's doctor initially refuses, he explains that the right type of blood is needed—Ruth shares the "right type" with escaped criminal George Leach, who provides the blood and saves her life.[33] Comic strips also furthered knowledge of blood typing. In a 1943 panel from the popular comic strip "Terry and the Pirates," wounded American soldiers and prisoners of war receive blood transfusions in a field hospital. Although the sergeant knows the men carry their blood type designations on their dog tags, he doesn't know the blood type of a newly captured female prisoner, until one of the soldiers explains that she carried a card from an American hospital where she received tetanus injections and blood typing.[34]

Popular knowledge about the blood types diffused slowly in the first four decades of the twentieth century. The biological differences in human blood intensified with the discovery of other blood groups that possessed clinical significance. Perhaps the greatest of these was another discovery by Karl Landsteiner and his associates that human blood could be divided into two group based on the presence or absence of what would come to be called the Rh factor.

The Rh Factor

Knowledge of the four major ABO blood groups was nearly four decades old when Karl Landsteiner and other workers made a dramatic discovery. In 1940 Landsteiner and Alexander Weiner, a young New York physician, described a new blood factor created by injecting rabbits and guinea pigs with the red blood cells of rhesus monkeys. This antibody reacted strongly when mixed with the blood of most human beings. They named this the Rh factor for the Rhesus monkeys that supplied the initial bloods. Discovery of the Rh factor promised to resolve one of the ongoing mysteries in blood transfusion: why did some recipients experience the distress, discomfort, and even death despite the fact that they received the "right type" of blood?

In the 1920s and 1930s Landsteiner had continued his work on the blood types. In 1927 he and Philip Levine described another system of blood groups, which they called the M, N, and P system. This blood group system was observed when they injected rabbits with human red blood cells and then tested the human red blood cells with the antibodies made in the rabbit's body. With another colleague, Landsteiner pursued the evolution of blood types in the anthropoid apes and monkeys and their similarities to human blood. Alexander Weiner, who first met Landsteiner as a medical student in 1929, worked with the Rockefeller researcher on various factors in ape and monkey blood, when they discovered that the anti-rhesus immune sera they developed reacted with blood from nearly 85% of white people tested. These people were called Rh positive. The remaining 15% were said to be Rh negative; their blood did not possess the blood factor. The discovery of the Rh factor did much to explain why some transfusions produced adverse reactions even when the ABO typing was correct.[35]

The Rh factor also proved enormously significant in resolving another clinical puzzle that confronted mothers and obstetricians. This puzzle concerned the disease known as erythroblastosis fetalis or hemolytic disease of the newborn. This condition occurred when a mother's blood was incompatible with the blood of her fetus. Physicians noted that women who had experienced stillbirths or with other children who developed the disease were more likely to develop the condition in subsequent pregnancies. When tested for the presence of the Rh factor, physicians learned that many of these mothers were Rh negative, their babies were Rh positive, and the mother's immune system was defending itself against this foreign presence.[36]

How could this knowledge be mobilized to save American babies? One way to prevent Rh incompatibility in childbirth was to insure that Rh-incompatible couples did not marry and have children. Legislators in Illinois and New York moved swiftly to act on the newly discovered Rh factor and its potential harms. In 1945, the Illinois legislature entertained a bill to require prospective marital partners to undergo a blood test to ascertain whether they had "conflicting blood types" (Rh factor).[37] In 1947, the New York legislature considered a bill making the test for a "negative Rh factor in the blood mandatory of married couples."[38] Presumably armed with this knowledge, couples could decide not to marry and to seek another marital partner whose blood would be compatible. The following year New York Republican Senator Thomas Desmond sponsored a bill to require Rh blood tests in all pregnancies. In 1949, the New York State Health Department, headed by Dr. Herman Hilleboe who endorsed the legislation, began providing a line on all New York birth certificates to indicate that an Rh blood test had been made."[39] The same year the New York legislature once again considered a bill to require Rh factor blood tests in pregnancy cases.[40]

Preventing the marriages of Rh-incompatible men and women was one way to prevent miscarriages, stillbirths, and diseased infants. In the case of infertile couples, artificial insemination offered another means to avoid the problem. In their 1944 exhibit of 110 authenticated cases of artificial insemination presented at the meeting of the Medical Society of the State of New York, physicians Frances Seymour and Alfred Koerner described the careful steps taken before inseminating a woman with donor sperm. Not only did "the anonymous father" have to be "in perfect mental and physical health and of sound stock" and his "past performance in life" above the average in his chosen field, but the physicians explained that blood tests were necessary for both donor and recipient: "His Rh factor (a hereditary blood ingredient which was recently discovered in the rhesus monkey and which may result either in stillbirth or early death if it cannot united with the recipient's blood) must be determined. Blood of the two parents must match."[41] Thus compatibility of the blood became part of the effort to promote "eugenic births."

Unlike the ABO blood grouping, the Rh factor and its role in maternal and fetal health was rapidly disseminated to popular audiences. In the context of the postwar 'baby-boom,' American popular media embraced the medical developments that saved the lives of babies. In 1949, the United States Children's Bureau included the information about the Rh factor and the potential complications in a revised edition of "Prenatal Care," as part of the effort to help women with the question "will my baby be normal?"[42] In the American Medical Association's magazine for lay audiences, Elizabeth Sturns described her experiences in "My 'RH factor' baby." In 1947, her newborn son Raymond underwent a 2-hour exchange transfusion that "gave the baby victory in his fight for life." In extensive detail, Sturns explained the Rh factor, sensitization through transfusion and/or pregnancy, and the potential risks of incompatibility. When she miscarried in July 1937, Sturns explained, she had no idea of the "near tragic effect" it was to have on her life. After losing another pregnancy in 1942, she delivered a premature infant in 1943, who did not survive. After her husband's return from Okinawa in 1945, she visited her obstetrician, who tested her for the first time for Rh sensitivity. When she conceived another child in 1947, her doctors were ready to perform the exchange transfusion that saved her son's life. Sturns expressed skepticism about plans to make the marriage of incompatible men and women illegal, but she endorsed the plan to require testing of all pregnant women for their Rh status and their potential sensitization.[43]

The Rh factor was also quickly integrated into the blood tests used in cases of disputed paternity. Although the use of blood tests to exclude paternity had been introduced in Germany in 1924, the use of blood groups to identify children began in the United States in 1930. In an infamous case of "baby-switching" at a Chicago hospital, a number of experts were called in to place the babies with the right parents. Only blood tests, however, established which baby belonged to which group of parents—as a process of exclusion, the doctors ruled that the Watkins couple (both blood type O) could not have a baby with blood type A. This pronouncement did little to assuage the Bambergers, who were persuaded that they had the right baby despite the blood evidence. Serologist Alexander Weiner offered an extensive discussion of this case and underscored the fact that the babies had in fact been switched at the hospital. This case, and the highly disputed paternity case of celebrity Charles Chaplin (who, despite the blood evidence, was declared the father of Joan Barry's child), made headlines around the country. In 1934, courts in New York State began accepting evidence from the blood groups, although many state courts refused to consider such evidence (California, for example, only accepted such evidence in 1953). By the late 1940s, however, many American courts accepted that findings from the ABO groups could provide evidence of exclusion of paternity.[44] The new knowledge about the Rh factor diffused more rapidly in court cases involving disputed paternity. By 1947, Weiner had performed some 200 tests of Rh blood groupings to resolve cases in which putative fathers disputed their parentage (cases of disputed maternity were extremely rare). In one case before the Court of Special Sessions of New York City, Weiner confronted an unmarried woman who charged a man with the paternity of her child using the evidence from blood groups, specifically the Rh factor. The complainant, he noted, who "had previously denied contact with anyone but the putative father" recalled her experience with another man. In this case, the man accused of paternity was cleared.[45]

The Rh factor, like the ABO blood groups, also made its appearance in popular fiction and film. In his 1959 novel, *The Final Diagnosis*, writer Arthur Hailey used the discovery of the Rh factor and its role in infant deaths as the crucial divide between a young pathologist and an older doctor, less familiar with the introduction of blood tests and other procedures that could save infants. When the wife of a young intern at the hospital becomes pregnant, the older doctor does not perform a test to determine her Rh sensitization. Shocked by his ignorance of latest medical technique, the younger doctor discovers the problem with the Alexander baby when he is born prematurely. The young doctor orders an exchange transfusion, but it is not enough to save the frail, tiny infant. The young doctor is able to work out how the baby's mother was sensitized by an earlier transfusion. In one of those surprising twists of fate beloved by novelists, it becomes clear that the young doctor's own father had transfused the woman in 1949. Despite the fact that the Rh factor had been discovered in 1940, only 10 years later did all hospitals and doctors perform Rh cross matches before transfusion: "Naturally David Coleman's father could not be blamed, even if the hypothesis was true. He would have prescribed in good faith, using the medical standards of his day. It was true that at the time the Rh factor had been known, and in some places Rh cross-matching was already in effect. But a busy country G.P. could scarcely be expected to keep up with everything that was new. Or could he?"[46] When the novel became the basis of a Hollywood film (*The Young Doctors*, 1961), actor Ben Gazzara played the young doctor who is stunned by his elder colleague's refusal to test for Rh sensitization. In the film version, the Alexander baby survives the exchange transfusion, but not before demonstrating to the older doctor (played by Frederic March) that he should retire from the medical profession.

The discovery of the Rh blood group sparked renewed interest in blood groups. New laboratory methods for the detection of differences in blood groups produced a dramatic increase in the number of blood group antigens. To describe or identify all the new blood groups systems with their specific red cell antigen would make, in the words of hematologist Louis Diamond, "as dull reading as the catalogue of ships in Homer's Iliad."[47] More significant than their names and discoverers was the realization shared by many physicians that these hitherto unknown red-cell markers could have not only clinical consequences but could also be used in identifying both individuals and ethnic groups. One of the first observations about the Rh blood factor, for example, was the extent to which Rh negativity varied among groups. Blood tests on large groups of New Yorkers revealed that roughly 15% of Americans of European descent tested negative for the Rh factor. Roughly 5% of the New Yorkers of African descent tested negative for the Rh factor, and those from Asia even lower—from 0% to 2%. In addition to the Rh factor, other clinically significant blood groups identified in the 1940 and 1950s, including the Kell (discovered in 1946) and the Duffy systems (identified in 1950), varied along racial and ethnic lines. The increasing importance of transfusion as a medical intervention and the discovery of these new, clinically significant blood groups prompted calls for rethinking the selection of blood donors in transfusion.

Blood Groups and Biologic Differences

In the 1940s, blood researchers soon realized that working with the Rh group required more than the simple division of individuals into those with the factor (Rh+) and those whose cells did not possess the factor (Rh–). The so-called "Rh factor" actually involved a number of different antigens, some with greater clinical significance than others. Hematologist Peter D. Issitt has noted that the Rh blood group system "represents the most complex polymorphism of human red cell markers and one of the most complex of all human polymorphisms."[48] Given the extent of the variations in the Rh and ABO blood groups, some questioned the role of such variation in health and disease. In 1945, geneticist E. B. Ford speculated on the biologic role of the variations in blood groups. "A valuable line of enquiry, which does not yet seem to be have been pursued in any detail," Ford noted, "would be to study the blood group distributions in patients suffering from a wide variety of diseases. It is possible that in some conditions, infectious or otherwise, they would depart from their normal frequencies, indicating that persons of a particular blood group are unduly susceptible to the disease in question."[49] Ford seemed unaware that in fact some physicians had already sought to correlate disease and blood groups.

In the 1920s and 1930s, studies that compared the distribution of the blood groups in cancer, syphilis, malaria, epilepsy, whooping cough, scarlet fever, tuberculosis, toxemia of pregnancy, and polio appeared in the medical press. Several physicians noted that individuals with Type AB blood were overrepresented in positive Wassermann tests for syphilis, and that persons with Type O blood were underrepresented. But there was little consensus about the reliability of these often-conflicting reports, and much speculation held that they represented an inadequate sample size rather than a durable finding. In 1929, Laurence Snyder, a member of the National Research Council's Committee on Blood Grouping, reported his findings from his own laboratory about the distribution of blood groups among "normal Americans" and those with a pathologic condition "Conflicting reports constantly occur, some workers claiming an excess of group A, some of group B, some of group AB, and still others of group O, while many investigators find a normal distribution," Snyder explained. "Under such conditions, no abnormal distribution can as yet be accepted as final, and it seems likely that a normal distribution will eventually be demonstrated for these conditions."[50]

Despite skepticism about the reliability of such associations, some researchers continued to seek linkages between disease and blood group or between behaviors and blood group. These investigations produced often strange observations, including the report that hangovers (from alcoholic indulgence) were worse in people with blood type A, that group B individuals defecated with greatest frequency, and group O possessed the best teeth. After extensive blood testing on military personnel, one German investigator concluded that persons with group O blood possessed less satisfactory strength of character and personality, that persons with group B blood were impulsive, and that persons with A blood were "especially suitable for 'goal-keeper jobs.'" Other blood workers reported relationships between blood groups and homosexuality, lesbianism, sadism, and flat feet.[51]

The discovery of the Rh factor prompted similar efforts to link the factor and blood incompatibility to a particular disease state or outcome. In 1944, some linked the Rh gene to a "significant amount of feeblemindedness." Herman Yannet and Rose Lieberman collected blood from 109 mothers visiting their children at the Southbury Training School in Connecticut. In a group of some 56 mothers, the number of those who were Rh negative was twice the rate of the frequency of the factor in the general population, and 11 of the 14 children of these mothers were Rh positive.[52] The potential linkage of feeblemindedness to Rh incompatibility prompted zoologists Laurence Snyder, Murray Schonfeld, and Edith Offerman to test the blood of "feebleminded children" and their mothers at the Ohio Institution for the Feebleminded in 1945. Their studies confirmed the finding of much higher rates of Rh incompatibility between the mothers and children tested.[53] In 1948, physicians at New York University College of Medicine called attention to the link between Rh incompatibility and cerebral palsy. "An Rh-negative mother giving birth to an Rh-positive child develops in her blood antibodies to that child's blood. The antibodies tend to destroy the child's blood, and he is born with severe hemorrhage and jaundice and certain portions of the brain are destroyed. If the child survives, he usually has a rigidity type of cerebral palsy."[54]

The search for linkages between blood groups and disease continued in the 1950s and 1960s. In 1964, psychologists Raymond Cattell, H. Boutourline Young, and J.D. Hundleby published their findings about blood groups and personality traits in the *American Journal of Human Genetics*. This work, supported with grants from the National Institute of Mental Health and the Wenner-Gren Foundation, correlated blood group with personality traits in four groups of "boys of Italian stock," (in Rome, Palermo, Florence, and Boston). Cattell's group found that boys with blood type A were more "premsic" (sensitive, intuitive, refined) and boys with types O, B, and AB "more harric" (tough-minded, less sensitive, objective)."[55] Prominent hematologists, including Alexander Wiener, bluntly dismissed such research: "It seems a shame that an important scientific journal like the *American Journal of Human Genetics* has wasted valuable space on an article of such poor caliber. The only consolation is that the article is probably harmless, because few readers will take it seriously." If Wiener rejected such work, other investigators continued to seek linkages. With funding from the Public Health Service, psychiatrists at Duke University linked manic depression with blood group O; other psychiatrists pursued the association of the ABO blood groups, Rh factors, and the MN blood group and schizophrenia. In 1962, two Johns Hopkins physicians, whose work was funded by the Tobacco Industry Research Committee, reported correlations of ABO and Rh blood groups in smokers and nonsmokers. (Nonsmokers had a "significant excess" of groups B and AB).[56] Amid the flurry of reports about side effects of the newly licensed oral contraceptives in the late 1960s, Hershel Jick, an assistant professor of medicine at Tufts University School of Medicine, linked blood type to the formation of blood clots. In 1969, Jick reported that risk of developing a blood clot in the lung (pulmonary embolus) was three times higher in women with types A, B, and AB combined than in women with type O blood. The findings by American, British, and Swedish physicians prompted an editorial writer in the British medical journal *Lancet* to advise that women with blood groups "other than O who practice oral contraception run an appreciable risk—a risk which some may wish to weigh for themselves."[57]

In the 1950s, two British researchers offered evidence that stomach cancer occurred more frequently in individuals with blood group A. Their results were based on a large group of individuals, and the results confirmed by other investigators. The controversy raged over the association between blood group and gastric function (especially gastric secretion) but, by 1996, immunobiologist George Garratty observed "It seems hard to dispute that cancer of the stomach occurs more frequently in group A's compared to group O. If one reviews all the published work of associations of ABO groups and malignancy, one is impressed that, overall, group A predominates over group O, especially if one reviews data from the largest studies, or when smaller studies, on a particular malignancy, have given similar results when reported by many difference investigators."[58] Garratty concludes that Wiener and others were wrong to dismiss so readily the associations between ABO groups and disease because of the increasing evidence that the antigens that give rise to blood differences are not merely artifacts but play an important biologic role in the body and in the red blood cell itself.

Certainly, some physicians continue to assert the importance of blood groups in diet and nutrition. In the 1990s, naturopathic physician Peter D'Adamo built on his father's research to create "The Eat Right for Your Type" diet and cookbook. D'Adamo traced the dietary needs of each of the ABO blood types to human evolutionary patterns, from type O (for oldest), to type A (for agrarian), type B (for balance), and type AB (for modern, representing the recent intermingling of type A Caucasians and type B Mongolians). By eating the right foods associated with your blood type, D'Adamo claimed that one can be healthier, live longer, and achieve an ideal weight. Other physicians extend D'Adamo's use of blood types to explain not only diet, disease, and nutrition but also "sexual compatibility" based on blood types. Obstetrician-gynecologist Steven Weissberg offers an analysis of President John F. Kennedy's blood type (the only American president to have AB blood) and his relationships with women, including Jacqueline Bouvier (blood type O) and Marilyn Monroe (also apparently possessed of the rare AB blood type). Although such analyses strike many as laughable, a number of products cater to people who "eat right for their type," including specialty teas for individual blood types.[59]

In the Cards

The recognition that human blood could be classified into different groups received enormous impetus from American entry into World War II and the American Red Cross's campaign to procure blood for the Armed Forces. In 1939, as the American military considered adding the soldier's ABO blood type to his metal identification tag, authorities encouraged civilians to know their own blood type, to note it on the identification card they carried, and even to have their blood type "tattooed on your arm or, less usefully but more symbolically, over your heart."[60] David Hellman, a volunteer in the Civilian Conservation Corps camp in Solon Iowa, a program established by President Franklin Roosevelt in 1932, informed the Director of the Public Health Service that he had "Type 2" blood when he wrote offering to serve as a "human guinea pig."[61]

In cities and towns across the United States, as Americans were exhorted to give their own "blood sacrifice" for the war effort, one tangible outcome of their participation was receiving a wallet-sized card that identified them by name and blood group. In 1944, for example, the optimistically named Honolulu Peacetime Blood Bank issued cards to individuals stating their ABO blood group. The printed cards had no indication for Rh status, but the back of the card emphasized that "blood from all races is equally good!" The card contained printed information explaining that people with type O blood were "universal givers"; they could give blood to people with O, A, B, and AB blood. The card explained that people with type AB blood were "universal receivers."[62] In 1945, the blood bank of Queens County, New York, issued identification cards for its blood donors with spaces for name, address, blood type, and Rh factor. "All persons typed have, in addition to their own type and Rh factor, the names of six persons of their acquaintance of the same type and Rh factor on their identification card. All of this saves valuable time at the critical moment and does away with the unnecessary confusion and loss of time trying to locate a donor of the proper type."[63]

The war's end did not bring an end to the need for blood and the identification of blood type. Although he deplored the "hysteria" surrounding atomic warfare and the "fanciful tales of total destruction and creation of a race of monsters and misfits," Brigadier General James P. Cooney, representing the Atomic Energy Commission, nonetheless supported the plan for mass blood typing of civilians, in which the blood type of every person was tattooed on an exposed body site like the wrist.[64] (Cooney may have been familiar with the tattoos used by the Nazi SS troops, whose members were distinguished by tattoo marks in their armpits.) Other civil defense planners, as they readied for a "Hiroshima-like attack" on an American city, contemplated the need for every citizen to wear a "dog-tag" identifying the individual by name, address, and blood type. Carleton Simon, a member of the New York Association of Chiefs of Police, claimed credit for civilian dog tags in 1949, when he noted that such tags would be useful "in saving lives in serious accidents." In 1950, the veterans' organization AMVETS launched a drive to distribute 150 million "atomic radiation-resistant plastic tags" by presenting President Harry Truman with his own civilian defense tag. This tag identified him as having Type O, or "the universal type" (it did not carry his Rh status). AMVETS awarded the second such tag to actress Doris Day, as part of the drive to convince Americans to wear such tags to meet "the tremendous needs of whole blood that would follow in the wake of atomic bombing."[65] That same year, the Public Health Service's Chronic Disease Division proposed mass blood typing of American citizens: "If atomic warfare, or even bombardment by high explosives, resulted in sudden and extensive civilian causalities," the agency recommended, "citizen's knowledge of their blood types would save many lives."[66] Other cities and states adopted their own programs for mass typing and identification tags. In Maryland, the proposal to furnish metal dog tags bearing their name and blood type to boys, and metal bracelets with similar information to girls, was abandoned when civil defense authorities conceded that children traded such things, that older boys might give their tag to their "best girl," and older girls might bestow their bracelets to their "favored beau." Still, when the Gallup Organization polled Americans about "dog tagging all civilians," they found that 86% of Americans believed it would be a good idea to have information about names and blood types in case of a nuclear attack. Some 45% of those polled granted that such a law would be difficult to enforce.[67]

In Chicago, civil defense planners proposed a tattoo instead of a dog tag. When a *Chicago Tribune* reporter interviewed five men outside the Today Theater about the plan to tattoo every resident's blood type under their arm in case of an atomic attack, all five endorsed the idea. "Blood typing should be done not only in preparation for atomic attack but in cases of accidents and injuries," noted law student Francis Byrne. Both he and Harry Cohen, a salesman, expressed concern that women would prove less cooperative with the plan because of the tattoo site. "The tattoo should be put in a less conspicuous place than under the arm," Byrne explained, "because many women will object because of strapless evening gowns."[68]

There were other reasons to reject the possibility of mass blood typing. Such prominent blood specialists as Alexander Wiener warned that mass blood typing did not ensure accuracy. During World War II, Wiener explained, 10% of the dog tags worn by American soldiers were wrong. Fortunately, according to Wiener, "no one took the dog tags seriously." Wiener's warning about trusting such information was echoed by other blood bankers. When the California legislature considered adding blood type information to all drivers' licenses, blood banker Elmer Jennings warned that "no hospital would dare give transfusions on basis of information on a driver's license." By 1960, most of the interest in mass blood typing had dissipated, reflecting concerns about the cost and complexity of implementing such a program and the growing recognition that developments in nuclear weaponry made the prospect of surviving a "Hiroshima-like" attack less likely.

Medicine's "Most Exclusive" Club

If all blood types were equal, some were certainly rarer than others. Some Americans learned that they possessed unusual blood types when they or a family member required blood for transfusion. When Dorothy Sanders needed surgery to repair a leaky mitral valve (a blood-intensive operation in which the surgeons requested some 20 pints of fresh blood), the New Jersey woman discovered that she was AB negative, one of the rarer ABO types. Unable to line up the necessary blood, her family learned about the National Rare Blood Club, an organization sponsored by the Knights of Pythias. Founded in 1864, the Knights were a quasi-Masonic organization with links to blood rituals. In 1959, the nonsectarian fraternal organization organized the Rare Blood Club and, by 1961, claimed some 900 members, all of whom possessed the "rare blood types," including A negative, B negative, O negative, AB positive, and AB negative. The Rare Blood Club provided blood free of charge to patients who, like Dorothy Sanders, needed large quantities of blood for transfusion.[69]

The other alternative for patients who possessed rare blood types was self-donation, banking one's own. In the 1950s, the National Institutes of Health and the United States Navy began freezing the blood of individuals with rare blood types. In 1956, the Naval Hospital separated blood into fractions, bathed the red blood cells in glycerol (as a type of antifreeze), and froze the preparation. When needed, the cells could be reconstituted and used for transfusion. Such preparations were necessary for patients with extremely rare blood subgroups. When physician Morten Grove-Rasmussen needed blood for a surgical procedure on a child at the Massachusetts General Hospital in 1959, he discovered that the child's blood type (ABO and subgroups) had been identified in only five people in the United States and 11 people in the world. (In some ways, these rare subgroups were iatrogenic—the individuals had been sensitized through transfusions.) Concern about the subgroups prompted the formation of reference program files, which maintained registries for unusual sensitizations and subtypes.

Possessing a rare blood type could confer a financial windfall. In the 1950s and 1960s, some Americans discovered that their blood contained unusual antigens that made it valuable for creating blood typing serums. In 1961, Clearborn F. Parker, a food processing supervisor in Fort Worth, Texas, learned that he had a genetic blood disease, hemochromatosis (a condition in which the blood contains excessive iron that can damage the pancreas and liver). When he underwent treatment for the disease (bloodletting), his doctors discovered that his serum was particularly useful for creating Rh typing serum (he was Rh negative but had mistakenly received Rh positive blood during an earlier surgery on his spine). When his doctors proposed giving him more Rh positive blood to stimulate the production of more antibody, Parker agreed to undergo the risks of blood incompatibility to produce more serum. His physicians offered him $300 and free medical care for the typing serum sufficient for some 7 million Rh typing tests.[70] In Detroit, Joseph Thomas, employed on the assembly line at Chrysler, learned that his blood contained an unusually high concentration of a rare antibody—anti-Lewis B—which made his blood attractive to doctors and medical suppliers. He signed a contract to supply his blood on a regular basis to a Florida biologic firm for approximately $1500 a quart (for an annual income of roughly $12,000). In addition to the money and notoriety of his "precious blood," Thomas was offered a small role in the ABC television program *The Immortal.* This dramatic series opened with the following narration: "This man has a singular advantage over other men. Ben Richards is immune to every known disease, including old age. Periodic transfusions of his blood can give other men a second, a third lifetime, perhaps more." (Again, and perhaps not surprisingly, a greedy billionaire seeks to kidnap the man and use his blood to live forever.)[71]

What did American make of the biochemical differences inscribed in their blood types? Public support for the campaigns for mass blood typing suggests that many accepted it as a matter of fact. Blood typing could aid American response to atomic attacks. It could also prove useful in other disasters when blood was needed immediately. Blood typing may have also lost of some of its mystery through its introduction into the science curriculum in American public schools. Science teachers began using simple and inexpensive equipment for students to perform tests on their own blood.

With sera (anti-A and anti-B) purchased from the Gradwohl Laboratories in Saint Louis, one Illinois high school teacher introduced blood typing during the unit on Mendelian genetics. Students used glass slides, pipettes, a lancet for pricking the finger, alcohol, cotton, saline solution, and a microscope to determine their own blood types and those of their class mates. Not only did students perform the tests on their own blood, but many students apparently obtained blood samples from family members. Some students wrote to family members in the armed services (whose dog tags contained the information about their blood type) in order to flesh out the family tree.[72] Humorist Dave Barry has observed that "if you surveyed a hundred typical middle-aged Americans, I bet you'd find that only two of them could tell you their blood type, but every last one of them would know the theme song from the Beverly Hillbillies." This observation tells us more about popular culture than it does about the diffusion of information about the blood types. Certainly, the routine blood-typing exercises in high school science classes have stopped due to concern about blood-transmitted diseases and anxiety about liability. It is possible that, during the middle decades of the twentieth century and with the memory of wartime blood collection and the experience of high school science experiments fresh in their minds, many more Americans knew their blood type then than do now.

In postwar fiction, authors made reference to blood types in a number of imaginative ways to reinforce themes of both similarity and difference. In her novel *Member of the Wedding* (published in 1946), Southern author Carson McCullers's young protagonist reflects about donating blood to the Red Cross: "she wanted to donate a quart a week and her blood would be in the veins of Australians and Fighting French and Chinese, all over the whole world, and it would be as though she were close kin to all of these people."[73] Here, blood is seen as a vehicle for bringing people together, uniting them in kinship. John Oliver Killens's 1954 novel *Youngblood* similarly suggested a new model of kinship wrought by blood. The novel focuses on the efforts of a young, black working-class man to organize the first labor union in Georgia. When Joe Youngblood is shot by a white supervisor for protesting unfairly low wages, the hospital refuses to treat him (hospitals were segregated by race). The black doctors begin to organize transfusions for Youngblood. None of his "blood relatives" share his type O blood. One nonrelated black man with the same blood type offers blood for the first transfusion, but Youngblood needs more. A poor white man, Oscar Jefferson, learns about his fellow worker's condition and, with considerable reluctance, considers giving blood: "But giving his blood, a white man's blood, and letting it mix with a black man's blood was more than he had counted on." When Oscar makes it to the wounded man's home, he asks the doctor "Do white blood mix with colored?" "There's no white blood and there's no black blood," Doctor Riley said. "All blood is red-blood. The only difference is in the different types.

Blood doesn't know any color line." Oscar's blood type is not compatible, but his 17-year-old son, Junior's, is compatible. The "pale-face, chunky shouldered white boy" stretches out next to the large black Youngblood, as the blood flowed from the boy to the man. Youngblood dies soon after from his injuries and the failure to be admitted to the City Hospital. But things are changing. In the second to last sentence of the novel, a man reassures Youngblood's widow "There's going to be a reckoning day right here in Georgia, and we're going to help God hurry it up."[74]

In 1964, Senator Barry Goldwater donated a pint of blood to the Red Cross, but insisted to newspaper reporters that none of his blood should be used for New York Governor Nelson Rockefeller (who opposed Goldwater for the GOP presidential nomination). When he was asked whether his blood would turn a man into a conservative, Goldwater replied "I know of several liberals I'd like to give transfusions. I would do it every day if I could pick the liberal radical who would get it." According to the newspaper account, Goldwater had supplied some 90 pints of blood between 1944 and 1964. For the record, he was A-negative.[75]

Notes

1. Pauline M.H. Mazumdar, *Species and Specificity: An Interpretation of the History of Immunology* (Cambridge: Cambridge University Press, 1995), 3.

2. Markus Figl and Linda E. Pelinka, "Karl Landsteiner, the Discoverer of Blood Groups," *Resuscitation* 63 (2004): 251–254. See Mazumdar, *Species and Specificity*, for Landsteiner's centrality to the study of difference in blood.

3. G. Garratty, W. Dzik, P.D. Issitt, D.M. Lublin, M.E. Reid, and T. Zelinski, "Terminology for Blood Group Antigens and Genes—Historical Origins and Guidelines in the New Millenium," *Transfusion* 40 (2000): 477–489.

4. William L. Moss, "Studies on Isoagglutinins and Isohemolysins," *Bulletin of the Johns Hopkins Hospital* 21(1910): 63–70.

5. See Philip Levine and Eugene M. Katzin, "A Survey of Blood Transfusion in America," *Journal of the American Medical Association* 110 (1938): 1243–1248.

6. A.D. Farr, "Blood Group Serology—the First Four Decades (1900–1939)," *Medical History* 23 (1979): 215–226.

7. Ludvig Hektoen, "Isoagglutination of Human Corpuscles," *Journal of the American Medical Association* 48 (1907): 1739–1740.

8. William Pepper and Verner Nisbet, "A Case of Fatal Hemolysis Following Direct Transfusion of Blood by Arteriovenous Anastomosis," *Journal of the American Medical Association* 49 (1907): 385–389.

9. George W. Crile, *Hemorrhage and Transfusion: An Experimental and Clinical Research* (New York: D. Appleton, 1909), 308.

10. Walter V. Brem, "Blood Transfusion with Special Reference to Group Tests," *Journal of the American Medical Association* (July 15, 1916); see George W. Crile, *Notes on Military Surgery* (Cleveland: William Feather Co., 1924), 49.

11. Don Dunham, "56 Years after Transfusion He Finds Blood Was Wrong," *Cleveland Press*, 18 Sep. 1962, p. 1. Clipping from George Crile Papers, Case Western Reserve.

12. Reuben C. Ottenberg, "Reminiscences of the History of Blood Transfusion," *Mount Sinai Journal of Medicine New York* 4 (1937): 164–171. See William C. Schneider, "Blood Transfusion between the Wars, "*Journal of the History of Medicine and Allied Health Sciences* 58 (2003):187–224.

13. It remains a complex issue. As of 1996, a reported 300 blood-group antigens have been detected on the surface of the red blood cell membrane; see George Garratty, "Association of Blood Groups and Disease: Do Blood Group Antigens and Antibodies have a Biological Role?" *History and Philosophy of Life Sciences* 18 (1996): 321–344.

14. Henry M. Feinblatt, *Transfusion of Blood* (New York: Macmillan, 1926), p.31.

15. I. S. Ravdin and Elizabeth Glenn, "The Transfusion of Blood with Report of 186 Transfusions," *American Journal of the Medical Sciences* 161 (1921): 705–722.

16. Bertram M. Bernheim, *Adventure in Blood Transfusion* (New York: Smith & Durrell, 1942), 93.

17. Sanford B. Hooker, "Transfusion of Blood," *New England Medical Gazette* (Feb. 1917): 79–87.

18. E.H. Fell, "Report of 500 Blood Transfusions," *Surgery* 4 (1938): 253–60; Robert Bates, "Experiences of a Blood Transfusion Team," *Surgery, Gynecology & Obstetrics,* 65 (1937) 545–549.

19. John Harper and Welker C. Byron, "Influence of Diet on Blood Grouping," *Journal of the American Medical Association* 79 (1922): 2222–2223.

20. Laurence H. Snyder, *Blood Groups in Relation to Clinical and Legal Medicine* (Baltimore: Williams and Wilkins, 1929), 22–23.

21. M. Gundel, "The Blood of a Criminal," *Literary Digest* (7 May 1927): 87; "Urges Blood Tests to Stop Mismating," *New York Times,* 22 Sep. 1923, p. 3.

22. Geoffrey Keynes, *Blood Transfusion* (London: Hodder and Stoughton, 1922), 84.

23. Ivan Calvin Waterbury, "Blood as Clue to Parentage," *New York Times,* 15 Jan. 1922, p. 75.

24. Louis Schwartz, "Full-Blooded Donors," *Hygeia* 8 (1930): 1109–1112.

25. Clennie E. Bailey, "Blood—Confusions about Transfusions," *Hygeia* 12 (1934): 404.

26. "107 Transfusions Fail to Save War Veteran," *New York Times,* 16 Jul. 1926, p. 15.

27. George Lee Dowd, Jr., "Gives 42 Quarts of Blood to Save 86 Lives," *Popular Science Monthly* (1928): 34.

28. "Japan Is Urged to select Diplomats by Blood Type," *New York Times,* 25 Jun. 1937, p. 11.

29. "Asks Blood for Hudson Grauert," *New York Times,* 20 Aug. 1938, p. 30.

30. Dorothy L. Sayers's short story, "Blood Sacrifice," first appeared in 1936, in the *London Daily Mail.* The story first appeared in an American edition as part of her collection entitled *In the Teeth of the Evidence* (New York: Harcourt Brace, 1940).

31. Carlton Williams, *Emergency Nurse* (Philadelphia: Penn Publishing, 1940), 87–88. See "3 Weeks More of Life Suggested as Gift," *New York Times,* 15 Dec. 1935; and "Many Offer Blood to Ailing Actress," *Los Angeles Times,* 26 Jun. 1945, p. A3.

32. Milton Propper, *The Blood Transfusion Murders* (New York: Harper & Brothers, 1943), 14.

33. See entries for each film in the American Film Institute On-line Catalogue.

34. "Terry and the Pirates," Milton Caniff, 1943.

35. David R. Zimmerman, *Rh: The Intimate History of a Disease and Its Conquest* (New York: Macmillan, 1973) provides an excellent account of the discovery of the Rh factor.

36. Alexander S. Wiener, "History of the Rhesus Blood Types," *Journal of the History of Medicine and Allied Sciences* 7 (1952): 369–383.

37. See "Medical Legislation," *Journal of the American Medical Association* 127 (1945): 721. Also see "Observations on Sensitization to the Rh Factor by Blood Transfusion," *American Journal of Clinical Pathology* 15 (1945): 280–285.

38. "State Law Asked for Blood Tests," *New York Times,* 9 Jul. 1947, p. 27.

39. "State Bill to Ask Rh Test for Blood," *New York Times,* 24 Dec. 1948, p. 11.

40. "Safety Standards for Flats Sought," *New York Times,* 11 Feb. 1949, p. 14.

41. "Case for Eugenics," *New York Times*, 14 May 1944, p. E9. Also see Edith Potter and J. Robert Willson, "Artificial Insemination as a Means of Preventing Erythroblastosis," *Journal of the American Medical Association* 127 (1945): 438–439.

42. Catherine Mackenzie, "Thoughts Now Out in the Open," *New York Times*, 5 Jun. 1949, SM48.

43. Elizabeth Daws Sturns, "My 'RH Factor' Baby," *Hygeia* 27 (1949): 458–459; 489–491.

44. Shari Rudavsky, "Separating Spheres: Legal Ideology versus Paternity Testing in Divorce Cases," *Science in Context* 12 (1999): 123–138, is the best source on the science and cultural impact of paternity exclusion by blood tests.

45. Alexander Wiener, *Blood Groups and Transfusion* (1943), 391. See also "Rh Blood Test Accepted in Parentage Case; Justice Rules Husband is Not the Father," *New York Times*, 21 Jul. 1947, p. 19.

46. Arthur Hailey, *The Final Diagnosis* (Garden City, New York: Doubleday, 1959), 258.

47. Louis Diamond, "History of Blood Transfusion," in Max Wintrobe, ed. *Blood, Pure and Eloquent: A Story of Discovery, of People, and of Ideas* (New York: McGraw-Hill, 1980). p. 698.

48. Peter D. Issitt, "The Rh Blood Groups," in *Immunobiology of Transfusion Medicine* ed. George Garratty (New York: Marcel Dekker, 1994), 111-148, on pp.111–112.

49. G. Garratty, "Blood Groups and Disease: a Historical Perspective," *Transfusion Medicine Reviews* 14 (2000): 291-301, on p. 291.

50. L.H. Snyder, *Blood Groups in Relation to Clinical and Legal Medicine*, p. 106.

51. Otto Prokop and Gerhard Uhlenbruck, *Human Blood and Serum Groups* Trans. John L. Raven. (London: Maclaren and Sons, 1969), 691.

52. "The Rh Gene as a Cause of Mental Deficiency," *Journal of Heredity* 35 (1944): 133–134.

53. Laurence H. Snyder, Murray D. Schonfeld and Edith M. Offerman, "The Rh Factor and Feeble Mindedness," *Journal of Heredity* 36 (1945): 9–10.

54. N.S. Haseltine, "Doctors Find Rh Factor May Cause Cerebral Palsy," *Washington Post*, 11 Sep. 1948, p. 1.

55. R.B. Cattell, H. Boutourline Young, and J.D. Hundleby, "Blood Groups and Personality Traits," *American Journal of Human Genetics* 16 (1964): 397–402. See also Raymond Cattell, C.J. Brackenridge, J. Case, D.N. Propert, A.J. Sherry, "The Relation of Blood Types to Primary and Secondary Personality Traits," *Mankind Quarterly* 21 (1980): 35–51.

56. B.H. Cohen and C.B. Thomas, "Comparison of Smokers and Non-Smokers: The Distribution of ABO and Rh (D) Blood Groups," *Bulletin of the Johns Hopkins Hospital* 110 (1962): 1–7. For Wiener's dismissal, see A.S. Wiener, "Blood Groups and Disease," *American Journal of Human Genetics* 22 (1970): 476.

57. "Blood Type Found Factor in Pill Hazards," *Medical World News* 10 (1969): 17.

58. G. Garratty, "Association of Blood Groups and Disease," p. 332. See Maurice Sievers, "Hereditary Aspects of Gastric Secretory Function," *American Journal of Medicine* 27 (1959): 246–255.

59. Peter J. D'Adamo, *Eat Right for Your Type* (New York: Putnams, 1996); for JFK, see Steven M. Weissberg and Joseph Christiano, *The Answer Is in Your Bloodtype* (Lake Mary, FL: Personal Nutrition, 1999).

60. "Identification Tags May Carry Blood Type Data," *Science News Letter* 36 (1939): 280.

61. David Hellman to Office of the Director, Public Health Service, RG 443, NIH 1930–48 General Records, Box 46, f. He, National Archives.

62. Card, in author's possession.

63. "Identification Card for Blood Donors," *Journal of the American Medical Association* 128 (1945): 225.

64. "Health Group Hits Atomic War Fears," *New York Times*, 8 Jun. 1950, p. 11.

65. "Truman Gets a Tag to List Blood Type," *New York Times*, 22 Nov. 1950, p. 8; "AMVET Drive for Blood-Type Tags Given Boost," *Los Angeles Times*, 6 Mar. 1951, p. A2.

66. "Blood Type Program for U.S. Proposed," *Washington Post*, 24 Oct. 1950, p. B9.

67. "Poll Favors Dog Tags for Bomb Attacks," *Los Angeles Times*, 25 Sep. 1950, p. 8. "Kids Swap Things, So Blood-Type Dog-Tag Is Abandoned," *Washington Post*, 6 Jan. 1958, p. A1.

68. "The Inquiring Camera Girl," *Chicago Daily Triune*, 3 Aug. 1950, p. 15.

69. Theodore Irwin, "Medicine's Most Exclusive Club," *Today's Health* 39 (1961): 34–37, 88. Information on the activities of the Rare Blood Club are sketchy; the Knights of Pythias apparently have retained no records of the group's work, and it is no longer in existence.

70. "Blood Money," *Time* 78 (1961): 91–92.

71. "The Precious Blood of Joe Thomas," *Ebony* 26 (1971): 72–74. "Blood Money," *Newsweek* 76 (17 Aug. 1970): 77.

72. Mary Creager, "Blood Typing—A Study in Genetics," *The Science Teacher* 13 (1946): 14–15, 61.

73. Carson McCullers, *The Member of the Wedding* (Boston: Houghton Mifflin, 1946), 23.

74. John O. Killens, *Youngblood* (New York: Dial Press, 1954), 547 for Oscar and the doctor; p. 566 for the last paragraphs. For a very different take on the biopolitics of blood types, see Donna Haraway's "Universal Donors in a Vampire Culture: It's All in the Family: Biological Kinship Categories in the Twentieth-Century United States," in William Cronon, ed., *Uncommon Ground: Toward Inventing Nature* (New York, Norton, 1995).

75. "The Blood Donor," *San Francisco Examiner*, 16 Jan. 1964, p. 5.

6

Medicalizing Miscegenation
Transplantation and Race

"Americans," noted historian David Hollinger, "have mixed in some ways and not others, and they have talked about it in certain ways and not others." Hollinger was referring to the American experience of "amalgamation," the word generally used before the Civil War to describe race mixing and, after 1863, "miscegenation," a word introduced by an anonymous American to characterize "mistaken mixtures" between the races.[1] In American history, intimacies across the color line have a long and complex history, punctuated by violence, legislation, and Supreme Court decisions. This chapter explores a different kind of physical intimacy across racial lines, the surgical transfer of tissue—skin, bone, organs—between whites, blacks, and other people of color.

Some of these transfers involved external tissue, especially the skin. The visibility of skin grafting between individuals of differing pigmentation attracted surgeons inasmuch as it promised to shed light on the biologic differences between the races and the stability of skin pigmentation. Although many surgeons described these grafting attempts, their efforts did not resolve longstanding questions about human variation and racial distinctiveness. In addition to external tissue, surgeons grafted internal tissues and organs, including sexual organs (ovaries and testicles), kidneys, and, in the 1960s, in the "ultimate operation," hearts. Unlike blood, which was plentiful, hearts and kidneys were difficult to acquire for transplantation. Whereas some white Americans expressed concern about getting the "wrong color blood," in the case of heart transplantation, some American blacks voiced fears that their bodies would be more readily harvested for organs that would be used to save the lives of white patients. In the early years of heart transplantation, American experience resonated uneasily with the racial dynamics of apartheid South Africa, where surgeon Christiaan Barnard performed the first human heart transplant in December 1967. As the transplantation of hearts, kidneys, lungs, and other organs became more routinely successful in the last quarter of the twentieth century, and the waiting lists for these scarce organs longer and longer, concerns about their equitable allocation and the specter of racial preference have continued.

Skin Deep

Reading the signs of skin had long been a feature of American medicine. Racial differences in the skin and its pigment spoke to boundaries and surfaces of contact; it raised issues of similarity and identity, both assumed and assigned. The nature of skin color, its mutability, and even instability challenged racial categories. The prospect of altering the color of the skin, especially to bleach black skin white, excited medical imaginations. In the early twentieth century, some physicians conducted experiments with the recently discovered x-rays in an effort to eliminate dark patches on white skin. In 1903, newspapers quoted University of Pennsylvania physician Henry K. Pancoast's announcement that x-rays "could turn the complexion of the blackest man to a beautiful, soft, creamy white color."[2] One year later, a University of California undergraduate majoring in chemistry combined radium and the x-ray in an attempt "to turn the skin of a Negro white." Physicians in Boston and New York offered similarly sensational claims about the successful transformation of black skin into white skin using the burning/bleaching process of the x-ray.[3]

Surgeons had long been intrigued by the question of skin pigment. After the Civil War, as American surgeons grew increasingly interested in repairs of traumatic injury, burns, and wounds through skin grafting, they speculated about the fate of skin pigment. What happened when black skin was grafted onto a white person, or white skin onto a black person? Would the grafted skin remain the same color? Would black skin become white? Would white skin turn black? Many physicians attempted to resolve this conundrum. One of the first to explore these possibilities was surgeon Thomas Bryant.

In 1871, Bryant transplanted the skin from a black man to cover the ulcerated leg of a white man. Before doing so, he made explicit that he sought "full concurrence of both patients" for the procedure. At a time when few, if any, surgeons sought explicit permission for surgical procedures, Bryant explained that he had taken this unusual step because the grafting was one that he would not have permitted on his own person.[4] Bryant did not make explicit why he would not have permitted it on his own person. The risk of disease transmission existed, certainly, as well as the violation of the conventional distinction between white and black skin. Fascinated by the question of whether the pigmentation of the new skin would expand in its new resting place, Bryant transferred small pieces of skin from the black donor to the white recipient. To his surprise, his patient and donor "both were rather disappointed that the operation could not be repeated. They were firm friends, and the link I formed bound them closer."[5]

Many American surgeons described their own similar experiments. In 1872, when Delaware physician G. Troup Maxwell was called in to see "James Pearce, a Negro, who had been shot in the face by the accidental charge of a gun," he performed a series of skin grafts to prevent disfigurement. "Whilst making preparations for the operation," Maxwell reported, "the idea of grafting the skin of a white man upon a Negro occurred to me." He "obtained the consent" of his patient to remove two dime-sized piece of skin from his own (white) forearm and two pieces from Pearce's forearm, which he inserted into the man's wounded face. After the grafting, the "experiment" nearly ended in failure when the doctor's patient "got on a 'spree,' and whilst intoxicated, destroyed two of the four grafts." Two of the four grafts (one black, one white) continued to grow; the novelty of the procedure afforded the physician "a peculiar pleasure" to witness the growth of the white graft. After several weeks, the doctor reported, upon seeing his former patient at a distance that the white skin had lost its distinguishing characteristics.[6] Newspapers carried occasional stories about interracial skin grafts, such as the "interesting experiments" of John Ege, a physician in Reading, Pennsylvania, who, in 1891, described how exchanges of skin between white and blacks revealed that white skin grafted onto a black person remained white, while black skin grafted onto a white person became white.[7]

In 1895, surgeon Leonard Freeman lectured the members of the Denver and Arapahoe Medical Society about skin grafting and the color question. Cautioning his fellow physicians about "the peculiar ideas" of some surgeons who refused to use an anesthetic and "needlessly tortured" their patients, Freeman announced that "when the skin of a Negro was transferred to a white man, it soon loses its black color." Although black skin grew readily onto white skin, Freeman explained that "white skin cannot be transplanted to a Negro." He based his findings on reports in the medical literature and upon his own experiments, including grafts on "aged darkey with an old crural ulcer, probably syphilitic" and "the transfer of a piece of skin from a Negro's thigh to the sole of his foot, the black graft presenting a marked contrast to the surrounding light-colored skin."[8]

When he published the first American textbook on skin grafting in 1912, Freeman reported extensive experimentation with grafting skin between the races. "Under ordinary circumstances no one would think of transplanting the skin of a Negro to a white man, or the reverse"; the surgeon explained, "so that the question as to whether or not the skin will retain, under such conditions, its original color is of scientific interest only."[9] Most surprising to Freeman was the fact that the many grafts undertaken for "scientific interest only" had produced "strangely conflicting" results. That skin removed from one person and grafted upon another would grow was less important than determining whether the color of the donor skin would remain. Some surgeons claimed that although "skin from a Negro will grow perfectly well upon a white man, white skin will not do well upon the Negro." In the face of these disparate accounts, Freeman concluded that the evidence seemed to indicate that the color of the skin grafts eventually changed, sometimes over a period of weeks and months, to resemble the color of the recipient skin. (This was undoubtedly good news for those individuals who received grafts from frogs, chickens, pigeons, and Mexican hairless puppies (see Chapter 1).

That pigmented skin transferred to a white person eventually fades was also the experience of surgeons at Johns Hopkins Hospital. Plastic surgeon John Staige Davis described how he transplanted several "white whole-thickness grafts upon Negroes" at the Baltimore hospital and observed how these white grafts "became dusky" although the pigmentation process took considerable time. Davis noted that the transfer of Negro skin onto white skin did not result in dark pigment on the recipient, explaining

> In considering the loss of pigment in a black graft transplanted to a white person, and the acquisition of pigment by the white graft placed on a colored person, we must bear in mind the fact that sometimes both auto and iso white grafts become pigmented, and moreover, that both auto and iso black grafts at first lose their pigment, although the pigment subsequently returns.[10]

It may very well be that this skin grafting between the races represented a novelty for physicians, most of whom did not display Dr. Bryant's scruples about obtaining consent from both the donor and the recipient. It would not be surprising to discover that African Americans patients were subjected more often to these therapeutic experiments, involving either skin from different races or even different species. When Richmond surgeon Stuart McGuire treated a badly burned African American child in 1903, he explained that the child was too feeble to provide skin. Not only did the child's relations refused to donate material, but "no jail bird would volunteer as a victim," even with the prospect of parole. McGuire purchased a chocolate-colored pig for grafting. "The pig was brought in on one table, the pickaninny on another. Grafts were taken from the belly of the pig and planted on the back of the child." The pig-skin graft was only partly successful because the child removed the dressing and disturbed the new skin.[11]

In the popular press, the issue of interracial skin grafting generally appeared when African Americans were described as unwilling to aid one of their own race. When Bertha Reed, a badly burned "Negro girl 8 years old" needed skin for treatment of her injuries, the press reported that the child's mother and other "volunteers of her race" refused to provide the needed tissue, so white donors had volunteered.[12]

Perhaps the most sensational interracial graftings before World War II involved the transplantation of testicles. In 1918, Leo Stanley, physician in charge at California's San Quentin Prison, grew interested in the relationship between endocrine glands and behavior. His initial interest was the thyroid gland, and he experimented with the surgical removal of the "the obviously overdeveloped thyroid gland" of violent prisoners. He invited Chicago surgeon G. Frank Lydston to undertake testicular transplants at the prison; Lydston was an influential, if eccentric advocate of the surgery and had transplanted material to his own body. (He dramatically revealed his surgical enhancement to Chicago surgeon Max Thorek, lowering his trousers in the doctor's office to display his handiwork.)[13] Lydston's San Quentin surgery involved an executed Negro whose testes were grafted onto a 72-year-old white prisoner "with marked evidence of senility." Mark Williams, who received the testicular material from an executed African American man, reportedly experienced marked improvement. Following the surgery, Stanley described how the patient improved both physically and mentally:

> His eyes are brighter and he is more active mentally and physically than a man many years his junior. Appetite is excellent. He is anxious to be doing something of interest. Before operation he was naturally reticent, but now is positively emphatic. Summing the whole demeanor 5 days after operation, he has more "jazz and pep" and the increased energy of a man many years younger than he.

Even more extraordinary, Stanley noted how, for the first time, Williams was able to comprehend jokes. Williams received parole in 1924, apparently much benefited by his surgery.[14] Stanley performed other testicular transplants, including a "double transplantation from a Negro, aged 27" onto a "rather dull" white man aged 25. This young man similarly became more active following the surgery; he wrote "better letters, comprehended jokes, and had more sexual activity than before." Stanley used the testicle taken from a Mexican for a transplant in February 1919 to treat a 50-year-old white man whose testicles had atrophied following infection with mumps. In June 1919, the surgeon used the two testicles of "an Indian boy, aged 19" to treat an unmarried, 72-year-old man.[15] Executed Mexican and Japanese prisoners were the source of testicular material for several white men. Two of the recipients of such material were identified as "Negro." A 50-year-old man who received a crushing injury to his groin received testicular material from a Mexican man in September 1919. In a "Negro, age 45" Stanley surgically implanted ram's testes, inasmuch as human material was unavailable.

It is unclear what selection criteria, other than availability, influenced Stanley's selection of donors and recipients. It may be that Mexicans, Negroes, Japanese, and Indians (in the language of his day; today, Native Americans) were more likely to be executed by the state and their bodies made available for harvest. At the same time, it is impossible to ignore the psychosocial dimensions of sexual tissue from African American men in the 1920s with a surgery intended in part to restore sexual vigor. As Stanley pointed out, the "monkey gland" operation of Serge Voronoff was all the rage. Stanley would not be alone in equating African American men with monkeys and apes. In the 1920s, one scientific project with marked international interest was the possibility of interbreeding apes and humans. When Russian scientist Il'ya Ivanov proposed in 1926 to inseminate human "volunteers" with sperm taken from anthropoid apes, Edwin E. Slosson, director of the influential Science Service, a leading popularizer of science in America, circulated the information to American newspapers. A Detroit lawyer and amateur biologist, Howell S. England offered the sum of $100,000 to support the experiment, which he hoped would demonstrate the possibility that new species could develop and cement the fortunes of Darwinian evolution. Not everyone supported this undertaking, including the Ku Klux Klan, the self-styled defenders of racial (and species) purity.[16] Fortunately for all, this experiment in hybridization did not bear fruit.

The prospect of transferring body parts between the races appealed to some fiction writers. In 1931, author Charles Gardner Bowers spun a fantasy for readers of *Amazing Stories*. In "The Black Hand" he described how an artist developed gangrene in his injured arm. Faced with amputation, he agrees to purchase the arm of a man sentenced to die in state prison and allows his surgeon to transfer the prisoner's arm to his body. The prisoner, however, is not only a convicted criminal but a "Negro." "The thought of a black hand was revolting," the artist muses, "but the thought of no hand at all was like death itself." Not only does the artist ponder the shape and size of the hand, but speculates about the gradations of color: "Would the hand be large and awkward or would it be slender and sensitive? Was it coal black or only a light mulatto? Could he ever return to society with such a stigma?" After the arm graft is performed successfully, there is no biologic rejection of the foreign tissue (the author explains that the prisoner's blood types perfectly with that of the artist). But there is a powerful psychological rejection of the newly grafted flesh. The artist develops an acute aversion to blacks: imagining that Negro men pursue him to recover the arm, he savagely murders a number of "Negroes." Once committed to the Psychopathic Hospital, he is discovered dead in his cell. He has bled to death from a slashing wound to his white arm (committed by the black hand).[17] This fictional surgery relied on visible markers of racial difference, the transfer of a black arm onto a white body. But in the 1950s and 1960s, as surgeons forged ahead with the transplantation of internal organs—kidneys, lungs, and hearts—there would be no such visible sign of the racial origins of the donor organs. This created a new set of issues and anxieties for Americans.

An American Transplant Tragedy

In May 1968, surgeons at the Medical College of Virginia (MCV) performed their first heart transplant (sixteenth in the world).[18] From the body of a severely brain-damaged 56-year-old man, the surgeons removed a heart and placed it in the chest of a 53-year-old man. Amid the intense media interest in heart transplantation, officials from MCV did not initially identify either the donor or the recipient.[19] On May 28, 1968, a reporter from the *Washington Post* described the first American interracial transplant, one in which a Virginia "white" received a "Negro's heart" in a Richmond hospital.[20] Although Joseph Klett, the retired white executive who received Bruce Tucker's heart, lived only 7 days before he succumbed to massive rejection of the transplanted organ, the story surrounding Tucker's heart lived on. It became the focus of a lawsuit, an eventual judicial decision about the nature and determination of brain death, and a spur to legislatures to craft new statutes for defining death.[21] As the first legal case in the United States to challenge the conventional "definition of death" in the context of heart transplantation, citations to *Tucker v. Lower* appeared (and continue to appear) frequently in the bioethics literature.[22] But a curious thing happened in many of these discussions: the issue of race disappeared. Yet, the fact that the heart of an African American man was removed and placed into the chest of a white man was not incidental in 1968, in Richmond, and to members of Bruce Tucker's family.[23]

In May 1968, MCV transplant surgeons were eager to join the raucous race to transplant the human heart ignited by South African surgeon Christiaan Barnard in December 1967. The MCV surgeons were well acquainted with Barnard; the

South African had spent 3 months in Richmond in 1966. Working with transplant pioneer David Hume, Barnard assisted with the Richmond kidney transplants and learned how to manage the postoperative care for transplant recipients, including the study of rejection and the use of drugs to suppress the immune system. Barnard also had the opportunity to observe the heart transplant studies conducted in dogs by MCV surgeon Richard Lower. Even before he returned to Capetown to establish South Africa's first kidney transplant program, Barnard had begun preparations for human heart transplantation.[24]

On December 3, 1967, Barnard transplanted the heart of a young woman, extensively brain damaged in an automobile accident, into the body of Louis Washkansky. With little mention of the extensive laboratory animal research into heart transplantation conducted by Norman Shumway's laboratory at Stanford University, by Richard Lower at MCV, and by surgeon Adrian Kantrowitz in New York, Barnard ignited an astounding media frenzy as his famous patient, Louis Washkansky, lived 18 days before he succumbed to pneumonia. American transplant surgeons, stunned by Barnard's boldness in heart transplantation, quickly mobilized to join the heart transplant enterprise.[25]

Within days of the Capetown transplant, New York surgeon Adrian Kantrowitz performed the second human heart transplant.[26] On December 6, 1967, he transplanted the heart of an anencephalic infant into another infant (18 days old), but the child lived for only 6 hours with the new organ. One month later Stanford surgeon Norman Shumway performed the world's fourth heart transplant; his patient, Mike Kasperak, lived 15 days before he died. In Texas, surgeon Denton Cooley joined the transplant race in May 1968 (Cooley would go on to transplant hearts into 17 patients in the remaining months of 1968). In Richmond, MCV surgeons were eager for their opportunity to take part in transplant history. MCV surgeon Richard Lower (who was also Shumway's first resident at Stanford) believed that Barnard became interested in heart transplants when he visited MCV and witnessed the apparent simplicity of the surgical procedure.[27] MCV surgeons had a potential recipient—Joseph Klett, a retired executive with ongoing heart problems. But where would they get the necessary heart?

They located the organ in the body of Bruce O. Tucker, a middle-aged African American man and a long-time employee at a Richmond egg-packing plant. After a fall onto concrete, Tucker had been brought by ambulance to MCV. He was unconscious and unaccompanied by any friend or relative. At MCV, he underwent a craniotomy to relieve the pressure in his brain. He was placed on a respirator, which kept him "mechanically alive." The following afternoon, Tucker was evaluated by a neurologist, who offered the opinion that it was "very likely" that Tucker's condition was "irreversible" when he had been admitted the evening before. He received both anesthesia and oxygen to maintain his organs. When he was removed from the respirator, the surgeons waited for his breathing to stop. They called for the medical examiner to pronounce him dead—and available for organ harvest. Both his heart and kidneys were removed for transplant into other patients.[28]

The members of Bruce Tucker's family were not consulted about the decision to remove his heart and kidneys. His brother, William Tucker, did not learn from the surgeons or from the hospital staff that his brother's heart had been removed. The family was not informed that Tucker had been declared one of the "unclaimed dead"; this pronouncement made his body, under Virginia state law, available for medical use. Tucker and another brother, Grover Tucker, discovered their brother's role in transplant history from the undertaker, who received his brother's body for burial. The surviving Tuckers were especially distressed by the identification of their loved one as "unclaimed." They were disturbed at how quickly Bruce Tucker's status mutated from dead person to "unclaimed dead." In fact, Virginia law required a 24-hour waiting period for family or friends to come forward to claim a deceased loved one. Such a waiting period, however, would make his organs unusable for transplant. Within 1 hour of the state medical examiner's pronouncement that he was "unclaimed dead," surgeons made the incision into his chest to remove the heart.[29] Angered by these events, William Tucker retained a young African American lawyer, L. Douglas Wilder, and brought two lawsuits. One lawsuit sought $100,000 from the three MCV surgeons (Richard Lower, David Hume, and David Sewell) and from Dr. Abdullah Fatteh, a Virginia state medical examiner, on the grounds of "wrongful death, deprivation of property rights, insubstantial due process and 'mutilation' of the body without consent." The other, a federal suit, sought $900,000 dollars in U.S. District Court for deprivation of civil rights.[30]

Tucker's attorney explicitly identified race as a critical issue in the MCV heart transplant. A person with status in the community, charged Wilder, would not have been treated in the manner accorded Bruce Tucker. The hospital "pulled the plug because he was poor and black, a representative of the faceless masses."[31] Before the case came to trial, Wilder, who also served as the first black state senator in Virginia since Reconstruction, successfully opposed a bill in the 1970 Virginia state legislature that would have legalized the removal of organs for transplantation without permission from the family of the deceased. Wilder called on traditional wisdom in the African American community about so-called "night-doctors," who abducted black children for use in medical experiments. "They're not going to be taking the hearts of any white mayors," Wilder noted, "You know whose hearts they're going to be taking. If this bill passes, its going to be so that black mothers will tell their children, 'Don't go walkin' down by the Medical College at night or the student doctor's gonna get you.'"[32]

Despite Wilder and his client's claims, MCV surgeons maintained that race played no role in the decision to take Tucker's heart; the transplant, they insisted, would have proceeded in an identical fashion if a middle-class white man had been brought to the hospital in a similar brain-damaged state. Moreover, MCV chair of surgery David Hume suggested that giving people "free" care in a state institution should immunize the doctors. "Look," he told a reporter, "this [MCV] is a state-run institution and a large proportion of our patients are black. We've done some 235 organ grafts here, and none of the recipients has ever been charged doctors' fees or hospital costs. We should be the last ones to be picked on over racial matters."[33] It is difficult to gauge the accuracy of Hume's claim, given that the hospital's patient records are not accessible. However, because of the publicity surrounding the kidney transplants and the candor with which Hume and his surgeons discussed their cases, it seems likely that most of the kidney transplants undertaken between 1957 and 1968 were performed for the benefit of white recipients. In part, this reflected the surgical and immunologic preference for familial donors rather than cadaveric donors. In the first seven kidney transplants at MCV, the kidneys were given by an identical twin, a mother, two sisters, a brother, and a father. In one case, George Blanton, a white barber from Hendersonville, North Carolina, received a cadaveric kidney from a Negro man killed in a traffic accident. Blanton's body rejected this kidney, and he received a second kidney transplant with an organ donated by his mother.[34]

Tucker did not prevail in his lawsuit; an all-white, all-male jury deliberated little over an hour before they absolved the surgeons of wrong-doing and accepted a novel medical definition of death based on the loss of brain function.[35] Race relations certainly seem to have played a role in the subsequent heart transplants undertaken at MCV. On August 25, 1968 Richard Lower and his surgical team at MCV performed a heart transplant. Initially reticent to release the details in order "to protect the privacy of the organ donors and their families," the hospital later announced that a 43-year-old man had received the heart of a 17-year-old gunshot victim.[36] But, unlike the Tucker transplant, both the donor and recipient in the August transplant were African Americans. In subsequent news reports, the recipient was identified as Louis B. Russell, Jr., an elementary school teacher from Indianapolis. Russell became the thirty-fourth transplant recipient in the world when he received the heart of Clarence Robert Brown, who had been shot in the back of the head with a small-caliber pistol following an argument in a Virginia restaurant.[37] A Richmond radio station broke the news of the identity of the donor.[38] Although newspapers outside the Richmond area did not identify the donor's race, a front-page story in the *Richmond Times-Dispatch* described the gunshot victim as "Brown, a Negro."[39] When the parents of the boy expressed the desire to meet Russell, MCV arranged transportation for the family to the Richmond hospital where Russell was convalescing.[40] Russell went on to become one of the longest surviving heart transplant patients in the early cohort of recipients; he survived 6 years with the transplanted heart. After his death, in November 1974, the American Heart Association created the Louis B. Russell Jr. Memorial Award in 1976, to encourage greater outreach to minority and low-income communities.[41]

What difference did race make in the early years of heart transplantation? Was Tucker's race material to his selection as a heart source? Is it significant that Russell's race was not initially identified in news reports (and Brown's only rarely identified in print)? How did Russell's status as the "longest living American heart recipient" influence the role of race in heart transplantation? How did the racial politics of heart transplantation comport with similar issues of access and success in kidney transplantation? How did the lawsuit brought by the Tucker family influence the selection of subsequent donors?

Certainly, the Tucker case resonated with the specter of racial selection already excited by Christiaan Barnard's South African heart transplants. Even before he electrified the world in December 1967, when he performed the first human heart transplant, Barnard's surgeries in apartheid South Africa rippled with racial currents.

In October 1967, as he performed the first kidney transplants in Capetown, Barnard acknowledged the "overtones of racial integration in a limited physiological arena" when his white patient, Mrs. Edith Black, received the kidney of "a colored youth." The world press could not resist such headlines as "Mrs. Black Receives Black Kidney."[42] Positioned like many white South African doctors between a desire for recognition by the international medical community and the racial politics and privilege that facilitated his practice, Barnard claims to have hoped that his first heart transplant recipient would be "a Bantu with cardiomyopathy," but a South African colleague told him to forget it. "Our first patient will never be black or colored because overseas they will say that we are experimenting on nonwhites."[43]

Perhaps in an effort to downplay the racial overtones, Barnard's first patient, a white, Jewish man named Louis Washkansky, received the heart taken from the body of a 22-year-old white woman, Denise Darvall. In the blaze of media attention, reporters also noted how one of her kidneys was transplanted into a "colored boy" (or "mulatto" in some news reports).[44] But, in January 1968, Barnard decisively crossed the cardiac color line. The recipient, rather than a black African, was Philip Blaiberg, a 58-year-old white, Jewish dentist. The source of the transplanted heart was Clive Haupt, identified as "Cape Colored" in the South African racial caste system. As a reporter for the *Washington Post* explained for the benefit of American readers, Cape Coloreds were usually a "mixture of European, Hottentot, Asian, and Black African stock."[45] The racial dynamics of this surgery prompted worldwide comment. In England, a South African diplomat was quoted to the effect that the transplant of Clive Haupt's heart did not alter Philip Blaiberg's status as a white man under South African law.[46] In Uganda, the Deputy Foreign Minister, Vincent Rwamaro, expressed fears that a black African might be "dragged from his house to a hospital and his heart pulled out to save a dying white man." Apprehensive that blacks would serve as "spare parts for whites," Rwamaro insisted that white South Africans regarded black South Africans as less than human.[47] Still for the South African government and leaders of South Africa, the transplants, which catapulted Barnard to the world stage, represented a source of national pride, an "affirmation of the country as a first world contender among technologically capable developed countries."[48]

Amid the hubbub of the interracial transplant and the perception that black bodies were providing the raw materials for transplant, Barnard announced that a "black African" would receive a heart in a transplant operation. As he offered this news, Barnard also informed reporters that his "black African" candidate "was not mentally stable so he might not be suitable for the operation." He went on to explain that this patient would not be likely to comply with the demanding post-transplant regimen. "So, if the next patient is an African we will probably make some facilities available to keep him around for a few years."[49] Despite Barnard's announcement of plans to make a black African the recipient of the next heart transplant, his next recipient was a "white former policeman" in South Africa, who received the heart of a "pregnant black," whose family apparently only learned about the transplant after her death.[50] After protests about the use of "black donor hearts" and the "harmful" reporting of transplants in the media, Barnard announced in 1975 that his hospital would stop using blacks as donors.[51]

In the United States the news of Barnard's second transplant also resonated with a different kind of national politics, the politics of racial discrimination and the civil rights movement. Some American commentators interpreted the news of the Haupt donation as a sign of social progress: "the acceptance of the heart of a colored donor by a white patient, or the heart of a woman by a man, is a lesson in ethics as well as physiology . . . The dying South African accepted the heart of a colored man as eagerly as he would have the heart of a white man, and not even the most bigoted Afrikaners said a word."[52] But, in print, African Americans questioned Barnard's policies. In a letter to the *New York Times*, for example, Ellen Holly called for Barnard to use the organs of a white man to save a black man's life, noting "All I know is that, as a black, if I lived in South Africa, I would be terrified at the prospect of going into a white South African hospital with a major illness. I also know that because of the inadequacies of the bush hospitals I might have no other choice."[53] The editors of *Ebony* noted with evident pleasure how the transplant would enable the Cape colored man's heart to go places that Haupt himself had not been permitted to enter. "Haupt's heart will ride in the uncrowded train coaches 'For Whites Only' instead of in the crowded ones reserved for blacks. It will pump extra hard to circulate the blood needed in a game of tennis where the only blacks are those who might tend the heavy rollers to smooth the courts. It will enter fine restaurants, attend theaters and concerts, and live in a decent home instead of the tough slums where Haupt grew up."[54] But the editors cautioned that the use of black person's organs to save a dying white man in South Africa also raised fears that the practice would not remain in South Africa. "Many black people today in both the United States and South Africa," the editors noted, "fear hospitals because they believe that white doctors use black patients only for experimentation." This fear would lead families of potential black donors to refuse to authorize organ donation, because they believed that the doctors would "hurry a death" in order to finish a transplant.[55]

This fear was not limited to blacks. In Houston, a major center of heart transplantation, some called attention to the fact that dying Mexican patients were transferred to Houston hospitals where patients awaited a heart donor. In 1968, Maria Acosta, a 38-year-old Mexican woman with a severe brain hemorrhage, was transferred in an ambulance from a hospital in Yuma, Arizona to St. Luke's Hospital, where surgeon Denton Cooley ran a major heart transplant program. "No one says that Mrs. Acosta was actually taken from her Yuma hospital to St. Luke's for the specific purpose of being a heart donor. But this is certain: there are at present more than 30 potential heart recipients in St. Luke's; and some have been waiting as long as 3 months for a donor. Was someone playing God with Mrs. Acosta's life?"[56] In February, 1969, Mrs. Guadalupe Montez, the widow of a Mexican-American heart donor, instituted a million dollar lawsuit against Cook County Hospital in Chicago, alleging that her husband died as a result of "careless and negligent acts" in order to hurry a transplant operation.[57]

The Tucker lawsuit represented a transitional moment in the history of organ transplantation and the determination of death by new criteria involving the brain. But it also resonated with traditional medical practices involving low-income and minority patients. William Tucker remained convinced that the MCV surgeons killed his brother in order to take his heart. His attorney made reference to the undue haste with which the medical examiner declared Bruce Tucker to be "unclaimed dead." As Douglas Wilder emphasized in his closing arguments, Bruce Tucker belonged to the "faceless black masses of society." Because he was black and poorly dressed (and also because he had, according to various accounts, injured himself while drinking) he was declared "unclaimed."[58] Wilder angrily pointed out that the chief medical examiner of Virginia, Dr. Geoffrey T. Mann, had reassured him that his (Wilder's) body would never be declared "unclaimed" "presumably because he was plainly well dressed."[59] The determination that his brother's body was unclaimed particularly inflamed William Tucker. As the judge noted, when Bruce Tucker entered the hospital, his wallet contained a business card with the address of his brother's store (located within 15 blocks of the hospital). Moreover, William Tucker had called three times at the hospital seeking news of his brother with no success. Despite his efforts and the information on Tucker's person, the decision to identify his body as "unclaimed dead" was made.

The Tucker case has been hailed as a critical milestone in the history of brain death, but it also reflects Bruce Tucker's status as "socially dead" before he was pronounced physically dead by the medical examiner. Ethnographer David Sudnow chose the term "social death" to refer to the state in which a hospital patient "is treated essentially as a corpse, though perhaps still 'clinically' and 'biologically' alive."[60] Bruce Tucker entered the hospital without friends or family members. Even worse, in terms of medical decision-making about his "terminality" as a patient, he entered the hospital with alcohol on his breath and on his clothes. "The alcoholic patient," Sudnow concluded in his observational study of public hospitals in the late 1960s, "is treated by hospital physicians, not only when the status of his body as alive or dead is at stake, but throughout the whole course of medical treatment, as one for whom the concern to treat can properly operate somewhat weakly."[61] In the case of Bruce Tucker, physician concern about his recovery was colored by his race, socio-economic class, and alcohol use.

How did race influence the practice of heart transplantation? The information in both the medical and popular press was often sketchy and inconsistent. Clearly, some anxieties existed about the unequal burdens of transplantation. In 1968, when the American College of Chest Physicians Committee on Heart Transplantation recommended greater responsibility in media reporting of heart transplants, including that all donors remain anonymous, W. Montague Cobb, editor of the *Journal of the National Medical Association*, insisted that their endorsement of anonymity was premature. Cobb cited the practice of declaring some dead persons as "unclaimed" as a particular area of concern. "Minority and impoverished groups," Cobb explained, "would be the most likely to be affected by the policy of anonymity. Therefore, any approval of such a policy should be withheld until all aspects of the situation have been publicly explored in depth."[62] In 1970, Cyril Jones, a professor of surgery at the Downstate Medical Center in Brooklyn, New York, cited a report from the American Civil Liberties Union's ad hoc committee on civil liberties and organ transplantation, which claimed that, among the first 100 heart transplants, there were 64 black donors but only one black recipient.[63]

The registry of heart transplants maintained by the American College of Surgeons–National Institutes of Health (ACS-NIH) offered a somewhat different picture. In 1970, the ACS-NIH registry recorded heart transplants by the race of the donor and the recipient. Whites served as donors in 110 cases, and 113 white patients received hearts. Hearts were obtained from seven black donors, one "Oriental," and four individuals identified as "other." Nine blacks received a heart, as did one "Oriental." Only one "other" patient received a heart transplant.[64] In the United States, Ester Matthews, a 41-year-old Dallas housewife, became the first woman and the first African American heart transplant recipient. In June 1968, she received the heart of a 26-year-old white man. Doctors at Parkland Memorial Hospital had hoped to transplant the heart of a woman into Matthews, but the woman's father refused permission for the transplant.[65] Houston surgeon Denton Cooley reported in September 1968 a case in which a 2-month-old "Negro girl" received the heart of a 1-day-old white anencephalic infant.[66] At MCV, following the Tucker transplant, surgeon Richard Lower and his colleagues transplanted the heart from a young black man into Louis Russell, a black school teacher, who survived 6 years with the new heart until he succumbed to rejection. In October 1968, Lower transplanted the heart of a young black man (killed by a gunshot wound in the head) into a 19-year-old African American woman. One week later, Lower's team transplanted the heart from a white Norfolk policeman into a former Alexandrian police officer (also white). Lower did not cross the color line in cardiac transplantation after the Tucker controversy.

The controversy over Bruce Tucker's bodily remains reverberated in American popular culture and remained focused on the expropriation of black bodies, rather than on the need for increased minority access to the benefits of American high-tech medicine. On the heels of the Supreme Court decision (*Loving v. Virginia*) that found state laws against interracial marriage unconstitutional, films and novels mined the cultural possibilities of medical miscegenation. In the 1969 film *Change of Mind*, the brain of a liberal white lawyer dying of cancer is transplanted into the body of a recently dead black man. He finds that both his mother and his wife cannot accept his transformation, and the black man with the white man's brain seeks solace in the arms of the widow of the man who furnished the body for brain transplant. In 1970, Lawrence Louis Goldman's novel *The Heart Merchants* featured a transplant surgeon faced with a decision over which patient will receive the donor heart: "One man is old, rich, and white. The other is young, poor, and black. Which dying man will receive the heart transplant?" Complicating the issue of the transplant is the express wish of the father, who agrees to allow his son's heart to be used, but insists that his son's heart won't be "goin' in no nigger body!"[67] In the end, the young black man receives the heart transplant, but the heart does not function.

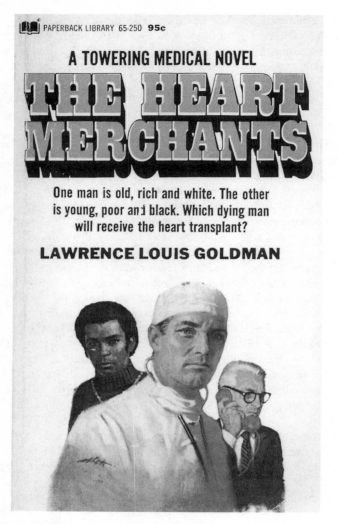

Figure 6.1 The racial politics of heart transplantation quickly became part of popular culture in such mass-market paperbacks as *The Heart Merchants* (Reprinted with permission of Hachette Publishing Group, Inc.).

In 1969, the young black comedian Dick Gregory played Carnegie Hall in New York City. In addition to riffs on the draft, Vice President Spiro Agnew, President Nixon, and the police, Gregory joked about interracial heart transplants. The one that ran the longest, he noted, "was a black heart transferred into a white patient. That heart would be goin' yet," Gregory continued, "if he'd eaten a little soul food." Warning the audience, comprised of mostly young, mostly white people, that blacks were not "goin' to be your spare parts," he called for transplants that could not be hidden: "I'd like to see a white cat get a black foot. Next summer, let him take that to the beach with him: Hey! They'd be yelling at him, 'take off your sneaker and come into the water.'"[68] The comedian could joke about interracial heart transplants and how blacks did not want to serve as "spare parts" for white people, but for others, this was no laughing matter. In 1974, Sandra Haggerty explained that most blacks rejected transplants because of their distrust of doctors who decide when you are dead. She quoted from an informal poll the range of black responses to transplantation: "You notice the heart transplants have all been from blacks to whites. I'd like to see a little reciprocation before I get on the bandwagon!" "No way! A brother's likely to go in the hospital with a cold and come out without a heart." "I just can't trust the Man. He's made it purrfectly [sic] clear whose life he values. No sense in me volunteering."[69]

Distrust of the white medical establishment has also been cited by Howard University transplant surgeon Clive Callender as one of the factors responsible for the lower rates of organ donation among African Americans. When he testified before the House Commerce Committee Subcommittee on Health and Environment in 1998, Callender reminded members of Congress that African Americans continued to wait twice as long as other Americans for kidney transplants. (In 2002, the waiting time for a cadaveric kidney was almost twice as long for an African American as it was for a Caucasian. Moreover, African Americans are less likely to have living donors.)[70] He pointed to a history of inequitable organ allocation, distrust of the medical establishment, and fear that signing an organ donor card would lead to erroneous or premature declarations of death. In 2002, the Hollywood film *John Q* featured actor Denzel Washington as a hard-working man engaged in a desperate struggle to ensure that his son will receive the heart transplant necessary to save his life. Many American filmgoers apparently identified with Washington's character as he confronted the harsh realities of managed care. Although the film generally received only tepid reviews, some reviewers praised the film for avoiding "the race card." Still, in the film, all the doctors and hospital administrators are white; the hero and his family, denied the necessary transplant, are black. Although the issue is not explicitly addressed, the skepticism about the medical establishment and its provision of care resonates with experiences like that of the Tucker family and the lingering resentment about differential treatment (or lack of treatment). As Nation of Islam minister Louis Farrakhan has caustically claimed, the failure of white society to control black-on-black violence provided a steady supply of organs: "When you're killing each other, they can't wait for you to die," Farrakhan announced at a rally, "You're good for parts."[71]

Black and White

In contemporary medical and surgical articles about transplantation, physicians and surgeons often make reference to the antiquity of ideas about transplantation. Although some begin with Adam's rib (an early form of tissue engineering), more often the authors recount the miracle attributed to twin brothers, Saints Cosmas and Damian, who lived in the third century A.D. These physicians performed the so-called "miracle of the black leg," in which they successfully replaced the gangrenous leg of a churchman with a limb taken from the body of a deceased African. When skeptics opened the grave of the deceased black man, they found the dismembered leg of the white man along with his body.[72] The miracle of the black leg attracted medieval and Renaissance painters, who imaginatively contrasted both the old and the new leg of the recovered church official. The images and discussion of the black leg miracle dramatically illustrated divine ability to replace old and diseased parts with healthy body parts.

The appearance of Cosmas and Damian in contemporary medical writings offers a vivid demonstration of medical and surgical, rather than divine, power. These depictions imply an optimism that race is no longer an issue in contemporary transplantation. No miracle is needed to unite the body parts of people from different races and ethnicities, when surgical expertise can restore injured and nonfunctioning bodies of whatever skin color or heritage. But race and reception of racial difference continues to fracture American society. In 2001, when Martha McNeil Hamilton donated her kidney to a friend and fellow journalist Warren Brown, the two recorded "the astonished reaction from so many people, blacks and whites alike" that a white woman had given a black man her kidney.[73] Times had changed, but perhaps a miracle would still be needed.

In 1990, when the father of Thomas Simons, a 24-year-old Ku Klux Klan sympathizer shot and killed by a black teenager, agreed to donate his son's organs, he stipulated in writing that the organs could be used in "white recipients only." Reports of this racial preference provoked different responses. Although the United States Office of Civil Rights declared that the practice of specifying the race of the recipient violated the 1964 Civil Rights Act, some transplant surgeons, including Dr. Clive O. Callender, a prominent black transplant surgeon and director of the Howard University Hospital Transplant Center in Washington, D.C., defended the transplant coordinator's decision to allow this racial preference. Callender explained to reporters that he had been in the reverse situation in which blacks donated organs, but only with the assurance that they would be transplanted into other blacks. "These were people from the South who had been discriminated against, and they felt blacks should get the first chance at organs because of that."[74] In spite of the mixed views about directing donation on racial grounds, the Florida Senate, in 1994, voted 37–0 to ban discrimination by organ donors and their families. The legislation allowed individuals to direct organs to members of their own families or friends, but prohibited restrictions on "the basis of race, color, religion, sex, national origin, age, physical handicap, health status, marital status, or economic status."[75]

The ongoing concern over racial disparities in transplantation donation and outcomes continues. Concerted efforts have been made to increase minority partic-ipation (African Americans, Hispanics, and Native Americans) in organ donation. In 1996, basketball superstar Michael Jordan joined a national campaign intending to increase the number of organ and tissue donors in the United States. A long-time star of the Chicago Bulls basketball team, Jordan appeared in several television and radio spots. In 1999, football star Walter Payton, a one-time candidate for a liver transplant, also endorsed campaigns to increase organ donations. Some commentators have noted that not even the enormous appeal of athletes like Jordan and Payton could overcome reluctance on the part of minority communities to donate organs.[76] People in these communities, according to one Gallup poll, were more likely to reject the definition of brain death, and be more likely to believe that the condition was reversible than those in white communities. Some transplant coordinators have identified the Tuskegee Syphilis Study as one of the chief reasons for minority suspicion about the transplant enterprise. "The Tuskegee experiments really damaged African Americans' trust in the medical community," noted the executive vice president of the Houston-based LifeGift Organ Donation Center, and "trust is the number one issue in organ donation."[77] But, as this chapter makes clear, the reasons for mistrust about organ donation and transplantation extend beyond the Tuskegee Syphilis Study. Bruce Tucker's family did not look to the syphilis study in rural Alabama for evidence of racism; they had plenty of experience in urban Virginia.

Notes

1. David A. Hollinger, "Amalgamation and Hypodescent: The Question of Ethnoracial Mixture in the History of the United States," *American Historical Review* 108 (2003): 1363–1390.

2. Bettyann Kevles, *Naked to the Bone: Medical Imaging in the Twentieth Century* (New Brunswick: Rutgers University Press, 1997), 49.

3. Charles D. Martin, *The White African American Body: A Cultural and Literary Exploration* (New Brunswick: Rutgers University Press. 2002), 150–153.

4. For a discussion of medical consent in late nineteenth-century America, see Susan E. Lederer, *Subjected to Science: Human Experimentation in America before the Second World War* (Johns Hopkins University Press, 1995).

5. Thomas Bryant, *The Practice of Surgery: A Manual* (London: Churchill, 1872), 436.

6. G. Troup Maxwell, "Grafting the Skin of a White Man upon a Negro," *Medical Times*, (1874): 37.

7. "The Black Skin Now White," *Wheeling* (W. Va.) *Register*, 19 Mar. 1891, p. 1.

8. Leonard Freeman, "The Thiersh Method of Skin-Grafting," *Denver Medical Times* 14 (1895): 421–431.

9. Leonard Freeman, *Skin Grafting for Surgeons and General Practitioners* (St. Louis: C.V. Mosby, 1912), 117–119.

10. John Staige Davis, *Plastic Surgery: Its Principles and Practice* (Philadelphia: P. Blakiston's Son, 1919), 94.

11. Stuart McGuire, "Method to Hasten Epidermization, with Special Reference to Skin Grafting," *Virginia Medical Semi-Monthly* 8 (1903–1904): 292–296.

12. "Graft White Skin on Negro," *New York Times*, 21 May 1908, p. 1.

13. Max Thorek, *A Surgeon's World: The Autobiography of Max Thorek* (Philadelphia: J.B. Lippincott, 1943), 174–191.

14. Leo L. Stanley, *Men at Their Worst* (New York: D. Appleton, 1943), 109–110.

15. L.L. Stanley and G. David Kelker, "Testicle Transplantation," *Journal of the American Medical Association* 74 (1920): 1501–1503. L. L. Stanley, "Experiences in Testicle Transplantation," *California State Journal of Medicine* 18 (1920): 251–253.

16. Kirill Rossiianov, "Beyond Species: Il'ya Ivanov and His Experiments on Cross-Breeding Humans with Anthropoid Apes," *Science in Context* 15 (2002): 277–316.

17. Charles Gardner Bowers, "The Black Hand," *Amazing Stories* (1931): 909–911, 923.

18. Susan E. Lederer, "Tucker's Heart: Racial Politics and Heart Transplantation in America," in Keith Wailoo, Peter Guarnaccia, and Julie Livingston, eds. *A Death Retold: Jessica Santillan, the Bungled Transplant, and Paradoxes of Medical Citizenship* (Chapel Hill: University of North Carolina Press, 2006), 142–157.

19. See "College Sets Report on Transplant," *Washington Post*, 31 May 1968, p. B9.

20. Victor Cohn, "Va. White Got Negro's Heart," *Washington Post*, 28 May 1968, p. B1.

21. There is an extensive literature on brain death; see, for example, Margaret Lock, *Twice Dead: Organ Transplants and the Reinvention of Death* (University of California Press, 2002); Stuart J. Youngner, Robert M. Arnold, and Renie Shapiro, eds., *The Definition of Death: Contemporary Controversies* (Baltimore: Johns Hopkins University Press, 1999); and Peter McCullagh, *Brain Dead, Brain Absent, Brain Donors: Human Subjects or Human Objects* (New York: Wiley, 1993). See also Martin S. Pernick, "Back from the Grave: Recurring Controversies over Defining and Diagnosing Death in History," in *Death: Beyond Whole-Brain Criteria*, Richard M. Zaner, ed. (Dordrecht and Boston: Kluwer Academic Publishers, 1988), 17–74; and Gary S. Belkin, "Brain Death and the Historical Understanding of Bioethics," *Journal of the History of Medicine* 58 (2003): 325–361.

22. See *Tucker v. Lower*, No. 2381 (Richmond, Virginia, Law & Equity Court, May 23, 1972).

23. Sarah D. Barber, "The Tell-Tale Heart: Ethical and Legal Implications of In Situ Organ Preservation in the Non-Heart-Beating Cadaver Donor," *Health Matrix* 6 (1996): 471. In both editions of the *Encyclopedia of Bioethics*, the entry for brain death (each written by Alexander Capron) mentions *Tucker v. Lower* but does not mention race. Margaret Lock discusses the Tucker lawsuit in "Inventing a New Death and Making It Believable," *Anthropology and Medicine*, 9 (2002), 97–115, but does not mention race. There are exceptions, however. Robert Veatch, for example, discusses race in his accounts of the Tucker case. See Robert M. Veatch, *Death, Dying, and the Biological Revolution* (Yale University Press, 1976), 21–25; Veatch, *Transplantation Ethics* (Georgetown University Press, 2000), 43–44.

24. Donald McRae, *Every Second Counts: The Race to Transplant the First Human Heart* (New York: Simon and Schuster, 2006), offers the most recent assessment of the heart transplant frenzy.

25. Christiaan Barnard and Curtis Bill Pepper, *One Life* (Toronto, Macmillan, 1969).

26. This enumeration counts as the first heart transplant surgeon James D. Hardy's chimp-to-human heart transplant in 1964. Different accounts assign the Virginia transplant a different number in the heart transplant chronology. Several popular histories of the heart transplants are available, including Tony Stark, *Knife to the Heart: The Story of Transplant Surgery* (Macmillan, 1996), and Nicholas L. Tilney, *Transplant: From Myth to Reality* (Yale, 2003).

27. Sara J. Shumway and Norman E. Shumway, eds. *Thoracic Transplantation* (Cambridge, MA: Blackwell Science, 1995), xi–xii.

28. Abdullah Fatteh, "A Lawsuit That Led to the Redefinition of Death," *Journal of Legal Medicine* 1 (July/August, 1973): 30–34.

29. R.M. Veatch, *Transplantation Ethics*, pp. 43–44.

30. "Seeks $1 Million in Mixed Heart Transplant Case," *Jet* 38 (11 Jun. 1970): 15.

31. "Civil Rights Questions Nag after Transplant Death Trial," *Medical World News*, 16 (Jun. 1972).

32. "Heart Snatch Case," *Richmond Afro-American*, 3 (June 1972): 1–2. For "night doctors," see Patricia A. Turner, *I Heard It Through the Grapevine: Rumor in African-American Culture* (University of California Press, 1993), 67–70.

33. See "Civil Rights Questions Nag after Transplant Death Trial," *Medical World News*, 16 (Jun. 1972).

34. See, for example, David M. Hume, et al., "Renal Transplantation in Man in Modified Recipients," *Annals of Surgery* 158 (1963): 608–644.

35. "Jury Rules in Favor of the Heart Team," (Richmond) *Journal and Guide*, 3 June 1972, p. 16

36. "Man, 43, Receives a Heart Transplant at Virginia College," *New York Times*, 25 Aug. 1968, p. 50.

37. See "Heart Donor's Killer Sought by Police," *Washington Post* 29 Aug. 1968, p. E18, which does not include mention of race. For identification of Russell by name (but not race) the following day; see "Latest Heart Patient, 43, Fed Day after Transplant," *New York Times*, 26 Aug. 1968, p. 8.

38. "34th Heart Transplant Aired," *Washington Post*, 25 August 1968, p. C2.

39. Beverley Orndorff, "Heart Transplant Performed at MCV," *Richmond Times-Dispatch*, 25 Aug. 1968, p. 1. In the numerous articles that appeared subsequently about Russell's successful transplant, the race of the donor is not mentioned. The only place the race of the Russell's donor was identified was in the *Times-Dispatch* article. My thanks to Jodi Koste for helping to locate this item.

40. "Teacher with Transplanted Heart Returns to Classroom," *Jet*, 27 Feb. 1969, pp. 46–52.

41. Diana Christopulos, *Time, Feeling and Focus: A Newly Designed Culture: The Evolution of the American Heart Association, 1975–1997* (American Heart Association, 2000). The first recipient of the award was a black nurse from Los Angeles, Winifred Ray Carnegie, 1977. Press Release, American Heart Association, 28 Jan. 1977, AHA materials.

42. C. Barnard & C.B. Pepper, *One Life*, p. 249.

43. C. Barnard & C.B. Pepper, *One Life*, p. 251.

44. C. Barnard & C.B. Pepper, *One Life*, p. 279 for Darvall's father's description of the kidney recipient. The "Two from One" was also reported in the *Chicago Defender*, December 16–22, 1967, p. 28.

45. "Another Heart Transplant: White South African Receives Cape Colored Man's Heart," *Washington Post*, 3 Jan. 1968, p. 1. Philip Blaiberg, *Looking at My Heart* (New York: Stein and Day, 1968). Long before the current heyday of reality TV, the NBC network sought to capitalize on intense interest in transplants; the network paid Philip Blaiberg $50,000 for exclusive rights to film his operation, and successfully sued when a photographer posing as a medical student sold photographs of the operation. See W. David Gardner, "The Heart Is a Lonely Hunter," *Ramparts* 7 (June 1969), 34–38.

46. "No Legal Significance." *New York Times*. 3 Jan. 1968, p. 32.

47. *The People* (Uganda), 6 Jan. 1968, p. 17.

48. Alexandra Niewijk, "Tough Priorities," *Hastings Center Report*, 1999, 42–50.

49. "Black African Due to Get Next Heart," *New York Times*, 9 Jan. 1968, p. 29.

50. See "A Pregnant Black was Heart Donor," *New York Times*, 8 Sept. 1968, p. 34; and "Heart Donor Was Unknown," *Washington Post*, 12 Sept. 1968, p. A3.

51. "Barnard Stops Using Black Donor Hearts," *Chicago Tribune*, 3 Feb. 1975, p. 4.

52. "Surgical Show Biz," *The Nation*, 206 (22 Jan. 1968): 100.

53. Ellen Holly, "Transplant Abuse," *New York Times*, 29 Sept. 1968, p. E11.

54. "The Telltale Heart," *Ebony* (March, 1968): 118.

55. Ibid.

56. Desmond Smith, "Someone Playing God," *The Nation* 207 (30 Dec. 1968): 719–721.

57. Charles Carroll, "The Ethics of Heart Transplantation," *Journal of the National Medical Association* 62 (1970): 14–20. See "Heart Donor's Widow Sues," *New York Times*, 9 Feb. 1969, p. 16.

58. The trial proceedings (the opinion; no transcript was prepared) did not include any information that drinking led to Bruce Tucker's injury. The judge published a lengthy analysis of Tucker but did not mention drinking as a precipitating factor. See A. Christian Compton, "Telling the Time of Human Death by Statute: An Essential and Progressive Trend," *Washington and Lee Law Review*, 31 (1974): 521–543. The ur-source for Tucker's drinking seems to be Lawrence Mosher, "When Does Life End?" *The National Observer* (3 June 1972). Several of the contemporary accounts, and recent popular and historical accounts, continue to mention Tucker's drinking as a precipitating factor. See for example Peter G. Filene, *Into the Arms of Others: A Cultural History of the Right-to-Die in America* (Chicago, 1998), 56–57.

59. "Heart Donor Was Dead," *Washington Post*, 18 May 1972, p. B3.

60. David Sudnow, *Passing On: The Social Organization of Dying* (Englewood Cliffs, NJ: Prentice-Hall, 1967), 74.

61. D. Sudnow, *Passing On*, p. 104.

62. "Withholding Names of Organ Transplant Donors," *Journal of the National Medical Association*, 60 (1968): 523.

63. Cyril J. Jones, "Medical Ethics and Legal Questions in Human Organ Transplantation," *Journal of the National Medical Association* 62 (1970): 12-13, 24; in the same issue, Charles Carroll, "The Ethics of Heart Transplantation," *idem.*, pp. 14–20, 24.

64. Registry Data, Richard Lower Papers, Box 6, folder: Transplant Registry, Archives, Tompkins-McGaw Library, Medical College of Virginia, VCU, Richmond, Virginia.

65. "Texas Negro Woman Dies after Implant," *Los Angeles Times*, 8 Jun. 1968, p. 6.

66. Denton Cooley, et al., "Human Heart Transplantation: Experience with Twelve Cases," *American Journal of Cardiology*, 12 (1968): 804–810.

67. Lawrence L. Goldman, *The Heart Merchants* (New York: Paperback Library, 1970), cover blurb, and p. 245.

68. McCandlish Philips, "Dick Gregory in an Hour at Carnegie," *New York Times*, 27 Nov. 1969, p. 51.

69. Sandra Haggerty, "Blacks' Attitudes about Heart Transplants," *Los Angeles Times*, 22 Jan. 1974, p. A7.

70. Joint Hearing of the House Commerce Committee Subcommittee on Health and Environment, June 18, 1998.

71. Trevor Corson, "Organ Rejection: Why Do Blacks Fear Organ Donation?" *American Prospect* (20 May 2002): 27–28.

72. See Dirk Schultheiss, et al., "Tissue Engineering from Adam to the Zygote: Historical Reflections," *World Journal of Urology* 18 (2000): 84–90, invokes both Adam and Cosmas and Damian.

73. Martha McNeil Hamilton and Warren Brown, *Black & White & Red All Over* (New York: Public Affairs, 2002): xx.

74. Jeff Testerman, "Should Donors Say Who Gets Organs?" *St. Petersburg Times*, 9 Jan. 1994, p. 1A.

75. Linda Kleindienst, "Organ Donation Bias Ban Passes," *Orlando Sentinel*, 31 Mar. 1994.

76. "Michael Jordan Is Volunteer Spokesperson for Organ and Tissue Donation," Press Release, Chicago, 17 Apr. 1996; available from TransWeb.org.

77. Patty Reinert, "Rebuilding a Shattered Trust," *Houston Chronicle*, 1 Dec. 1997.

7

Religious Bodies

For the life of the flesh is in the blood
Leviticus 17:11

Blood has long been a substance thick with meaning, magic, and symbolism. More than a red body fluid, blood also established relationships between humans and their gods, mediating between the heavens and the earth. In Mesoamerica, bloodletting rituals played a crucial role in religious governance. The ancient Mayans believed that human blood nourished and sustained the gods, and the shedding of blood opened the portal to the Otherworld. In the Aztec empire, the continuing welfare of the community demanded human blood sacrifice on a massive scale. Blood (and the flesh) have also played a profound role in the Christian tradition. For medieval theologians, blood established the true humanity of Jesus Christ, and his suffering and death—the shedding of his human blood on the cross—served to redeem humankind. This divine bloodshed, observed Pope Innocent III, enabled humans to enter into "the kingdom of heaven, whose gate the blood of Christ [had] mercifully opened for his faithful." The blood of Christ retained its physicality in Catholic ritual. In 1215, the Fourth Lateran Council ruled that the wafer and wine consecrated by a priest at the altar underwent transformation into the literal body and blood of Jesus Christ (transubstantiation). During the same period, accusations of ritual murder against Jews and witches were similarly steeped in blood symbolism and sacrifice—the innocent Christian infant or child murdered for blood necessary to occult rituals and arcane evils.[1] In many of the popular histories of blood transfusion mention is often made of the effort to save the aged Pope Innocent VIII. In the late fifteenth century, as the elderly Pontiff lay dying, a Jewish physician allegedly bled three young Christian boys to supply vital blood to the dying man. Blood from the boys, who died shortly after their bloodletting, was then used to prepare a draught. Although the ailing Pope did not survive, the story of this incident survived long after.[2]

In the twentieth century, religious beliefs about flesh and blood retained their power to influence nations and individuals. Some orthodox Jews, for example, refused to accept blood transfusions from non-Jews, and women in religious institutions apparently refused to accept blood from male donors. (The "special needs" of these women led the Blood Transfusion Betterment Association in 1938 to develop a small list of women blood donors.)[3] For the Jehovah's Witnesses, a religion that took root in late nineteenth-century America, passages from the Bible rendered blood transfusion unacceptable to believers. The group's refusal to allow blood transfusion for adults and especially infants, children, and pregnant women, created tensions with the American medical community, who turned to the courts to overturn these refusals. In so doing, the medical community confronted a number of issues. What are the limits of religious freedom when lives are at stake? Do adults have the right to refuse life-saving measures on "nonrational," religious grounds? Can parents decline life-saving transfusions on behalf of their infants and children? Over the course of the twentieth century, the answers to these questions have varied. Although the political circumstances may change (consider the last days of Terri Schiavo, whose death, in 2005, was marked by religious and moral controversy), there seems to be a consensus that adults in America retain the legal right to refuse even life-saving medical treatment except in special circumstances (pregnancy, diminished capacity, etc.).[4] Religious responses to blood transfusion, especially those of the Jehovah's Witnesses, continue to influence the ways in which the procedure is performed in the United States. The large number of court cases and the steadfast rejection of transfusion by Witnesses influenced American surgeons to attempt surgical procedures without using transfusion, prompting much new information about the uses of blood in surgery, trauma, and other medical conditions.

Flesh, like blood, and its transfer from one person to another, raised questions for both religious authorities and believers. What were the implications, for example, of transplanting tissues and organs if you believed that, on the day of divine judgment, you would experience the physical resurrection of the body? Whose body would be resurrected? Would such a body have the old or the new body parts and, even more importantly, would it matter? Early in the twentieth century, Catholic theologians debated the doctrinal issues posed by mutilating a healthy body (by removing an ovary or cornea) for the benefit of another. Other religious traditions expressed reservations about medical uses of the dead body (for both dissection and organ harvesting). This chapter considers the ways in which religious thinkers and religious beliefs shaped American transfusion and transplantation.

Blood Is the Life

Certainly, the best-known religious objections to blood transfusion have come from the Jehovah's Witnesses. This religious tradition stemmed in large part from the ministry of a wealthy Pittsburgh businessman, Charles Taze Russell. Brought up in the Presbyterian Church, in 1872, Russell formed a society that published tracts based on Biblical exegesis that anticipated the end of the world. (Even though the anticipated year—1914—came without ushering in the Second Coming of Christ, the sect continued to prosper with a revised date for the end of days). By 1909, when Russell relocated his society's headquarters to Brooklyn, New York, some 27,000 individuals subscribed to the group's journal *Zion's Watchtower*. By 1942, the number of Jehovah's Witnesses (the name was officially adopted in 1931) had grown to 115,000. After World War II, the movement grew even more rapidly; in 1984, the sect claimed more than 2.6 million followers.[5] In 2002, 1 million Jehovah's Witnesses lived in the United States, with an estimated 6 million worldwide.[6]

Unlike such other indigenous American religious traditions as Seventh-Day Adventism and Christian Science, the Witnesses expressed little initial interest in sickness and health.[7] After Russell's death in 1916, the editor of the second major Witness publication, *The Golden Age*, embarked on a campaign against orthodox medicine. Clayton J. Woodworth blasted the American medical profession as an "institution founded on ignorance, error, and superstition." As an editor, he sought to persuade his fellow Witnesses about the shortcomings of modern medicine, including the evils of aspirin, the chlorination of water, the germ theory of disease, aluminum cooking pots and pans, and vaccination. "Thinking people would rather have smallpox than vaccination," Woodworth wrote, "because the latter sows the seed of syphilis, cancer, eczema, erysipelas, scrofula, consumption, even leprosy, and many other loathsome afflictions."[8] This hostility toward regular medical practice was one element of the Witness response to blood transfusion.

The transfusion of blood, of course, predated the origins of the Jehovah's Witnesses. But the group took little official notice of the procedure before World War II. In December 1943, the Witness publication, *Consolation*, issued a sentinel warning with the description of a new vaccine against meningitis. The vaccine, made with blood from horses, was problematic because of "the divine prohibition as to the eating or partaking of blood," a failing that did "not appear to trouble the 'scientists.'"[9] Two years later, on 1 July 1945, the *Watchtower* denounced the movement of blood between bodies in transfusion as "pagan and God-dishonoring."[10] This wartime context may be crucial to understanding the emergence of the Witnesses' doctrinal ban on transfusion.

During World War II, as the American National Red Cross mobilized efforts to collect massive amounts of blood for the Allies, Red Cross officials, public relations people, and politicians construed blood donation on the home front as the patriotic duty of all healthy Americans (Negroes were, as an earlier chapter discussed, initially excused from this corpuscular responsibility). For this reason alone, blood donation may have aroused the suspicion of the Jehovah's Witnesses. In both World War I and World War II, the hostility of Witnesses to secular government created tensions with the American government. The refusal to support the war effort by serving in the armed forces led to the imprisonment of the sect's conscientious objectors. The Witness refusal to salute the American flag provoked many Americans, especially after the United States Supreme Court upheld a ruling that allowed school districts to expel Witness children who refused to salute the flag. (The Supreme

Court reversed this ruling in 1943.) After 4 years of national calls for Americans to donate blood for the war effort, the Witnesses rejected blood transfusion, citing passages from the Biblical books *Genesis*, *Leviticus*, and *Acts* that forbade the eating of blood.[11]

These Biblical passages dealt primarily with injunctions against eating the blood of animals. The Witness interpretation of this Biblical application to transfusion relied on an older understanding of the role of the blood in the body, namely that blood transfusion represented a form of nutrition for the body. The *Watchtower* article cited an entry from the 1929 edition of *Encyclopedia Americana*, in which blood was described as "the principal medium by which the body is nourished." But this description did not represent contemporary medical thinking. In fact, the description of blood as nourishment or food was the view of seventeenth-century physicians. That this represented centuries-old, rather than current, medical thinking on transfusion did not appear to trouble the Jehovah's Witnesses. In 1961, the Watchtower Bible and Tract Society issued *Blood, Medicine, and the Law of God*, outlining the Witness position on blood and transfusion. The author of this pamphlet returned to the original sources to buttress claims that blood represented nutrition, quoting among its sources a letter from the French physician Jean-Baptiste Denys that had appeared in George Crile's *Hemorrhage and Transfusion*. (The booklet did not mention that Denys's letter appeared in the 1660s, nor did it indicate that Crile's text had been published in 1909.) Denys's assertion that transfusion was "nothing else than nourishing by a shorter road than ordinary—that it to say, placing in the veins blood all made in place of taking food which only turns to blood after several changes" had been paraphrased by the author of the encyclopedia entry.[12]

Blood, Medicine, and the Law of God offered several other justifications for the ban on transfusion. According to the authors, God permitted only one arrangement in which blood could be used to save the life of another, the blood sacrifice of Jesus Christ. "The blood of Jesus was poured out on behalf of mankind, not by way of transfusion, which could have been administered to a few persons at most, but by means of sacrifice, and its benefits are available to all from among mankind who exercise faith in that divine provision."[13] Their stance on transfusion represented one "entirely religious, based on the law of God," but the Witnesses also offered some contemporary medical authorities to illustrate that transfusion was performed too readily, undertaken without compelling reason, and erroneously viewed as benign.

What perils lurked in a bottle of blood? For the Witness, many serious dangers awaited. They were ready and able to cite contemporary medical authorities who expressed concerns about the careless administration and overuse of blood transfusions. "There is probably no biological product in medical therapy that carries with it more possibilities of dangerous error than blood," observed Emanuel Hayt, attorney for the Hospital Association of New York State. "Blood is dynamite!" blasted blood banker Lester J. Unger in 1960. "It can do a great deal of good or a great deal of harm."[14] Sources of dangerous error included the possibility of mistakes in blood typing, accidents in which blood was mislabeled, and the transmission of such blood-borne diseases as syphilis and malaria. Drawing on the newer knowledge of transfusion, the Witnesses called attention to the potential for transfusion reactions when the subgroups of the Rh antigen were mismatched, and to the dangers of life-long sensitization to the Rh factor. They described the difficulties and dangers of syphilitic blood donors: "Most blood banks do not even ask donors if they have syphilis, because it is an embarrassing question and they know full well that they cannot expect a truthful answer. People who engage in sexual promiscuity are not honorable, and very few of them are going to volunteer an account of their deviations until they are forced to do so to regain their own health."[15] These were only some of the risks associated with blood transfusion.

The quality of the blood used in transfusion similarly represented a potent source of danger, for it was donated by prisoners and alcoholics compelled to sell blood for money. Just as sexual deviants who failed to disclose their tainted blood, Witnesses contended that men in prisons and alcoholics on the street often did not report their hepatitis infections. "Criminals in jail are given the opportunity to donate their blood. For example, the *New York Times* of April 6, 1961, reported: "Inmates of Sing Sing Prison at Ossining Will Give Blood to the Red Cross Today." A commendable act? Perhaps not as beneficial to their fellow man as the community is led to believe."[16] It was not just the threat of such diseases as hepatitis that made the blood of prisoners and alcoholics questionable. Some Witness publications suggested that more than microbes could be transmitted in the transfusion. Calling upon a durable belief in humoral pathology, they quoted homeopath Alonzo Shadman's claim about the transfusion of blood: "The blood in any person is in reality the person himself. It contains all the peculiarities of the individual from whence it comes. This includes hereditary taints, disease susceptibilities, poisons due to personal living, eating, and drinking habits . . . The poisons that produce the impulse to commit suicide, murder, or steal are in the blood."[17] Brazilian surgeon Americo Valerio also served as an authoritative source regarding blood transfusion: "Moral insanity, sexual perversions, repression, inferiority complex, petty crimes—these often follow in the wake of blood transfusion."[18] Such arguments echoed earlier beliefs about the transmission of extraphysical qualities in blood transfusion, arguments that remained alive and well in the era of heart transplantation.

The Witness opposition to blood transfusion roiled the medical profession, especially the surgeons. The issues raised by the ban on transfusion—allowing patients to reject life-saving treatment—were not new in American medicine. At the turn of the century, Christian Science had sorely tested American physicians, who looked to the courts in cases of so-called "Christian Science suicide" (involving adults who refused orthodox medical interventions) or "Christian Science homicide" (the death of a child whose parents refused life-saving treatments in lieu of Christian Science healing).[19] What was new at mid-century was the social standing of the medical and surgical professions. In the wake of therapeutic advances like transfusion and the stunning success of such "miracle" drugs as penicillin, the medical profession possessed greater confidence that they had life-saving measures to offer, and they were prepared to compel patients to receive these therapies. In so doing, they received material assistance from hospital officials and the judiciary.

In the 1950s, newspapers reported a slew of cases in which Witnesses resisted blood transfusion for themselves or their family members. In 1951, Chicago newspapers described the refusal of one Jehovah's Witness couple, Darrell and Rhoda Labrenz, to authorize a transfusion to treat their newborn daughter's blood condition (she was diagnosed with erythroblastosis fetalis, a serious condition of infancy produced by the incompatibility of the mother and infant's Rh antigens). Unable to persuade the Labrenzs to allow transfusion, the hospital filed a petition asking the court to appoint a guardian for the child. Three physicians testified that blood transfusion was essential to save the child's life and/or prevent lifelong mental impairment (what the doctors termed "imbecility"). Despite their pleas that the transfusion violated God's law, the couple lost custody of their daughter, and a court-appointed guardian allowed the transfusion to occur. Following the transfusion and the child's recovery, the couple regained custody of their daughter. Contending that their rights as parents had been violated, the couple appealed the transfusion order. In March 1952, the Illinois Supreme Court upheld the lower court ruling, noting that the infant's welfare trumped the religious beliefs of the parents.[20] Two years later, in 1954, the parents of Thomas Grzyb refused to allow a transfusion for Rh-associated anemia and their 9-day-old infant died in a Chicago hospital before a court-order for transfusion took effect. Illinois health officials called for changes in state law to permit the court to intervene immediately when the child's life was threatened by parental rejection of "scientific medical treatment."[21]

The Rh factor and its associated complications (anemia and erythroblastosis fetalis) prompted similar challenges to medical authority in other states. In 1952, a Juvenile Court in Missouri declared a 12-day-old infant, Janet Lynn Morrison, a ward of the court when she was diagnosed with severe anemia associated with Rh incompatibility. Physicians believed that delaying transfusion increased the risk of mental impairment and death, but her father, a Jehovah's Witness minister, argued that his religious beliefs were constitutionally protected. Granting that zealous adults might possess the right to risk their life by extreme fasting for religious reasons, the judge ruled that those same adults did not possess the right to refuse food to their children. "Youth, who constitute the hope of racial survival and progress, is of vital concern to the very life of the nation."[22] In 1955, physicians in Englewood, New Jersey informed Louis and Gloria Bertinato that a transfusion was necessary to treat their infant because of Rh sensitization. The physicians obtained a court order to transfuse the child., who survived. The couple's third child suffered a similar problem; in this case, no court order was obtained to compel a transfusion, and the infant died. In 1961, as Gloria Bertinato awaited the birth of her fourth child, the New Jersey child welfare department sought to obtain custody of the Bertinato fetus in order to be able to perform a transfusion immediately after birth. At the 1961 hearing, the Bertinatos did not dispute the medical indications for transfusion. Their objection was solely religious; as Jehovah's Witnesses, they could not approve a transfusion. The couple did acknowledge that "if the transfusions were ordered by the court—a matter beyond their control and against their wishes—they would nevertheless accept the child into their home as their child."[23] The New Jersey courts were not the first to offer legal protection to the unborn children of Jehovah's Witnesses. In 1960, a judge in Danville, Indiana authorized two physicians to perform a blood transfusion to save the unborn child of Richard Smock and his wife. The two were Jehovah's Witnesses; like the Labrenzs and the Morrisons, the Smocks were Rh incompatible.[24]

Jehovah's Witness parents opposed blood transfusion for children not only for Rh disease. When Ralph Dubose experienced complications from his appendectomy in 1953, his parents permitted the transfusion recommended by the hospital physicians. But the boy's parents balked when doctors ordered another transfusion. Citing their religious beliefs as Jehovah's Witnesses, they withheld approval for the second transfusion. Doctors at the Sydenham Hospital appealed to the New York Society for Prevention of Cruelty to Children for help. The child welfare agency brought the parents to court, and they were found guilty of neglect. The court-ordered transfusion took place, and the boy's life was "saved."[25] Court-ordered transfusion did not save all Witness children. When 3-year-old John Perricone was hospitalized in 1961 with a heart defect, his parents refused permission for a blood transfusion. Fifteen minutes after the hospital superintendent received temporary custody of the child, the boy received a blood transfusion. He died 4 hours later.[26]

Adult Witnesses presented different issues for physicians. Did competent adults have the right to their religious beliefs, even in the face of death? This was a moral issue that continued to challenge both doctors and patients. As Philadelphia surgeon William T. Fitts noted in 1959, members of the faith "constitute a growing religious order which very sincerely forbids blood transfusion for its members. In fact, the members of this society believe that if they submit to transfusion, they will lose all opportunity for life after death and will be ostracized by their associates for the remainder of this life."[27] Confronted with an adult Witness patient at the Hospital of the University of Pennsylvania, the surgeons agreed to treat the patient without recourse to transfusion. They offered two rationales for this unusual respect for patient autonomy in the late 1950s. Acknowledging that the easiest course would be to deny treatment altogether, the surgeons explained that their hospital was better equipped to treat the complications that might develop in the face of a no-transfusion policy. Moreover, they cited what might be called a "golden rule": "we believed that if we treated the patient as we ourselves wanted to be treated, we should accede to his wishes." This agreement apparently created widespread discussion among the hospital staff; the surgeons were "both vigorously denounced and stoutly defended" for their unusual willingness to accommodate a Witness patient who denied a scientifically based medical intervention. In light of the lack of professional consensus, the surgeons convened an unusual panel of "experts" to discuss the issues, including Fitts; his chief surgical resident; the chair of Penn's department of surgery, I. S. Ravdin; the chair of the department of medicine; the Chaplain of the University of Pennsylvania; and Laurence H. Eldredge, who lectured the medical students on medical jurisprudence.

Fitts's patient was a 34-year-old man with colon cancer. This man agreed to the surgery only after the surgeons promised that they would not use blood to treat him. When the patient developed complications and began to bleed severely, his surgeons begged him to reconsider his stance; they spoke to members of the Witness community and to the man's wife, who told them "that she would rather see him dead because if he were given a transfusion he would have no future life and no peaceful life on this earth if he recovered." The patient did not receive a transfusion, but fortunately he did stop bleeding and his hemoglobin (blood carrying oxygen to the tissues) began to climb. He was subsequently discharged from the hospital. What prompted this extraordinary consideration for the patient's wishes in the 1950s? There were certain features in this case that suggest that the Penn surgeons extended this courtesy to their patient because they were, to some extent, able to identify with the patient. The patient was apparently a man of a similar age who was able to articulate his beliefs in a compelling manner. Moreover, his wife and fellow believers fully supported his decision. This unanimity allowed the surgeons to proceed. Faced with an adamant refusal to permit the surgery without the promise, his surgeons reasoned that the patient would not survive without the surgery, but he might survive without the transfusion. Ravdin, the chairman of surgery, noted, "it is almost physically impossible to give a transfusion unless one is wanted."[28] This is also a case in which the patient survived—whether the surgeons would have convened their panel of experts and published the proceedings had the patient died remains a matter of speculation.

In the 1950s, physicians in Brookhaven, New York; Haverhill, Massachusetts; and Flemington, New Jersey did not intervene when their Witness patients (two women and one man) refused to authorize blood transfusion. Mary Bohnke experienced postsurgical shock but, despite foregoing transfusion, she was discharged from the hospital. Elizabeth Denno, a "43-year-old mother," did not survive her hospitalization for a bleeding ulcer, after she refused to accept "feeding upon the blood of a fellow man."[29] In this same decade, physicians in Atlanta, Georgia and Downey, California appealed to the courts when their adult Witness patients did not permit transfusions deemed essential to life. In 1958, a 19-year-old woman suffering with a ruptured spleen required a blood transfusion. Patricia Armstrong was a Jehovah's Witness, as was her husband. The Juvenile Court intervened in the case at the request of Armstrong's mother, who did not share her daughter and son-in-law's opposition to transfusion. There were other reasons for overruling Armstrong's refusal. She was the mother of a 20-month-old child, and she was pregnant with her second child.[30] American courts proved willing to compel medical treatment for pregnant women. But family opposition could also influence the outcomes for men who refused transfusion on religious grounds. In 1960, when an Atlanta man, 35 years old and a hemophiliac, was injured in a construction accident, he reportedly lost nearly 80% of his total blood volume. Both he and his wife refused to authorize transfusion. His father-in-law sided with the physicians but, as he lacked legal standing, the judge explained that he could not authorize a transfusion against the patient's wishes. The older man tried a different tactic; he approached the Fulton County Court of Ordinary to declare his son-in-law mentally incompetent and requested that he be named his guardian. At a hastily convened hearing, doctors testified that the massive blood loss had injured the patient's brain and adversely affected his mental processes. Despite his daughter's continuing opposition to the blood transfusion, B. E. Langley was named as guardian and immediately authorized transfusions. (The patient was expected to receive 12 transfusions.) Here again, family opposition seemed to play a role in overruling religious objections to blood transfusion.

To ensure that they would not receive blood transfusion, some Witnesses as early as 1950 began carrying a card in their wallet or purse that stated "No blood transfusion."

As one nurse explained in a 1950 *Watchtower* article, "it is becoming more prevalent to give blood transfusion during quite simple operations, and the only knowledge the patient may have of it is when asked to have friends and relatives replace it in the blood bank." The nurse advised her fellow Witnesses to add an exclusion clause to the hospital release contract they received when they signed a permit for operation. She also explained: "I carry an identification card in my wallet marked "No blood transfusion" in red ink and bearing my signature."[31] Whether an exclusion clause or a wallet card insisting that blood transfusion not be performed would have averted such cases as the one discussed above is less clear. Physicians and hospital administrators, not surprisingly, did not readily accept the refusal of patients to receive medical therapies regarded as life-saving. American physicians were trained to intervene, to apply medical technologies, to treat death itself as the enemy. Moreover, they were persuaded of the tremendous benefits of the therapies they offered. But they were also concerned about the medico-legal consequences of failing to observe the standard of care. This included responsibility for injury or death when physicians respected the patient's refusal, as well as the surgeon who "laboring under anxiety for his patient's welfare and despairing of what he regards as intemperate behavior in someone resigned out of misguided piety to a preventable death" administers blood without the permission of the patient or guardian. Recognizing that such transfusion had "doubtless taken place on innumerable occasions, and without generating overt recriminations or legal repercussions," New York physician David Schechter observed that transfusion without consent was a technical battery, for which physicians could be liable, especially in cases of a bad outcome.[32]

Table 7.1 Court Involvement in Cases of Transfusion and Jehovah's Witnesses

	Name	Age	City/State	Court-Ordered Transfusion
1951	Cheryl Labrenz	infant	Chicago, IL	Yes
	Jonathan Shelton	3	Brooklyn, NY	Yes
1952	Grace Marie Oliff	20	Odessa, TX	No
1953	Ralph Dubose	13	New York, NY	Yes
1954	Thomas Grzyb, Jr.	infant	Chicago, IL	No/infant dies
1955	Gail Bertimato	infant	Englewood, NJ	Yes
	David Siems	infant	Chicago, IL	Yes
1956	Linda Tanksley	2	Richmond, CA	Yes
1957	Mary Bohnke	40	Brookhaven, NY	No
	Ronnie Graves	12	Nashville, TN	Yes
1958	Philip Peace	19	Flemington, NJ	No
	Eliza.Denno	43	Haverhill, MA	No/dies
	Steven Siems	infant	Chicago, IL	Yes
	Patricia Armstrong	19	Downey, CA	Yes
1959	Linda Yorinko	6	Atlantic City, NJ	No
1960	Samuel David Hogan	35	Atlanta, GA	Yes
	Smock	fetus	Danville, IN	Yes
1961	John Perricone	3	Jersey City, NJ	Yes/child dies

To avoid legal responsibility for allowing the refusal of transfusion, hospitals adopted a policy of written waivers that served to indemnify institutions and medical personnel for failing to perform the recommended medical treatment. In November 1958, the Board of Trustees of the American Hospital Association adopted a formal resolution concerning the treatment of members of religious faiths that prohibited the transfusion of blood. They supplied a printed form entitled "Refusal to Permit Blood Transfusion" that included a waiver that released the hospital and the doctors from responsibility in the case of a bad outcome when blood transfusion was not performed. The form read:

> I request that no blood or blood derivatives be administered to _____
> _____ during this hospitalization. I hereby release the hospital, its
> personnel, and the attending physician from any responsibility whatever
> for unfavorable reactions or any untoward results due to my refusal to
> permit the use of blood or its derivatives and I fully understand the
> possible consequences of such a refusal on my part.[33]

In the 1960s, American courts continued to confront the right of competent, adult patients to refuse life-saving treatments. In 1962, when Jacob Dilgard entered a New York hospital with gastric bleeding, his physicians recommended blood transfusion. As a Jehovah's Witness, Dilgard declined to accept the transfusion; when the hospital superintendent took the issue to court, the judge refused the order to administer an involuntary transfusion, ruling "it is the individual who is the subject of a medical decision who has the final say and that this must necessarily be so in a system of government which gives the greatest possible protection to the individual in the furtherance of his own desires." A year later, in Washington, D.C., a young African American woman, a Jehovah's Witness who had suffered a ruptured ulcer, refused a transfusion. A lawyer for Georgetown Hospital sought a court order to administer a transfusion and was refused. The lawyer appealed to the Appeals Court, which issued an order for transfusion. When Mrs. Jessie E. Jones recovered, she filed suit in the U.S. Court of Appeals asking that the order for involuntary transfusion be set aside. The Court of Appeals refused to rehear the case, and the United States Supreme Court declined to review the lower court's decision.[34]

Jessie Jones was "25 and colored" and the mother of a 7-month-old son when she was brought to Georgetown Hospital in 1964. She had already lost more than two-thirds of her blood, and the doctors believed that transfusion was essential to save her life. Her husband explained that as a Jehovah's Witness he opposed blood transfusion, but he also said that "if the court ordered the transfusion, the responsibility was not his."[35] When Judge J. Skelly Wright attempted to interview the patient, she was barely able to speak. After meeting with doctors, the President of Georgetown University, and the patient's husband, the judge ordered a transfusion. The judge offered three arguments for his decision. First, the state did not permit parents to refuse on religious grounds life-saving treatments for their children; similarly a husband could not, on religious grounds, forbid treatment to his noncompetent wife. Pointing to the state's interest in children and to the patient's infant son, the judge suggested that the refusal to permit blood transfusion would result in the "most ultimate of voluntary abandonments," the loss of his mother. The judge also explained that the patient had placed a burden—both legal and ethical—on the physicians at Georgetown Hospital. The judge addressed only in passing the protection from civil liability that a waiver signed by the patient would grant the physicians, pointing out that such a waiver (as the card carried by Jehovah's Witnesses) did not guarantee immunity from criminal prosecution. In the District of Columbia, deaths that followed the failure to provide proper medical care were considered manslaughter. Dallas Wallace, the "overseer of Washington's Jehovah's Witnesses," stated that this decision was the first time a court had declined to accept an adult's refusal of transfusion.[36]

Judge Wright's violation of Jones' religious freedom produced mixed reviews. While some lauded his courage in acting "on the side of life," other commentators, especially other religious commentators, expressed concern about the implications of the decision.[37] Jehovah's Witnesses, not surprisingly, were critical of the decision. The violation of Mrs. Jones's religious freedom, Witnesses warned, should alarm other religious sects. "Should the Christian Scientist be forced to submit to any type of medical treatment against his will? Should Catholics be ordered to comply with birth control regulations? Should the doctors be ordered to save the mother rather than the child in the case of a difficult birth?" These appeals to religious liberty were not ignored by other believers.

The Catholic press raised questions about the implications of the Georgetown decision (even though the transfusion took place in a Catholic hospital) and the vagueness of the reference to "normal medical procedures" administered to save a life. "There are many 'normal medical procedures' in use today that would violate seriously the consciences of religious believers of various persuasions, including Catholics. Among them are sterilization and so-called therapeutic abortion. Who knows what other procedures in medicine may be legalized and come to be considered 'normal' in the future?"[38] Some Catholic theologians examined blood transfusions for adult Witnesses in the context of the Catholic distinction between *ordinary* versus *extraordinary* means to preserve life and health. For Jesuit writers like John Ford, the use of blood transfusion could be considered "an extraordinary means to preserving life to which he is not objectively obliged by the moral law." Ford distinguished between the state's lawful power to prevent a person from taking his or her own life and what he identified as an "affirmative legal duty to make use of highly developed surgical techniques in order to prolong" an earthly existence. "To kill oneself," Ford concluded, "is one thing. Not to avail oneself of surgery is quite another."[39]

The American Catholic Church had a well-developed tradition of moral guidance in medicine and nursing. Between the years 1880 and 1930, the number of Catholic hospitals increased in the United States, part of the enormous investment in hospital building across the nation. Catholic hospitals, physicians, and patients grappled with the issues raised by new techniques in medical and surgical practice. One of the most troubling dilemmas physicians faced in the late nineteenth century was the decision to intervene surgically in cases of difficult births. With improved techniques for caesarean delivery, for example, came difficult decisions about risking maternal life in order to save the life of the fetus. In 1884, George Shrady, editor of the New York-based *Medical Record*, noted that the Holy Office of the Catholic Church ruled that the procedure of craniotomy (perforating the fetal skull so that the contents could be withdrawn from the woman's body) could no longer be taught in

Catholic medical schools.[40] In the subsequent decades, Catholic writers offered guidance on a range of medical issues, including euthanasia, abortion, birth control, artificial insemination, eugenic sterilization, lobotomy, and vivisection.

Catholic theologians had seemingly little difficulty with the transfusion of blood, but some were quick to seize on the moral implications of the Rh factor. "The Rh factor has no moral value," observed Jesuit educator Alphonse M. Schwitalla. "It is a biological reality, comparable in practically all respects, as far as morality goes, to any one of literally thousands of substances occurring in the human body, each effecting a biological result in the biological economy of the organism." Nonetheless, Schwitalla warned that the presence or absence of the Rh factor offered the "occasion or excuse" for activities and behaviors that violated Catholic medical ethics, including contraception, abortion, radical obstetrics, and "preferential mating involving the conduct of engaged couples or those who might plan to be engaged."[41] Among the arguments the former dean of the St. Louis University Medical School offered against using the Rh factor as a rationale for contraception was the likelihood of "pathological offspring or a stillbirth." Schwitalla noted that many mothers who had lost children as a result of Rh incompatibility went on in subsequent pregnancies to bear healthy infants. Moreover, the clinical success in treating Rh disease as a result of early diagnosis and intensive management obviated the need, in the Jesuit's opinion, for contraception or "therapeutic" abortion. Schwitalla further questioned the need for radical obstetrics in response to Rh-sensitized mothers: "even though Cesarian [sic] section under certain conditions is ethically and morally permissible, it must still be regarded as an unusual obstetrical procedure which requires medical justification as the basis for its moral justification." Here again Schwitalla offered citations to the medical literature, including a 1946 editorial in the *Journal of the American Medical Association*, which cautioned physicians that "the handicap of prematurity" was rarely outweighed by "the alleged shortcomings of exposure to the damaging actions of maternal Rh antibodies."[42] The ability to predict outcomes of potential Rh-incompatible couples was further compromised by the emerging complexity of the Rh factor and "the occurrence of a complicated allelomorphic series of seven mutations in the Rh gene." The hundreds of possible combinations of the Rh allelomorphs illustrated the futility of medical advice about human mating; Schwitalla insisted that it certainly could not justify the warning that an Rh-negative girl who had received blood transfusions should forego marriage to an Rh-positive man. The available evidence for the potential of Rh sensitization, however, made it incumbent upon Catholic physicians to avoid the "indiscriminate use of blood" in young women, to transfuse young women with Rh-compatible blood, and to refrain from using injections of blood into the muscles.[43] Villanova College professor Charles McFadden offered similar advice in his textbook on medical ethics for Catholic nurses, even as he offered a new warning about Rh sensitization. The discovery that anti-Rh agglutinins could be transmitted in the breast milk to an infant prompted the warning that mothers of infants who developed erythroblastosis fetalis refrain from breast-feeding their infants insofar as the substances secreted in the milk and absorbed in the stomach could lead to the further destruction of the infant's Rh-positive blood cells. Writing in 1951, two Catholic physicians continued to minimize the risks associated with the Rh factor and pregnancy. In their guide to the medico-moral issues in matrimony faced by priests, physicians, nurses, and hospital administrators, Otis Kelly and Frederick Good explained how antibodies—described as "Nature's method for recovery"—formed in response to transfusions or injections of Rh-incompatible blood, how most such antibodies formed only in later pregnancies, and even advised the use of the "rhythm method" of contraception for those women who developed antibodies in their fifth pregnancy. Like earlier writers, these authors insisted that Rh incompatibility offered no justification for a "therapeutic abortion," or what one author identified as "therapeutic euthanasia." The two also cautioned, as did a number of lay writers, that much of the alarm over the Rh factor had been overblown, explaining that the factor was used too often to explain miscarriages without documentation of the Rh incompatibility between mother and father. They advised parents and potential parents to await further refinements in medical knowledge of the Rh factor and its treatment.[44]

Like American Catholics, members of the Mormon Church did not challenge the medical utility of blood transfusion, but their religious beliefs influenced their use of the procedure. In the late nineteenth century, the Church of Latter Day Saints (LDS), founded in 1830 by visionary Joseph Smith, began sending some of its young believers to attend orthodox medical schools in the Eastern United States, where they received training in "scientific medicine." In 1902, the Church opened a state-of-the-art hospital in Salt Lake City, which offered the latest in scientific medical and surgical treatments.[45] In 1943, the LDS Hospital opened a blood bank, one of the first in the intermountain West and the second largest in-hospital blood bank (after the blood bank at the Johns Hopkins Hospital).[46] The longstanding Mormon teaching about white racial superiority and concerns that even one drop of "Negro blood" might render a man unacceptable to enter the lay priesthood prompted the hospital's blood bank, like the blood banks in the American South, to maintain separate blood stocks for whites and blacks.[47] In 1978, after decades of controversy, the Church announced that "all worthy male members of the church may be ordained to the priesthood without regard for race or color." Shortly after this public directive, Consolidated Blood Services for the intermountain region announced for the first time an agreement to provide blood bank services for a group of hospitals with previous LDS connections, including LDS Hospital, Primary Children's and Cottonwood Hospitals in Salt Lake City, McKay-Dee Hospital in Ogden, and Utah Valley Hospital in Provo. Although the maintenance of separate blood stocks for whites and blacks had reportedly been abandoned by the 1970s, reporters described how some patients, who expressed concern about receiving blood from black donors, continued to receive the reassurance that this would not happen.[48]

The Morality of Organic Transplantation

For Catholics, blood transfusion and even skin grafting did not represent mutilations of the human body. Blood and skin taken to benefit another person involved substances readily replaced by the individual, and their transfer seldom endangered the wholeness and integrity of the body. More severe mutilations of the body's integrity were considered permissible in Catholic teaching; a mutilating operation undertaken to excise a diseased organ was therapeutic. Catholic theologians considered the mutilation of healthy organs without a sufficient medical rationale a violation of Church teaching. Georgetown University scholar Thomas O'Donnell, for example, explained that the transfer of one part of a person's body to another part of the body was permissible when the entire body benefited as a result. Even if the operative procedure was undertaken for purely cosmetic reasons, the principle of totality permitted the procedure so long as the risk was not disproportionate to the benefits and provided the surgery was not undertaken for an immoral reason. (O'Donnell cited an example of a dangerous criminal undergoing a cosmetic procedure to escape detection as an example of an immoral mutilation.)[49] Catholic teachings similarly permitted the use of materials taken from "lower animals" and transferred to human bodies when the intention was to benefit the individual patient. When Pope Pius XII addressed the Italian Association of Donors of the Cornea in 1956, he distinguished between permissible and morally objectionable "zooplastic transplants." "The transplantation of the sexual glands of an animal to man is to be rejected as immoral," the Pope explained. The transplantation of a cornea from an animal to a human being however "would not raise any moral difficulty if it were biologically possible and were warranted." The Pope also endorsed the removal of body parts from a dead human for transfer into a patient, provided it was acceptable to the family of the deceased and performed with "the respect that is due the body of the dead." These transfers all entailed "static" rather than vital tissue transplants. Acknowledging that the morality of this type of transplant—the transfer of the part of one living human to another human being—remained morally uncertain, the Pope limited his discussion to corneal transplants involving dead humans and animal bodies. Pius XII provided considerable material for the discussion of medical ethics for, in addition to his address to the Donors of Corneas, he addressed blood donors (1948), midwives (1951), histopathologists (1952), geneticists (1953), urologists (1953), military doctors (1953), and delegates to the Congress of the World Medical Association (1954).[50]

In the United States, the morality of organ transplantation had been the subject of ongoing analysis by Catholic theologians. One of the earliest contributors to this discussion was a young Catholic theologian who addressed the morality of "organic transplantation" in his 1944 doctoral thesis at Catholic University. Bert Cunningham offered two examples—ovarian transfer and corneal transplantation—of the tremendous advances in medical science that facilitated such surgery. Although the casual transfer of ovarian tissue from one body to another had been mostly eclipsed by developments in hormonal replacement therapy, Cunningham described how physicians in Philadelphia provided ovarian transplants to patients who had failed other therapies and who had "proper partners to swap ovaries." Surgeon M.J. Bennett performed such a surgery on two patients in Philadelphia's Hahnemann Hospital in 1935. After ensuring that his patients shared the same blood grouping, he removed the ovary from one young woman and transferred it into the abdominal cavity of her younger sister. Her older sister received one of her younger sibling's ovaries.

The two recovered from the surgery and Bennett claimed a remarkable benefit; the obese, older sister lost more than 100 pounds, her thin, younger sister put on healthy weight. Four years later, the two sisters were both "happy, healthy, and married." More than 80 women underwent this kind of surgery in Philadelphia in the 1940s.

These surgeries involved the mutilation of women's bodies, but were they morally acceptable in Catholic teaching? Could an individual allow himself or herself to be directly mutilated for the benefit of another person? Cunningham argued that such mutilations were acceptable if they met three conditions: proportionate benefit to the individuals, no grave threat to life for the donor, and the maintenance of reproductive potential in the donor. (In other words, it was immoral to transfer an ovary removed to produce elective sterilization in a patient.) Cunningham grounded his defense of organic transplantation in the principle of the common bond of human nature and in the unity of the individual in "the mystical body of Christ."[51]

Cunningham offered a similar analysis of "keratoplasty," the restoration of a "clear window" to enable a blind person to see. One leading proponent of this surgery was ophthalmic surgeon Ramon Castroviejo, who, in 1941, reported the results of corneal grafting in some 400 animals and 200 human beings.[52] Although this Columbia-Presbyterian eye surgeon had attempted to use animal corneas to restore sight in humans, Castroviejo reported greatest success with human corneas. These human corneas could be obtained from an eye removed because of a serious injury, but this supply was obviously limited. Castroviejo turned to the bodies of newly dead adults and infants. As in other transfers of body parts and fluids, timing was crucial; Castroviejo, for example, preferred to harvest corneas within 12 hours of death. (In San Francisco, one solution to the supply problem was to obtain premortem pledges from individuals willing to allow the removal of their corneas. In 1941, a California man, Theodore Olsen, organized what he called the Dawn Society to act as a "clearinghouse" to make corneas available.) Taking the eyes of the dead, who had authorized such a removal or with the permission of family members, posed few problems in Cunningham's analysis. But his correspondence with Ted Olsen revealed that some people had volunteered their corneas for donation while still alive. In these cases, most offers came from people "who mistakenly believed that the [Dawn] Society bought eyes for extraordinary prices."[53] These offers were refused, in part because surgeons feared subsequent court actions. But the religious question remained: if a donor of sound mind and legal capacity (the donor must be an adult, and if married, a woman required the permission of her husband) authorized the removal of a cornea to benefit a fellow human being, would this be a mutilation in Catholic theology and therefore illicit?

In some respects this question was not a new one, for it had arisen in the context of Serge Voronoff's testicular transplants. Catholic theologians had come squarely down against the transfer of either human or animal sex glands because of the stated intention of such operations, namely the restoration of sexual powers. More than that, however, in cases where young men offered one of their testicles for donation or sale, such an operation constituted a mutilation in Catholic terms, and one for which there was no contribution to the good of the whole body. Unlike the case of skin grafts or blood transfusions, these gonadal grafts did not regenerate; nature could not repair the loss of such an organ or the diminution in natural vigor that the individual had earlier possessed. But Cunningham questioned whether this assumed defect of "virile integrity" was absolute and whether the desire to benefit materially the body of another made such donation acceptable (provided the male donor retained his fertility). Cunningham outlined several scenarios in which such donations could occur with Church approval.

In the case of a young child who lost sight in both eyes following an accident, a mother's decision to donate one of her own corneas to restore the sight in one of her son's eyes was an acceptable mutilation. "If one may undergo a direct mutilation for the sake of the neighbor, any neighbor, it would seem, a fortiori, that a mother may submit herself to such an operation for the sake of her child. For the ties of charity are certainly more binding relative to those united to us by blood." In the case of a young riveter whose eyes were badly damaged by flying steel splinters, the offer from a prisoner serving a life sentence to allow one of his corneas to be used to restore the sight of the worker, Cunningham pronounced such an offer not only acceptable but commendable. Even though such an operation would render the prisoner totally and irreparably blind, the sacrifice of the cornea represented an atonement to society. The prisoner, Cunningham concluded, was "not needed by anyone." But the riveter was a husband and father, "the restoration of his sight would return him to a state of normal living." This rendered the prisoner's donation a heroic charity and a morally permissible act.[54] In 1956, when he addressed an Italian assembly, the Pope did not endorse these two scenarios, preferring to restrict his remarks to corneal transplants taken from the dead (and with the permission of the deceased and families).

At the Hour of Our Death

Using the dead body as a source of organs, skin, or tissue became more problematic as transplant surgeons extended their surgeries beyond corneas, sex glands, and kidneys. Perhaps more than any other organ, the heart and its transfer from one person to another provoked intense discussions and debates about the nature and determination of death. An individual can survive without sex glands and corneas, and with only one kidney. But the transfer of the heart between bodies guaranteed the death of the donor. Heart transplantation raised questions about the determination of death and the nature of life itself. The new surgery required a redefinition of death and the emergence of a new category for the legally dead—the brain dead.

In 1964, Mississippi surgeon James Hardy performed the first human heart transplant. He removed the heart from Boyd Rush, a 68-year-old retired man living in a trailer park in Hattiesburg, and replaced it with the heart of a chimpanzee that he had acquired from a fellow transplant surgeon. Rush's sister authorized the heart operation, apparently without the slightest understanding of what a heart transplant was and who would supply the new heart. (The operative permit that she signed mentioned that a "suitable heart transplant" would be performed if her brother's heart had failed.)[55] The chimpanzee's heart could not support Rush's circulation and, after little more than an hour, Hardy abandoned the effort to keep the heart alive. Hardy's pioneering heart transplant, like his pioneering lung transplant a year earlier, received little public attention. The media storm ignited by Christiaan Barnard's human-to-human heart transplant was a different story.[56]

In December 1967, Barnard, an American-trained heart surgeon working in a small hospital in Capetown, South Africa, electrified the world with the announcement that his patient, Louis Washkansky, had received the heart from a 22-year-old woman who had sustained a severe brain injury in an automobile accident. When Denise Darvall's father authorized the removal of his daughter's heart (and other organs) for transplant, he probably did not realize that his dead daughter would become the poster child for what the media dubbed "the ultimate operation." In magazines, newspapers, and television programs, the photographs of the surgeon, donor, and recipient flashed around the world. When Louis Washkansky recovered from the anesthesia following the transplant surgery, he told his nurses "I am the new Frankenstein." The reference to Mary Shelley's novel (banned in apartheid South Africa in 1955 for its immoral content) appropriately captured the disquiet and discord created by the union of the living and the dead, although her story of the making of a monster contained little or no reference to the sources of bodies and fluids used for the "new Adam."[57] Soon after the publicity surrounding the Capetown transplants, "donors became cloaked with anonymity as the ambiguity of their condition drew attention," and photographs and names of donors like Darvall disappeared from the media and medical journals.[58]

The rush to heart transplants precipitated by Barnard's success (Washkansky lived for 18 days, Barnard's next patient, Philip Blaiberg, lived for 18 months) provoked legal, moral, and religious discussions about death, dying, and the new definition of "brain death." It was not clear how and in what circumstances a person could become legally dead and legally available as a source of tissue for transplantation; even the surgeons shared in the linguistic and conceptual confusion fostered by the reinvention of death. At a 1966 conference devoted to "Ethics in Medical Progress: With Special Reference to Transplantation," Thomas Starzl, a surgeon who would become world famous for liver transplants, illustrated some of the confusion when he noted "I assume that when kidneys are removed from 'living cadavers,' only one organ is removed, so that the patient is not thereby killed."[59]

How did this debate affect religious responses to organ transplantation? In some religious traditions, the definition of death did not involve the brain. "Brain death," as the new term suggests, entails the death of the whole brain, including the brainstem. Although many countries adopted this new definition, several countries did not. Israel, China, and Japan, for example, do not accept this definition, in part because the religious traditions of Buddhism, Shinto, and conservative Judaism do not privilege the brain. In these traditions, death is a gradual process; for some conservative Jews, the body of the individual cannot be disturbed until respiration, circulation, and the heartbeat have ceased.

The religious issues raised by the prospect of organ transplantation, however, transcend the definition of death. They partake of issues relating to bodily integrity and respect. For some Christians, heart transplants did not pose spiritual or moral problems. When the Reverend J.L. Lundberg, a close associate of preacher Billy Graham, was asked about heart transplants in 1969, he explained that the "physical organ of the heart is not involved in the relationship of the individual to the Savior. The heart transplant is not a ticket to immortality, though it may prolong a person's life on earth for a few years."[60] But some Christian believers took the resurrection of the dead more literally. Although denominations such as the African Methodist Episcopal Church endorses organ transplantation as consistent with the church's embrace of love and charity, some individual members of the Church have reported that they reject organ donation because of their own ideas about bodily resurrection. When the day of judgment arrives, some believers describe the importance of "going to Jesus whole."[61] Even though each of the main branches of Christianity—Catholics, Protestants, and Orthodox—endorse organ donation, it seems likely that some members of these faiths share similar beliefs about the physical resurrection of the body and the importance of being whole on Judgment Day. Each of the governing bodies of these religions has also expressed concern about the economic implications of buying and selling organs.

In the United States, the three branches of Judaism—Orthodox, Conservative, and Reform—have adopted similar views. In 1990, the Rabbinical Council of the Conservative branch encouraged all Jews to carry signed cards and express the willingness to help others in need. Still, for some Jews, the definition of brain death remains highly controversial and colors the interpretation of the duty to donate organs and other tissues. In the early days of heart transplantation, some Orthodox thinkers were more hostile to heart transplantation; one eminent authority characterized such surgeries as "double murders" insofar as they required the desecration of the "dead body" and the experimental nature of the procedure endangered the life of the recipient. Three decades later, some Orthodox Jews do not accept the criteria of brain death as signifying death in Jewish law. The removal of organs from a "brain-dead" body becomes unacceptable. These thinkers point to some of the debates over the moral and biologic status of brain death that have continued into the twenty-first century.[62]

For many reasons, Islamic thinkers have only in the last three decades addressed the issues—moral and religious—posed by organ donation, organ harvest, and transplantation. Like Jewish religious scholars, Islamic jurists have been divided over the morality of organ transplantation. The key text for Muslims, the Quran, for example, does not mention transplantation, and there are different interpretations of Islamic obligations and responsibilities that arise from the canon of Islamic law. Some more traditional Islamic scholars, representing a minority position, have noted the sanctity of the body and human life in Islam. If the body and its parts are gifts from God, they are not available for donation. The removal of organs and tissues from a dying or dead person, these commentators argue, violates human dignity and the sanctity of human life, which cannot be reduced to a means to an end. Finally, these scholars invoke verses from the Quran "to support the view that cutting human bodies and removing body parts is altering God's creation, which is not allowed."[63] The majority of Islamic scholars and commentators on medical ethics share the view about the sanctity of the human body and the Islamic belief that God's laws exist for the betterment of human society. These laws sanction the use of organs from one person to save the life of another. Most also express reservations about the commodification of body organs and the black market in kidneys which adversely affects the most vulnerable members of the community. Finally, Islamic scholars have debated the definition of death which allows the early removal of organs from the body, and there remains no consensus about the moral status of brain death.[64]

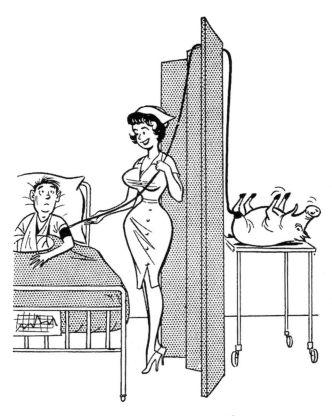

"Sorry, we can't disclose the identity of a donor with *your* type blood."

Figure 7.1 In 1955, the use of a pig as a blood donor was comic, but in some religious traditions, using animal parts or fluids in human bodies was transgressive (Source: Meyer H (comp.): *Let's Play Doctor!* [New York: Shepsel Books, 1955], 39).

Brain death is an important consideration when the source of donor organs is human. But what if the source is an animal? In one celebrated case of cross-species transplantation, the decision to implant the heart of a baboon into a human infant reflected religious beliefs about evolution, or more precisely, the rejection of evolutionary theory. On October 26, 1984, surgeon Leonard L. Bailey and his colleagues at the Loma Linda University Medical Center placed the heart of a 7-month-old baboon into Baby Fae, a newborn with hypoplastic left heart syndrome. Baby Fae lived for 20 days with the baboon heart before she succumbed to heart and kidney failure stemming from the rejection of the animal tissue. The Baby Fae case received enormous media attention: physicians, surgeons, ethicists, and other social commentators voiced a spectrum of opinions about this cross-species transplant effort, including concerns about the lack of prior peer review of the research protocol, the quality of parental consent, the issue of animal sacrifice, and the violation of the species boundaries between animals and humans.

Religious traditions have played an important role in the societal response to the new surgeries of transfusion and transplantation. In the case of transfusion, the belief that blood represents life has led one sect, the Jehovah's Witnesses, to refuse transfusions and the use of whole blood. (It has similarly raised questions about the use and acceptance of donor organs that might contain the blood of an individual.) The refusal to accept what physicians and surgeons deemed life-saving care compelled legal challenges to individual autonomy, which became a notable focus for the emerging discipline of bioethics. At the same time, respect for patient refusal to permit blood transfusion encouraged surgeons and physicians to limit the use of blood in surgery and treatment, thereby potentially improving the welfare of all patients. (As we continue to learn more about the immunologic complexity of blood, we may someday regard the transfusion of blood between persons as entirely misguided, much like the "heroic bloodletting" by leeches and lancets in the early nineteenth century.)

The movement of body parts between persons and animals similarly reflected religious beliefs about bodily integrity, responsibility to others, and the respect due to the dead. For many Americans, these were questions of both Church doctrine and individual beliefs about the afterlife. Albeit with early trepidation, most mainstream American religious traditions—Catholic, Protestant, Jew, and more recently, Islam—have accepted organ transplantation as consistent with their commitments to advance the welfare of others and express love and charity for their fellow human beings. In the United States, the Catholic faith sponsored the earliest systematic engagement with moral dimensions of organ transplantation, including the mutilation of the healthy body for the benefit of another. But by the 1960s and 1970s, all major religious traditions adopted formal stances about the value and conditions of transplantation.[65]

Notes

1. Uli Linke, *Blood and Nation: The European Aesthetics of Race* (Philadelphia: University of Pennsylvania Press, 1999), 101; for blood libels, see pp. 145–153.

2. Geoffrey Keynes, ed. *Blood Transfusion* (London: Simpkin Marshall, 1949), 3. See G.A. Lindeboom, "The Story of a Blood Transfusion to a Pope," *Journal of the History of Medicine* 9 (1954): 455–459.

3. De Witt Stetten, "The Blood Transfusion Betterment Association of New York City," *Journal of the American Medical Association* 110 (1938): 1248-1252, on p. 1249.

4. See George Annas, "The Case of Terri Schiavo," *New England Journal of Medicine* 352 (2005): 1625–1626.

5. Ronald L. Numbers and Darrel W. Amundsen, ed. *Caring and Curing: Health and Medicine in the Western Religious Traditions* (New York: Macmillan, 1986).

6. D. John Doyle, "Blood Transfusions and the JW Patient," *American Journal of Therapeutics* 9 (2002): 417–424.

7. Ronald L. Numbers, *Prophetess of Health: A Study of Ellen G. White* (New York: Harper & Row, 1976); Rennie B. Schoepflin, *Christian Science on Trial: Religious Healing in America* (Baltimore: Johns Hopkins University Press, 2003).

8. *The Golden Age* (1 May 1929): 502.

9. *Consolation* (December 1943).

10. *The Watchtower* (1 July 1945): 198–201.

11. The specific passages are Genesis 9:4; Leviticus 17:11–12; and Acts 15. See Richard Singelenberg, "The Blood Transfusion Taboo of Jehovah's Witnesses: Origin, Development and Function of a Controversial Doctrine," *Social Science and Medicine* 31 (1990): 515–523.

12. *Blood, Medicine, and the Law of God* (Brooklyn: Watchtower Bible and Tract Society of New York., 1961), 14.

13. *Blood, Medicine, and the Law of God*, p. 8.

14. Lester J. Unger, "Medicolegal Aspects of Blood Transfusion," *New York State Journal of Medicine* 60 (1960): 237–245.

15. *Blood, Medicine, and the Law of God*, p. 28.

16. *Watchtower* (15 Sep. 1961): 564.

17. Alonzo J. Shadman, *Who Is Your Doctor and Why?* (Boston: House of Edinboro, 1958), 132–33.

18. *Watchtower* (15 Sep. 1961): 564.

19. See R.B. Schoepflin, *Christian Science on Trial*.

20. See "Baby Receives Transfusion on Judge's Order," *Chicago Daily Tribune*, 19 Apr. 1951, p. C1; "Suit Asks Rule on Forced Care Given Rh Girl," *Chicago Daily Tribune*, 20 Jul. 1951, p. A12; "Parents Regain Infant Who Got Rh Transfusion," *Chicago Daily Tribune*, 5 May 1951, p. A5; and "Court Place Life of Child Above Religion," *Chicago Daily Tribune*, 21 Mar. 1952, p. A5.

21. "Death of Baby Denied Medical Aid Stirs Row," *Chicago Daily Tribune*, 15 Jan. 1954, p. 6.

22. Morrison decision cited in Joel Stephen Williams, *Ethical Issues in Compulsory Medical Treatment: A Study of Jehovah's Witnesses and Blood Transfusion* (Ph.D. dissertation, Baylor University, 1987), 121. Williams offers a detailed analysis of the hundreds of court cases involving transfusion refusals by Witnesses.

23. *Hoener v. Bertinato*, 171 A.2d 140 (NJ Juvenile & Domestic Relations Court, 1961).

24. "OKs Transfusion for Unborn Child Despite Parents," *Chicago Daily Tribune*, 14 Jan. 1960, p. 1.

25. "Boy's Life Saved by Transfusions as Court Bars Parents' Objection," *New York Times*, 10 Mar. 1953, p. 31.

26. "Boy Dies as Family Refuses Medical Aid," *New York Times*, 5 Mar. 1961, p. 59.

27. William Fitts, "Blood Transfusion and Jehovah's Witnesses," *Surgery, Gynecology & Obstetrics* 108 (1959): 502–507.

28. W. Fitts, "Blood Transfusion."

29. "Mother Refuses Transfusion, Dies," *Washington Post*, 30 Jul. 1958, p. A2.

30. "Judge Orders Transfusion for Dying Woman," *Los Angeles Times*, 4 Apr. 1958, p. B1.

31. "An 'Exclusion Clause' Recommended," *Watchtowe*r (15 Dec. 1950): 524. See Andre Carbonneau, *Ethical Issues and the Religious and Historical Basis for the Objection of JW to Blood Transfusion Therapy* (Lewiston, NY: Edwin Mellen Press, 2003), p. 20, and p. 144 for the current Advance Medical Directive that Witnesses are instructed to carry.

32. David Schechter, "Problems Relevant to Major Surgical Operations in Jehovah's Witnesses," *American Journal of Surgery* 116 (1968): 73–80.

33. *Hospitals* (1 Feb. 1959); the form also appears in *Blood, Medicine, and the Law of God*, pp. 50–51.

34. William J. O'Donnell, "Power of the State to Impose Medical Treatment," *Archives of Environmental Health* 10 (1965): 641–648.

35. Application of the President and Directors of Georgetown College, 118 U.S. App. D.C. 80; 331 F. 2d 1000, 1964.

36. The woman's race was not reported in the case, but the press identified her as either "colored" or "a Negro." See "Judge Here Orders Blood Transfusion for Woman Patient," *Washington Daily News*, 18 Sep. 1963; "Transfusion by Decree," *Christianity Today*, 11 Oct. 1963; newspapers clippings, Georgetown Hospital Records, Box 318, f. 3,

37. The *Washington Post* applauded his courage; see "Judge's Dilemma," *Washington Post*, 7 Feb. 1964. For a more critical response, see "Against Her Will," *The Sunday Star* (Washington D.C.) 9 Oct. 1963, clippings.

38. "Good Sense or Danger?" *New York Catholic News* (26 Sep. 1963), clippings file.

39. John Ford, "Refusal of Blood Transfusions by Jehovah's Witnesses," *Catholic Lawyer* 10 (1964): 212–226.

40. Joseph G. Ryan, "The Chapel and the Operating Room: The Struggle of Roman Catholic Clergy, Physicians, and Believers with the Dilemmas of Obstetric Surgery, 1800–1900," *Bulletin of the History of Medicine* 76 (2002): 461–494; and Kathleen M. Joyce, *Science and the Saints: American Catholics and Health Care, 1880–1930* (Ph.D. dissertation, Princeton University, 1995).

41. Alphonse M. Schwitalla, "The Moral Aspects of the Rh Factor," *The Linacre Quarterly* 14 (1947): 9–18. *The Linacre Quarterly* was the official publication of the Catholic Medical Guild.

42. Editorial, *Journal of the American Medical Association* (9 Nov. 1946): 581.

43. Donald H. Kaump, "The Rh Factor in the Hemolytic Disease of the Newborn," *The Linacre Quarterly* 14 (1947): 1–8.

44. Charles J. McFadden, *Medical Ethics* (Philadelphia: F.A. Davis, 1949), 178–192. See Frederick Good and Otis Kelly, *Marriage, Morals, and Medical Ethics* (New York: P.J. Kennedy, 1951), 100–104.

45. Lester E. Bush, Jr. "The Mormon Tradition," in Ronald L. Numbers and Darrel W. Amundsen, eds., *Caring and Curing: Health and Medicine in the Western Religious Traditions* (New York: Macmillan, 1986), 397–420.

46. Henry Plenk, ed., *Medicine in the Beehive State* (Salt Lake City: University of Utah Press, 1992), 493–494. See Newell G. Bringhurst, *Saints, Slaves, and Blacks: The Changing Place of Black People within Mormonism* (Westport, CT: Greenwood Press, 1981).

47. F. Ross Peterson, "Blindside: Utah on the Eve of *Brown v. Board of Education*," *Utah Historical Quarterly* 73 (2005): 4–20.

48. David Briscoe and George Buck, "Black Friday," *Utah Holiday* (July 1978): 39–40.

49. Joseph B. McAllister, *Ethics with Special Application to the Medical and Nursing Professions* (Philadelphia: W.B. Saunders, 1954), 240–247.

50. See Gerald Kelly, "The Morality of Mutilation: Towards a Revision of the Treatise," *Theological Studies* 17 (1956): 322–344.

51. Gerald Kelly, *Medico-Moral Problems* Part II (St. Louis: Catholic Hospital Association, 1950), 22–24; Bert J. Cunningham, *The Morality of Organic Transplantation* (Washington, D.C., Catholic University of America Press, 1944).

52. Ramon Castroviejo, "Keratoplasty," *American Journal of Ophthalmology* 24 (1942): 1–20; 139–155.

53. B. J. Cunningham, *Morality of Organic Transplantation*, p. 58.

54. B.J. Cunningham, *Morality of Organic Transplantation*, p. 106.

55. Jürgen Thorwald, *The Patients* (New York: Harcourt Brace Jovanovich, 1971), offers a lively, journalistic account from the patient's perspective of several innovative surgeries. When I interviewed Doctor Hardy in [2001], he continued to defend the "informed" nature of the authorization for the chimpanzee transplant. He received the chimpanzee from surgeon Keith Reemtsma, who was working at the Tulane University Hospital.

56. Interview with James D. Hardy; see James D. Hardy, *The Academic Surgeon: An Autobiography* (Mobile, AL: Magnolia Mansions Press, 2002).

57. Susan E. Lederer, "Transplant Nation: Heart Transplantation and National Politics in the 1970s," in Caroline Hannaway, ed. *Biomedical Research and the NIH* (forthcoming).

58. Margaret Lock, *Twice Dead: Organ Transplants and the Reinvention of Death* (Berkeley: University of California Press, 2002), 93.

59. G.E.W. Wolstenholme and M. O'Connor, *Ethics in Medical Progress: With Special Reference to Transplantation* (Boston: Little Brown, 1966), 155.

60. Joshua A. Perper, "Ethical, Religious, and Legal Considerations to the Transplantation of Human Organs," *Journal of Forensic Science* 15 (1970): 12.

61. John Gilman, "Religious Perspectives on Organ Donation," *Critical Care Nursing Quarterly* 22 (1999): 19–29.

62. R.D. Truog, "Is It Time to Abandon Brain Death?" *Hastings Center Report* 27 (1997): 29–37. See Aaron Mackler, "Respecting Bodies and Saving Lives: Jewish Perspectives on Organ Donation and Transplantation," *Cambridge Quarterly of Healthcare Ethics* 10 (2001): 420–429.

63. Ghulam-Haider Aasi, "Islamic Legal and Ethical Views on Organ Transplantation and Donation," *Zygon* 38 (2003): 731.

64. Mohammad Mehdi Golmakani, Mohammad Hussein Niknam, and Kamyar M. Hedayat, "Transplantation Ethics from the Islamic Point of View," *Medical Science Monitor* 11 (2005): RA105–109.

65. Courtney S. Campbell, "Religion and the Body in Medical Research," *Kennedy Institute of Ethics Journal* 8 (1998): 275–305.

8

Organ Recital

Transplantation and Transfusion in Historical Perspective

In late 2007 a Frenchwoman named Isabelle Dinoire smiled and expressed herself as "satisfied" with her surgery. This was no mean feat, for two years earlier, Dinoire had lost her lips, checks, chin, and most of her nose when she was catastrophically mauled by her dog. In November 2005 she underwent a fifteen-hour surgical procedure in which her surgeons replaced what remained of her face with one taken from a 46-year old brain-dead donor.[1] Although some critics expressed concern about the cost-benefit ratio of the surgery (tremendous risks for a non-life threatening injury), others worried about the psychological issues prompted by wearing another's face in light of the cultural and personal investment in this aspect of the body and its important role in identity.[2] Since Dinoire's spectacular recovery, there have been at least two other face transplants, and undoubtedly more to come.

Transplanting a human face was a new surgical procedure in 2005, but the concerns about its implications were not new. The face transplant provoked many of the same concerns about identity, ethics, and the "supply" problem created by the transplantation of glands, skin, bones, and other body parts in the first part of the twentieth century, what some might call the "pre-history" of organ transplantation. These were also among the concerns occasioned by moving blood between human bodies. Like transplantation, blood transfusion redrew the lines between self and other, and raised profound questions of identity and difference.

Both transfusion and transplantation have been hailed as miracles of modern medicine, and surely, many thousands of people in the United States and around the world survived because of these procedures. Along with these triumphs of medicine and surgery have come disappointments. The recent history of blood transfusion is an object lesson in how a medical procedure intended to improve the lives and health of patients can become the vehicle of disease and death. For hemophiliacs whose lives were adversely affected by the failure of their blood to clot, the discovery of clotting factors, especially factor VIII, transformed their lives on a day-to-day basis. Yet, the clotting factor concentrate they used to transform their lives was obtained from large numbers of blood donors whose blood was pooled in order to separate out the clotting factor. In 1982, the Centers for Disease Control reported that three hemophiliacs had developed a frightening new disease, acquired immune deficiency syndrome (AIDS). In 1985, the Food and Drug Administration licensed a test to screen for the retrovirus (human immunodeficiency virus; HIV) identified as the cause of AIDS. Unfortunately, by the time that systematic screening began, thousands of Americans with hemophilia, together with other blood transfusion recipients, had become infected with HIV. By some estimates, more than three-quarters of hemophiliacs treated before 1985 with factor VIII tested HIV-positive. The widespread infection of the hemophiliac community and the role of blood banks, pharmaceutical companies, and health foundations in delaying recognition of the threat in the blood supply prompted more than a decade of litigation and complex negotiations that produced some economic redress for those infected with HIV.[3]

Organ transplantation, too, partakes of what some commentators have described as "the dark side." References to the dark side appear most frequently in discussions of and explanations for the scarcity of donor organs and the numbers of people unwilling to give the ultimate gift. In the United States, where more than 60,000 people appear on waiting lists for donor organs, the problem of scarcity prompts a large number of potential solutions, including using animal organs, introducing cash bounties for donors and donor families, and campaigns for "presumed consent" laws whereby individuals are assumed to be volunteers for organ harvesting unless they formally opt out of the donation.[4] It is the procurement of organs, their retrieval from the bodies of the living and the dead, that has given rise to suspicion about the transplant enterprise. "Movies such as *Frankenstein, Bride of Frankenstein*, and *Coma*," writes psychiatrist Stuart Youngner, offer "grotesque portrayals of organ procurement which have captured the public imagination . . . There seems always to be lurking in the public consciousness a suspiciousness and paranoia that defies the rationality of medical science. Justified or not, we cannot afford to ignore it."[5]

To explain the cultural unease about cutting into the human body, some bioethicists have invoked a transhistorical resistance to organ donation. Reaching back to the tension in early Christianity between fears that God would reassemble a fragmented body on the Day of Judgment and terror that he would not, ethicist John Portmann draws on the important work of medieval historian Caroline Walker Bynum to explain how this centuries-old tension can explain "the psychological complexity of organ donation in a Christian or residually Christian culture."[6] Some medical anthropologists have drawn parallels between biologic resistance—the organism's response to cells that are not its own—and cultural resistance to the idea of harvesting body parts from one person to save the life of another. Anthropologist Donald Joralemon, among others, has argued that the success of organ procurement strategies requires "an ideological equivalent to cyclosporine to inhibit the cultural rejection of the [transplant] surgery and the view of the body it promotes. Perhaps the most extreme expression of the cultural rejection argument has been offered by literary scholar Leslie Fiedler. Organ transplant programs, argues Fiedler, do not succeed because of "an unsuspected secular scripture" that operates at the deepest level of our collective psyches. He identifies this secular scripture in four key texts from the nineteenth century: *Frankenstein* (1818), *The Strange Case of Dr. Jekyll and Mr. Hyde* (1886), *Dracula* (1897), and *The Island of Doctor Moreau* (1896). These enduring novels, in Fiedler's estimation, demonstrate how the twentieth century impulse to prolong life at any cost is "wrong, misguided—finally monstrous."[7]

This book, *Flesh and Blood: Organ Transplantation and Blood Transfusion in Twentieth-century America*, complicates assumptions about the resistance to organ transplantation and organ donation. The historical record of skin grafting and blood transfusion in the early twentieth century challenges the idea that Americans approached cutting up the body of themselves or others with great reluctance. On the contrary, the willingness "to be flayed alive" or "go under the knife" was celebrated in the popular press as emblematic of surgical possibility and promise. Americans brought their family members to donate material for them, they brought their animals or purchased animals for sources of tissue, and they proposed buying and selling human materials from prisoners, the needy, and others. Some writers not only reveled in the possibility of "spare parts surgery," but relished the image of "composite human frames," the union of the flesh of two or more bodies.

At the same time, however, *Flesh and Blood* demonstrates that whose body and whose body part or fluid was acceptable followed no simple or straightforward path. Issues of biologic difference and similarity oscillated over the course of the twentieth century. At the beginning of the century, the discovery of blood groups (by Landsteiner, Moss, and Jansky) argued for the universality of human blood despite outward appearances. But as immunologists and hematologists extended their analysis of blood and recognized its chemical specificity, issues of biologic difference prompted new considerations about the potential importance of outward appearances— especially in the late 1950s, when calls for same-race transfusions based on the distribution of red blood cell proteins roiled the blood bank communities.

Just what blood groups meant and how they could be harnessed to improve health outcomes continue to be debated. The discovery of the Rh blood factor demonstrates how new information about biologic incompatibility fostered calls for limitations on marriages (namely forbidding the marriage of Rh-incompatible couples to prevent poor outcomes for their children) and offered new impetus for eugenic artificial insemination. At the same time, the moral implications of the Rh factor and the apparent rationale it offered for abortion, birth control, and "unnatural fertilization" was challenged by Catholic theologians.

In addition to issues of difference and individuality, blood transfusion called on the cultural imagination of donors and recipients. Just as it had in the seventeenth century, the transfusion of blood in the first half of the twentieth century, especially between people of dissimilar backgrounds, challenged the stability of identities grounded in blood. What did it mean to receive blood from someone of a different sex, religion, race, or even political affiliation? Although some recipients reportedly relished their new constitutions (like the "Hebrew merchant" who received blood from a young man claiming to be descended from Irish kings), others apparently did not (one woman "so unpleasant that none of her family would donate" was angry to learn that she had received blood from a prizefighter, but it wasn't clear whether this resulted from his occupation or his sex). What did it mean to serve as a blood donor, especially in the early twentieth century, when it involved being surgically cut open and intimately linked to the body of a person—friend or stranger—perilously close to death? What animated donors to undergo risk and discomfort, and what prevented others from participating?

Finding definitive answers to such questions is also neither simple nor obvious. At a fundamental level, it raises questions about what kind of evidence would enable us to know about cultural resistance and the extent to which it was shared by many Americans. Certainly, the willingness to undergo blood donation and/or blood transfusion suggests that some Americans privileged the medical potential over their cultural reluctance. Similarly, the willingness to embrace a broad range of materials for transplantation, from bodies of the living and the dead, the skin of pigs, pigeons, and dogs, and the sexual organs (both ovaries and testicles) from anthropoid apes challenges the assumption about what some bioethicists have called "the yuk factor" or more elegantly, if less memorably, "the wisdom of repugnance."[8] The history of medicine, and of organ transplantation in particular, defies assumptions that the repellent is a historically stable category, that what repels us today is necessarily what repelled us in the past and will certainly repel us in the future. For those who suggest that xenotransplantation (the use of animal organs in human bodies) is inherently repellent to human psyches, they would do well to contemplate photographs from the 1920s in which a wealthy male patient on the operating table is positioned adjacent to a smaller table on which an etherized chimpanzee lies, and the surgeons prepare to move testicles from one primate to another.

The performance of such surgeries must be understood within a cultural context in which the union of animal and human bodies and blood received imaginative treatment in popular film and novels. The 1926 film *Wolf Blood* (the plot should be obvious—it featured a lumberjack who needs a transfusion but no human donors are available, so the doctor places a wolf on the operating table and transfers its blood to the man, who believes he has taken on "wolf attributes") was only one of a slew of films released in the 1920s, 1930s, and 1940s that depicted the horrific encounter of human and animal body parts and fluids. The union of ape and human bodies particularly attracted film makers. In *The Ape Man* (1943), the scientist played by Bela Lugosi—best known for his role in *Dracula*—experiments with gorilla spinal fluid and comes to a bad end. The 1942 *Dr. Renault's Secret* also featured a scientist experimenting with gorilla fluids, and several films explored the transfer of human and ape brains. How should these films be read? Are they in fact evidence of cultural unease about the union of animal and human bodies? Or do they represent an effort to sensationalize the potential of such surgeries and to create unease?[9]

This book illustrates that one cultural function of films and novels (including the many others discussed here, from *The Degeneration of Dorothy* and *Youngblood* to *The Hero* and *Coma*) was to establish the surgical imaginary, a trajectory of possibility about remaking the human body. Such films, novels, early science fiction, and even the pulps (*Detective Weekly, Horror Stories*) provided representations of surgical science; the buying, selling, and stealing of blood and organs; and the social, cultural, and political implications of these techniques. This surgical imaginary, along with the practices of surgeons and patients in the first half of the twentieth century, argues that no history of organ transplantation can profitably begin with the "successful" transplants of the 1950s—most notably, the kidney transplants between identical twins in 1954 at the Massachusetts General Hospital, which inaugurated a new era in organ transplantation.

Transfusion and transplantation transformed American bodies, surgeons, and the cultural meaning of surgery. The developments in the sciences associated with transfusion and transplantation offered new vistas for biologic similarity and difference. In much the same way, the developments in human genomics demonstrate the tension between genetic similarity and genetic difference (for example, the advent of race-based pharmaceuticals like the heart drug Bi-Dil). These two surgical innovations—transfusion and transplantation—had profound implications for concepts of bodily integrity. The meanings of self, identity, and integrity have reflected particular historical situations and contingencies, as well as developments in medical science. Throughout the twentieth century, the technologies of transfusion and transplantation offered new opportunities and novel interfaces for probing the limits of biomedical innovation, reconsidering the nature of heroism and altruism, and reconceptualizing human individuality and community in an age of medical miracles.

Notes

1. Jean-Michel Dubernard et. al, "Outcomes 18 Months after the First Partial Human Face Transplant," *New England Journal of Medicine* 357 (2007): 2451–2460.

2. For an entire issue devoted to face transplantation, see the *American Journal of Bioethics* 4 (2004): 1–33.

3. Eric A. Feldman Ronald Bayer, eds., *Blood Feuds: AIDS, Blood and the Politics of Medical Disaster* (New York: Oxford University Press, 1999), 48–53. See Susan Resnik, *Blood Saga: Hemophilia, AIDS, and the Survival of a Community* (Berkeley: University of California Press, 1999).

4. For challenges to the scarcity issue, see the provocative work of Lesley A. Sharp, "The Commodification of the Body and Its Parts," *Annual Review of Anthropology* (2000); and "Commodified Kin: Death, Mourning, and Competing Claims on the Bodies of Organ Donors in the United States," *American Anthropologist* (2001).

5. Stuart Youngner, "Organ Retrieval: Can We Ignore the Dark Side?" *Transplantation Proceedings* 22 (1990): 1014–1015.

6. John Portmann, "Cutting Bodies to Harvest Organs," *Cambridge Quarterly of Healthcare Ethics* 8 (1999): 288–298.

7. Donald Joralemon, "Cultural Perspectives on Organ Transplantation," *Medical Anthropology Quarterly* 9 (1995): 335–356. Leslie Fiedler, "Why Organ Transplant Programs Do Not Succeed," in Stuart Youngner, et al., eds., *Organ Transplantation: Meanings and Realities* (Madison: University of Wisconsin Press, 1996), 56–65.

8. Ethicist Leon Kass is most closely associated with the "wisdom of repugnance," bioethicist Arthur Caplan introduced "the yuk factor" in 1987, in the context of using the organs of anencephalic infants as donors.

9. See Bryan Senn and John Johnson, *Fantastic Cinema Subject Guide* (McFarland, 1992), for more descriptions of the ape–human boundary crossing.

Acknowledgments

Transfusion was once hailed as "a miracle of resurrection." The theme of the miraculous has also been repeatedly invoked in the context of organ transplantation. But what sometimes may seem like a miracle is instead the product of persistence, dedication, energy, and empathy. In this respect, this book resembles the history of transfusion and transplantation, with their false starts, uneven developments, unknown trajectories, and hopes and success. In this endeavor, I have greatly benefited from the help of many, many people, and take this opportunity to express my gratitude for their generous aid and assistance.

I am especially appreciative of the graduate students whose research forays on the slightest of indications prompted such great results, especially Gretchen Krueger, Sally Romano, Kari McLeod, and Megan Glick. These students also generously read portions of the manuscript in its various iterations, offering valuable feedback and comments. I also thank Rana Hogarth, Ziv Eisenberg, and Justin Barr for their research assistance, as well as Patricia Johnson, Ramona Moore, Janis Wethly, and Barbara McKay for their efforts on my behalf.

My colleagues at the Pennsylvania State University College of Medicine in Hershey, especially David Barnard, David Hufford, Marshall Jones, Eric Juengst, Victoria Carchidi, and June Watson, supported my earliest interests in blood and its movement, listening to (seemingly) endless stories about the tenor Enrico Caruso, his donors, and his concerns about his lost "Italian identity." My colleagues at Yale University, especially Daniel Kevles, Bettyann Kevles, Bruno Strasser, Bill Summers, Cindy Connolly, and the members of the Yale Center for Bioethics, similarly endured and graciously responded to musings about why was blood stored in a "bank" rather than another kind of storage facility and other intriguing (at least too me) questions. I am also grateful to Dr. Edward L. Snyder, professor of laboratory medicine at the Yale School of Medicine and director of the Yale-New Haven blood bank, who generously read portions of the manuscript and attempted to instruct me in the intricacies of blood antigens.

I also benefited from the opportunity to present aspects of *Flesh and Blood* at history of science and medicine colloquia at the University of Pennsylvania, Duke University, Harvard University, Indiana University, the University of Wisconsin, the University of Michigan, the Johns Hopkins University, the New York Academy of Medicine, Vanderbilt University, the University of California San Francisco, the University of Manchester, and the Wellcome Library in London at a wonderful conference organized by Kim Pelis. In the spring of 1998, a fellowship at the Shelby Cullom Davis Center for Historical Studies at Princeton University enabled me to pursue the use of animal parts in human bodies, where I also benefited from the valuable insights of Mary Fissell (also a Fellow) and Angela Creager.

Librarians and archivists have greatly facilitated this work. I am especially grateful to the warm reception and liberal aid I received from Jodi Koste at the Medical College of Virginia archives, from Richard Nollan at the University of Tennessee Health Science Center Library, from David A. Juergens, archival manager at the Rowland Medical Library at the University of Mississippi Medical Center, who also assisted me in interviewing surgeon James D. Hardy. A generous grant from the Rockefeller Archive Center enabled me to use the papers of Karl Landsteiner, Cornelius Packard Rhoads, and others. John Erlen at the University of Pittsburgh Health Sciences Library generously arranged for me to meet surgeons who were among the first generation of American heart transplanters. At the Yale School of Medicine and at the Hershey Medical Center, librarians and inter-library loan specialists, especially Toby Appel, Susan Wheeler, and Esther Dell, helped me to locate obscure pamphlets, rare books, arcane editions and images with ease and expertise.

I have been buoyed on this project by the collegiality of colleagues near and far, especially Janet Tighe and Barron Lerner, who read the manuscript in its entirety and gently attempted to persuade me about the error of my ways (I naturally resisted.) My wonderful sister-in-law Ann Lederer also read the manuscript, and provided valuable comments and the perspective of an enormously intelligent lay reader. I also thank John Parascandola, Suzanne Junod, Aya Homei, Dorothy Porter, Janet Golden, Charlotte Borst, Arleen Tuchman, Todd Savitt, Keith Wailoo, Julie Livingston, and Margaret Humphreys for provoking my thinking in productive and valuable ways. With persistence and good humor, David Diaz reminded about the strangeness of the quest to understand flesh and blood.

This book is dedicated to my children, who provide daily instruction in the importance of compassion, intelligence and mirth. Gregory, Eric, and Emma each contributed in their own ways to the project; together with their father, Mark, they are tangible reminders that, in the words of Henry David Thoreau: "We are all sculptors and painters, and our material is our own flesh and blood and bones."

Index